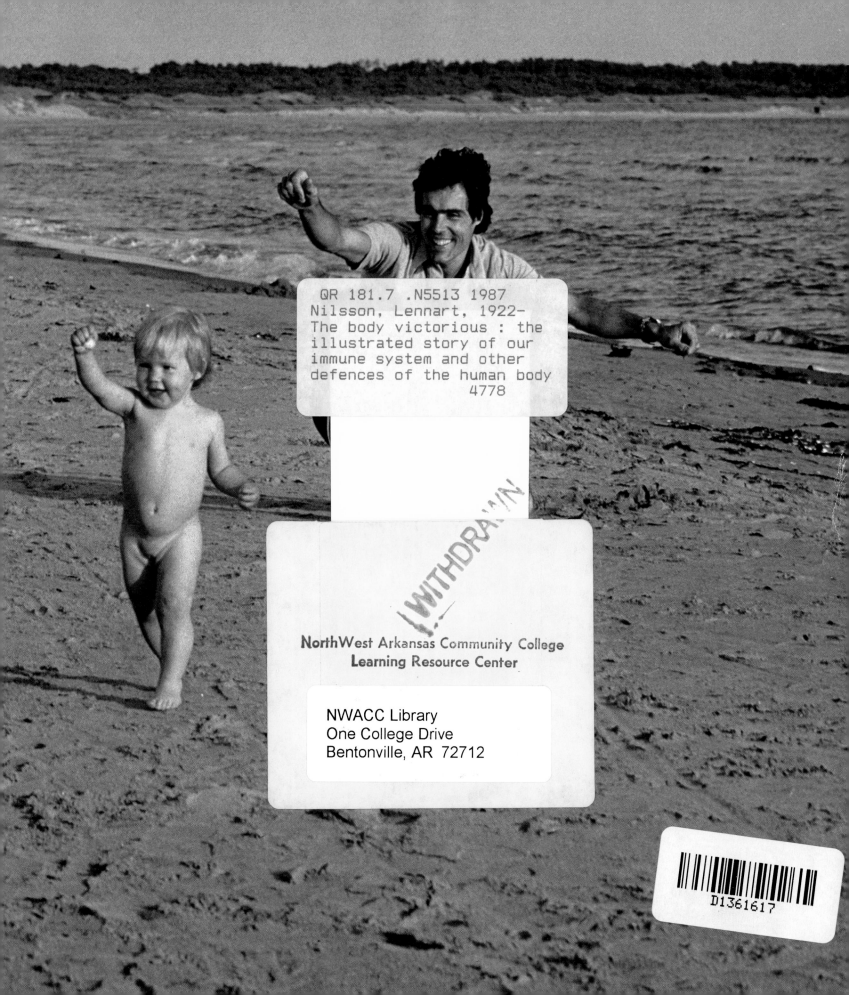

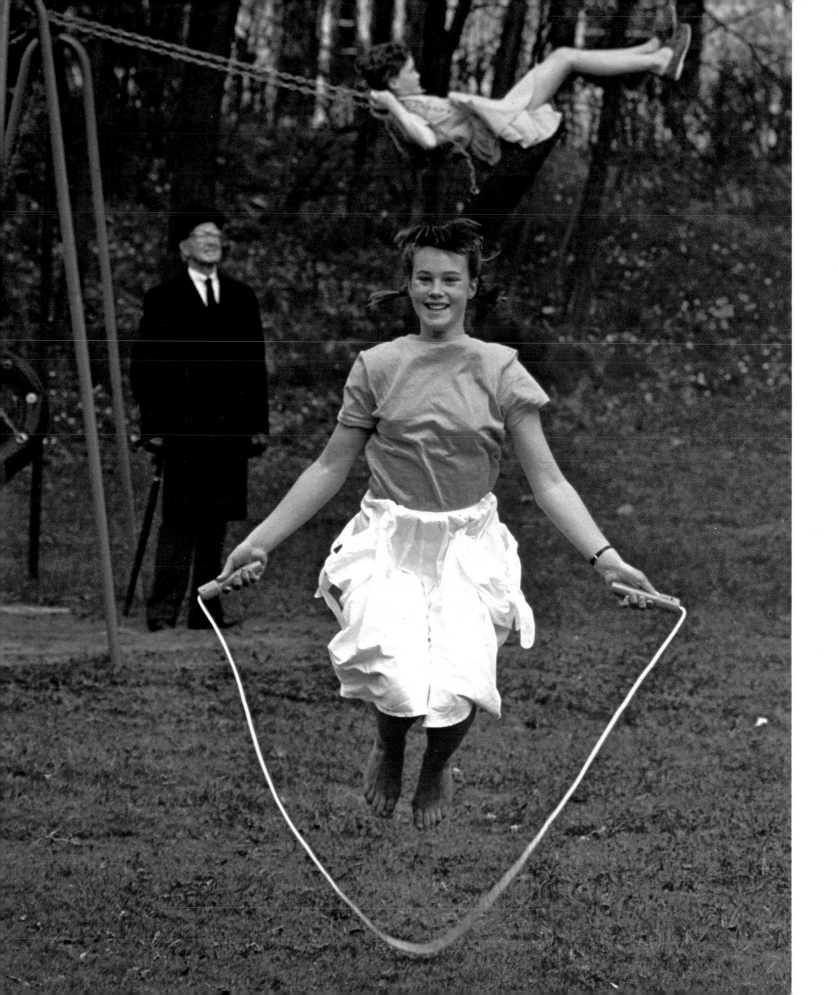

The Body Victorious

The illustrated story of our immune system and other defences of the human body

Lennart Nilsson

in collaboration with
Jan Lindberg

Text by Kjell Lindqvist and Stig Nordfeldt
Translated into English by Clare James

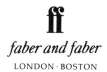

faber and faber
LONDON · BOSTON

EDITORS:
Bo Streiffert, Lars Svensson
DESIGN:
Bo Berling
DRAWINGS:
Urban Frank
TYPESETTING:
Ljungbergs, Köping
LITHOGRAPHY:
Litoteam AB, Gothenburg
PRINTED AND BOUND BY:
Arnoldo Mondadori Editore S.p.A.
Verona, Italy

Original edition first published in Sweden 1985
First published in the United States of America 1987
First published in the United Kingdom 1987
by Faber and Faber, 3 Queen Square, London WC1N 3AU

Boehringer Ingelheim International GmbH, Ingelheim, West Germany, owns the copyright to the following photographs: Page 7 (pictures 1, 4, 5, 6, 7, 10, 12), 18, 19, 23, 25 (pictures to the right), 26, 29, 30, 31, 48, 49, 53, 54, 55, 56, 57, 58, 59, 60, 61, 62, 63, 64, 65, 66, 69 (below to the left), 70, 71, 76, 77, 78, 79, 80, 81, 86, 87, 90, 91, 92, 93, 94, 95, 98, 99, 100, 101, 102, 103, 104, 105, 106, 107, 110, 111, 114, 115, 116, 117, 127, 128, 129, 130, 131, 132, 133, 138 (pictures 1 and 3), 141 (the two below), 142, 143, 147 (the three below), 162, 163, 166, 167, 168, 169, 170 (the two below), 171, 172, 173, 174, 175, 184, 185, 187, 188, 189, 191 (top), 192 (the two below); the front cover (the lymphocyte picture), the back cover (herpes virus).

British Library Cataloguing in Publication Data

Nilsson, Lennart
    The body victorious: the illustrated
    story of our immune system and other
    defences of the human body.
    1. Immune response
    I. Title II. Lindberg, Jan
    616.07'95   QR181
    ISBN 0-571-13832-2

Contents

Acknowledgments by *Lennart Nilsson*   8
Foreword by *Jan Lindberg*   9
Threats to mankind   10

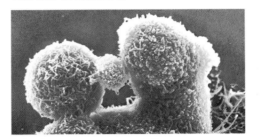

The immune system   18

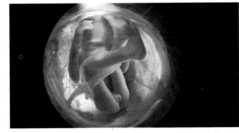

Immunity in the newborn child   32

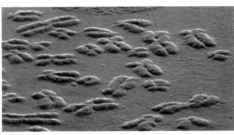

Chromosomes   40

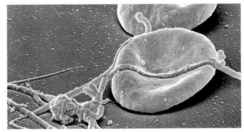

Blood clotting   48

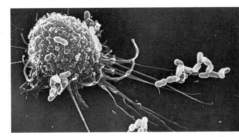

Bacteria   70

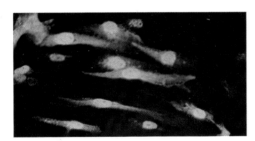

Viruses   86

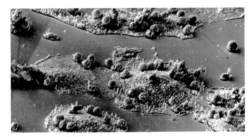

Cancer   94

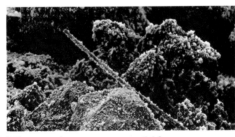

The respiratory tract   110

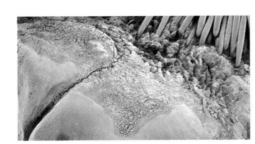

Teeth   148

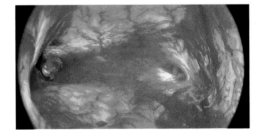

The digestive tract   162

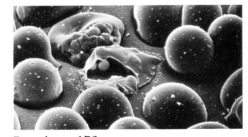

Parasites   176

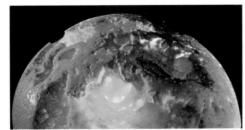

Autoimmune disease   184
The future   190
Credits   195
Index   196

ACKNOWLEDGMENTS

The planning of this book, which provides glimpses of everyday processes in the human body—but ones that are impossible to observe without highly advanced technology—began as long ago as the early 1970s. *The late Jan Cornell, director at Albert Bonniers Förlag,* and *Dr. Jan Lindberg* initiated the book; *Kjell Lindqvist, Bo Streiffert,* and *designer Bo Berling* are responsible for the final draft and layout. I thank them for their inspiring and high-quality cooperation. Kjell Lindqvist and *Stig Nordfelt* wrote the vivid and coherent captions to the photographs.

Naturally, bringing the book to completion has taken a long time, since it deals at length with the immune system of the human body—a field in which research is undergoing vigorous expansion and new discoveries are being made all the time. In the course of the work, new medical discoveries have been made which, in turn, new and improved technical aids have made it possible to photograph.

Many people—both scientists and others—have generously contributed both material and advice. I would like to give warm thanks to all those who in any way helped with the pictures and the production of the book. A complete list of all the persons and institutions who have helped me in my work appears at the end of the volume. I would particularly like to thank the scientists and other employees at *Boehringer Ingelheim International GmbH, Ingelheim-am-Rhein,* West Germany. Without the generosity of Boehringer Ingelheim, a large number of pictures could undoubtedly never have been taken.

Lennart Nilsson

NOTE: Throughout the translation the word "billion" is used in the British English sense of one million million rather than the American sense of one thousand million.

Foreword

Mankind is but a tiny detail in the vast biological system which controls all life on our planet. Man fancies himself the crown of creation, and believes that he can dominate and manipulate his biological surroundings at will. Around him, he sees multifarious biological threats. Animals and plants which have in some way disturbed or threatened the world of human beings have been vigorously decimated or eradicated. Thus—sometimes in an incredibly short time—man has succeeded in disturbing the finely tuned ecosystems that took nature eons to construct.

Through increasing technical skills, man has now acquired the ability to threaten his own existence. Chemical insecticides and weedkillers, and waste products, have damaged the forests, killed lakes, and made even the rain dangerously acid. The contamination has led to a change in the nature of disease. Numerous people are incurably injured by harmful working environments.

In daily life, man thus encounters constant threats of the most varied nature. But he has at his disposal—inbuilt at various levels—a miraculous system of defensive barriers. For example, in order for bacteria and viruses to enter the body, they must first pass the protective barricades constituted by skin, membranes, and various secretions. If the invaders manage to cross these barriers, they are confronted by other defence systems that employ methods still incompletely understood by science—but which we know break them down or prevent them from penetrating further into the body. Such defence systems have the power to imprint in their chemical memories the very code word characteristic of a specific invader at a particular time. The body's defences are thereby strengthened and better equipped in case the attack is repeated on a later occasion.

There are, however, states in which these physiological defence forces turn against the body's own tissues. These illnesses—the autoimmune diseases—remain an enigma. They can advance gradually, bringing various forms of insidious deterioration interrupted by periods when the illness appears to have been arrested.

Another threat to the body takes the form of a shortage of important elements essential for the clotting of blood, the fluid red tissue in our vessels, enabling it to coagulate and seal leaking, damaged tissues. A body which lacks this ability to protect itself is in grave danger, but many years' work have given man the capacity artificially to replace what is missing and thus correct an error which was once fatal.

There is no end to the threats to which we are perpetually exposed. The same applies to the defence mechanisms which nature has developed and refined over millions of years. Such defence systems first appeared in primitive organisms and were then adapted to various organisms in our biologically multifaceted world.

Nature is constantly reshaping its defences against man's sudden weapons. One example is DDT, which was supposed to eradicate malaria by killing all malarial mosquitoes. DDT proved not to be the trump card mankind hoped for: mosquitoes were killed, but resistant strains also evolved. Nature developed a new form of defence. Bacteria strains which are supposed to be knocked out with antibiotics sometimes develop insensitivity, and intractable infections result.

Lennart Nilsson has long been my close friend and much appreciated colleague. Together, we have repeatedly attempted to document the remarkable functions of the human body. By creating the photographs in this book, he has made yet another pioneering contribution. When they were taken, many of the processes depicted had hitherto never been amenable to biological study. It was only by research workers unselfishly sharing new scientific information that the pictures were made possible. Nor could they have been made if Lennart Nilsson had not devoted virtually all his waking hours to the work. Of all who helped, perhaps those who meant most in the gestation of this book were the scientists—and all the others who helped us—from Boehringer Ingelheim International GmbH, Ingelheim-am-Rhein, West Germany. Without the extremely valuable cooperation of Boehringer Ingelheim, it is doubtful whether a number of processes could have been documented.

What this book offers is a glimpse of processes until now hidden to science which, thanks to Lennart Nilsson's unique photographic skills and stamina, have for the first time been revealed to both specialists and the general public. The invisible in us has suddenly become visible.

Jan Lindberg

9

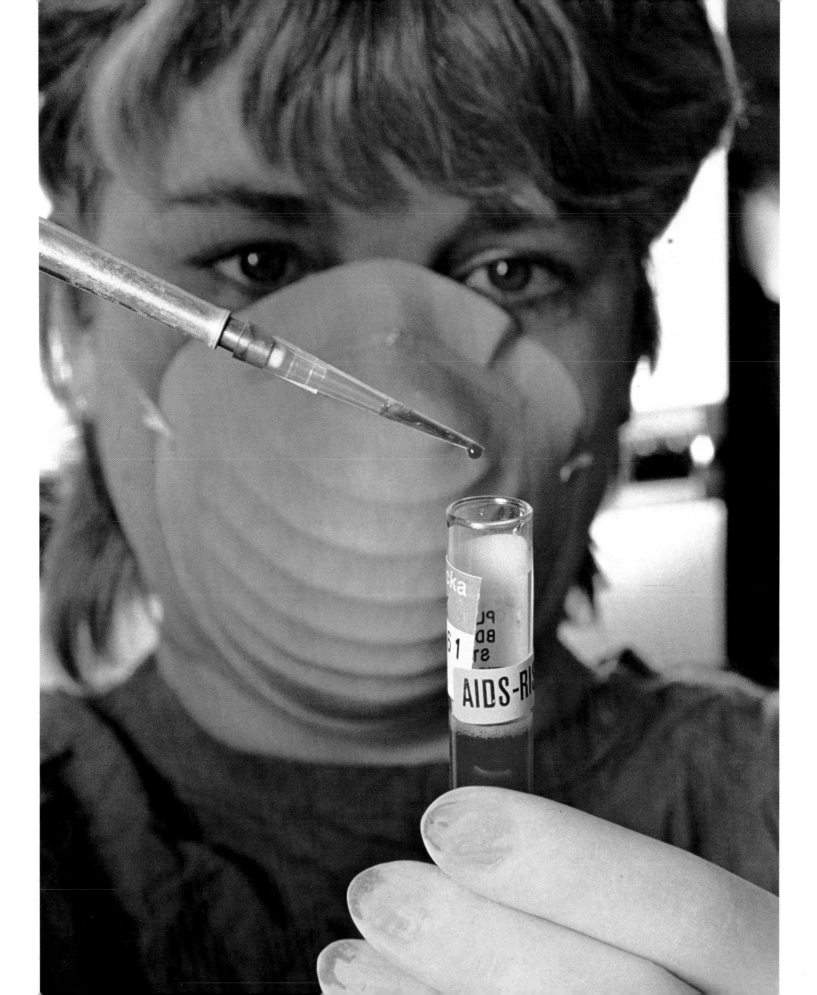

Threats to mankind

Four thousand million years went by before life diversified its basic pattern into the vast, rich array of forms we see today.

A million of these went by before man, a low-ranking inhabitant of the savannah, was transformed into a virtuoso of space.

In barely half a century, mankind, having finally learned to split the atom, brought all creation to the brink of destruction. In the era of nuclear missiles, life itself—everything with a genetic blueprint that can be damaged by radiation, from plants upward—suddenly hangs in the balance.

Never in his long history has man confronted such an overwhelming threat to his existence. What are natural disasters, hunger, predators, epidemics, small-scale conventional wars, or traffic fatalities compared with nuclear war?

The situation is inconceivable, beyond all reason. And yet it is highly characteristic of the human animal, for his innate aggression, while disciplined in everyday life by laws and regulations, is of a highly distinct kind. It permits him deliberately to kill individuals of his own species—something unique in the animal kingdom. Wild predators, who live by aggression and tend to be scorned for it, have instinctive psychological barriers against behaving as we do.

Mankind's ability to live in the shadow of total annihilation may stem from the fact that, as a species, man has always lived dangerously—and survived up to now.

In the beginning, there were leopards, lions, and hyenas; volcanic eruptions and earthquakes; heat and cold; thirst and hunger. With his learning capacity, intelligence, ingenuity, and ruthlessness, man taught himself how to avert most of these threats to life and limb.

Predators exist today only by the grace of man, confined to reserves. Our capacity to predict, and take precautions against, natural catastrophes is increasing. In large parts of the world, however, starvation is still a severe, and growing, problem. It need not exist but it does, a product of the uneven distribution of the earth's resources along with overpopulation.

Epidemic diseases, which made their appearance with population growth and concentration in villages and towns, are now more or less a thing of the past. Improved hygiene, vaccination, and antibiotics have relegated most of them to history's chamber of horrors.

The classic threats to man's existence are thus, broadly speaking, under control—with the major reservation that we now face the risk of nuclear war. Evolution has favoured our species. But the starting point—the body and its built-in defences—was also favourable.

With hindsight, we can claim that the recipe for our unparalleled evolutionary success was the combination of physical and mental attributes that we, and we alone, possessed. *Free hands* were a concomitant of *upright gait,* and they in turn brought fruitful interaction with the *expanding brain.* The brain developed the ability to analyse and foresee situations, to plan, organise and communicate. Our atavistic *reaction to stress*— the "fright, flight, or fight" response—guaranteed the mobilisation, at lightning speed, of all the body's resources. The *blood-clotting mechanism,* coagulation, saw to tissue repair after injury and prevented excessive blood loss. The *immune system* not only constituted a barrier against microbes but also disarmed poisons.

A brain more efficient than any other species'; free hands for wielding weapons and tools; innate sytems which automatically enhance the body's

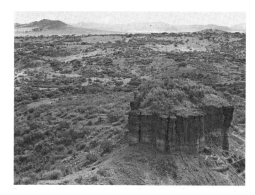

Olduvai Gorge in Tanzania. Here, erosion has laid bare the fossil remains of early man, including Homo habilis.

The reaper strikes off heads in the cabbage patch—an omen presaging a 16th-century plague epidemic. The illustration comes from a Swedish manuscript.

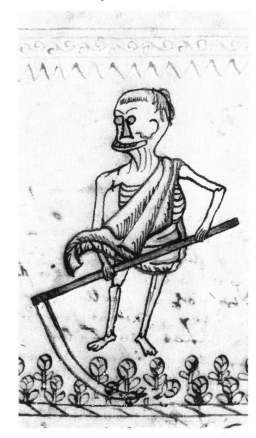

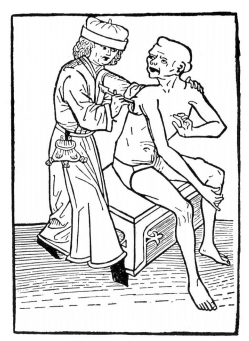

The medieval physician cuts off the boil-like swellings characterising the plague. With his creased clothes and unwashed hands, he spread infection. Below: *Today, the health of even sparse rural populations is monitored, as by this itinerant medical unit in Mozambique.*

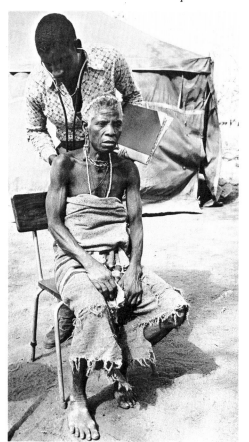

capacities, put a stop to bleeding, and defend the organism against microorganisms—this is early man in a nutshell.

However, evolution took its time to reach that point, as we can see if we turn the pages of paleontology. Fossil flakes from a dim and often controversial past show that many lines of prehuman development were curtailed—many prototypes ended in disaster or destruction. Nature seems to have worked on "Project Man" for something like fifteen million years before it began to succeed.

That was about a million years ago, with the appearance of *Homo erectus,* the upright hominid and leading survivor, on the East African savannah. A new species was established in the bloody arena of herbivores and large carnivores: a two-legged, ape-like figure, mediocre as regards physical strength and inferior to his competitors in all respects but one: *Homo erectus* could think.

Prehistoric man was both hunter and hunted. The leopard, slayer of baboons, was his principal enemy, but in hard times he was also eaten by the lion. His chances of survival must have been small, but he maximized them by fashioning simple weapons, staying in groups, and learning to outwit the big cats. Raining stones and spears on his opponents, running and taking refuge in the branches of trees, or barricading himself in caves, man made the most of his opportunities—he had to.

Without the extra impetus of his stress reaction, early man would have been no match for enemies that were many times faster and stronger. It was this reaction which, in a split second, put practically all his organ systems on red alert, preparing him for fight or flight, and, in the heat of the moment, gave him superhuman powers. We still have this response—but to modern man it is more of a curse than a blessing.

The alarm works as follows: When a threat appears, the sensory organs send signals to the brain. We see or hear something; we smell burning; we are bitten by a snake or stung by an insect. Whatever the stimulus, the result is the same: From the brain come impulses, via the portion of the nervous system beyond voluntary control, to the adrenal (or suprarenal) glands.

These glands, located on the kidneys, release the "disaster hormone" adrenaline. Conveyed throughout the body by the blood, it at once galvanises its target organs into action.

The heart is off to a flying start—"my heart was in my mouth," as the idiom has it. Its rate and throughput rise dramatically: instead of the normal five or six litres of blood a minute, the heart pumps out thirty to forty. Blood pressure rises.

At the same time, respiration increases, to boost the blood oxygenation rate. A tidal wave of fresh blood sweeps into the muscles, imparting maximum strength. Good supplies of oxygen and nutrients are necessary when the muscle cells spring into action.

The pituitary gland—the pea-sized gland on the underside of the brain which controls operations in the entire hormone system—reacts at times of stress to the impulses from the brain, ordering the adrenal glands to produce more cortisone. When this hormone reaches the liver, it "shovels" out more sugar (glucose). The liver also discharges fat into the blood—like glucose, fat is fuel for the cells.

All these reactions take place at tremendous speed: in a few seconds, the body is ready to act. When we have dealt with the threat, or fled to safety, the stress reaction subsides: muscle tension diminishes, the heart pumps more slowly, and breathing returns to normal.

The negative effects of the stress reaction in modern man are due to the fact that we rarely find an outlet for the extra strength it mobilises. We strike our fists on the table, but we do not stand up and fight. Stress at work, in traffic, or at home leads to raised blood pressure and excess fat and sugar in the blood, which

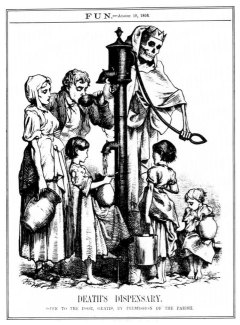

FUN.—August 18, 1866.

DEATH'S DISPENSARY.
OPEN TO THE POOR, GRATIS, BY PERMISSION OF THE PARISH.

The cholera bacillus is water-borne, and many of the major epidemics are spread from contaminated wells. In this woodcut, Death himself pumps up water, free of charge, for the poor.

Below: *blood testing, with a view to identifying elephantiasis carriers, at a hospital in Guinea-Bissau.*

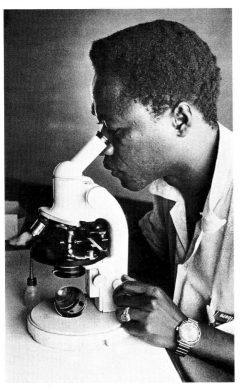

in time damage the blood vessels. Stress is a major cause of arteriosclerosis, which, in turn, underlies vascular spasms, heart attacks, and strokes.

For early man, the stress reaction was a precondition of life; for us, it is a serious threat to health.

Homo erectus was constantly on the move in the plains and woodlands, living on pickings from the large carnivores' kills or hunting his own prey, presumably small animals for the most part. Our relatively poor night vision may indicate that, as a species, we have long been active in the daytime, when our most dangerous natural enemies, the big cats, are inactive. The loss of fur and the development of sweat glands also supported this assumption, being beneficial to a creature which, in a hot climate, had to be out and about when the sun was up. Man's ability to rid himself of excess heat by means of millions of sweat glands gave him a clear-cut advantage over the fur-bearing animals. Like the modern Bushmen of the Kalahari, he could pursue his prey with persistence, in blazing sunshine: he was not forced to renounce the chase because of overheating. As a substitute for fur, man developed subcutaneous fat, which is both a food reserve and a form of insulation against cold. With irregular access to food, it was an advantage to be capable of building up one's fat reserve in times of plenty, and to live on one's energy capital in times of want.

On the other hand, naked skin is more vulnerable than a furry pelt. Surrounded by bushes, rough grasses, and the wild animals, a young human being must have bled regularly, indeed daily, from his wounds. An effective form of protection was needed, and this nature had provided: a highly complex process called *blood clotting* or *coagulation.* Clotting is the first stage in tissue repair. The tissue leak is plugged by a blood clot, or coagulum, which develops into a scab under which new skin forms.

The need for blood clotting arose early in the chain of development, and the coagulation mechanism has existed ever since multicellular life began. The complexity of clotting and the need for several checks and balances are due to the fact that blood clotting in the wrong place—for example, in a blood vessel—is as dangerous as unchecked bleeding. To perform its function of taking oxygen and nourishment to every cell in the body that needs them, the blood must flow easily. If it coagulates in a blood vessel, a dangerous clot (thrombus) is formed. A clot in a vital organ, such as the heart or brain, may cause death in a short time.

The healing of a superficial wound does not always go smoothly. Microorganisms of various kinds strive to intervene. Millions of bacteria, viruses, and fungi attack the nourishing tissue suddenly exposed.

It is then that the third of our innate survival systems, the *immune system,* is mobilised. Various types of white blood cells called feeding cells assail the intruders and enclose them inside their own cell bodies, quite simply eating them. Sometimes without delay, sometimes later, the body mobilises an in-depth defence force consisting of antibodies and a special commando unit of T-lymphocytes, including a group aptly termed "killer cells." It is these which track down their quarry in every nook and cranny of the body, and destroy it.

Early man on the savannah was thus well equipped to cope with the dangers he encountered. He had his hands free—and weapons in them. He had a brain with which to devise strategies. And he had three invaluable gifts from his previous development: the stress reaction, the blood-clotting system, and the immune system.

How did he live? What did he eat?

These are questions fundamental to his survival, but they are far from easy to answer. His encampments were swept away by winds and washed away by rains, many hundreds of millennia ago. His caves remain, and in them we find fossils

13

of human bones and of animals, sometimes marked with the stone flints he used for carving off the meat. The osteologist can study the wear pattern on early man's teeth surfaces and conclude that *Homo erectus* was an omnivore whose diet included sandy, enamel-scratching roots. The anthropologist can compare him with the nomadic hunter peoples of today and draw conclusions about his social behaviour.

If we wish to try to visualise *Homo erectus's* life-style—which enabled him to survive and, in due course, evolve into *Homo sapiens* and his successor of today, who might be called *Homo sapiens sapiens*—we must make use of information from many different scientific fields.

As early as a million years ago, mankind had learned to make simple, wedge-shaped stone tools. Their edges were a substitute for the fangs of carnivores: with these flints, man could cut through an animal's pelt to reach the meat. He also obtained protein by consuming insects, worms, birds, eggs, lizards, and amphibia. More easily available were the fruits and nuts of the woodlands and seeds from the wild forerunners of today's grains. Beneath the surface of the soil, primitive man found roots of various kinds.

Nutritionists or physiologists assessing this diet—with hunter peoples of today as their starting point—find it satisfactory in every way. It was varied and rich in nutrients. We may assume, however, that mankind's numbers increased slowly: nomadic life itself constitutes a brake on population growth. Food availability is limited, and the group cannot become too large.

A brain proportionally larger than that of other species and the propensity to live and hunt in groups compensated *Homo erectus* for his deficient speed and strength. He could organise hunting and self-defence, and he was able to develop a language of gestures and grunts which, tens of millennia later, were enriched with spoken and written communication.

And as human beings became more numerous they migrated in a centrifugal fashion out of East Africa, their original home.

Around ten thousand years ago, *Homo sapiens* underwent the revolutionary change in life-style that was, once and for all, to alter his course: the nomadic hunter (Paleolithic man) became a settled farmer (Neolithic man), and civilisation took a great leap forward.

What is remarkable is that this change took place at approximately the same time all over the world, although there can have been few connections between the small, widely dispersed groups of people. The period of migration was over; the ground was cleared, cultivation spread, and in an astonishingly short time Neolithic farmers had learned to grow crops and reap large harvests.

Now the problem of obtaining the day's rations was less formidable. Mortality rates declined, populations grew and individual farms fused, forming villages. As early as nine thousand years ago, the earliest town known to scholars, with thick walls, was built on the fertile banks of the Jordan River just north of the Dead Sea. Its name was Jericho.

This way of life, with its improved organisation and enhanced protection, was totally new. But at the same time a number of new threats to man's life and health came into being.

Parasites, bacteria, viruses, and other microorganisms play an insignificant role in human life as long as people are constantly on the move, ranging over wide areas in small groups. Fixed settlements and the concentration of people and domestic animals into limited areas, on the other hand, favour parasites. It is when people live in contact with their own refuse and bodily wastes that contagious diseases become a major problem. Infected material is borne by rainwater to the water supply. Flies and other insects carry bacteria and viruses

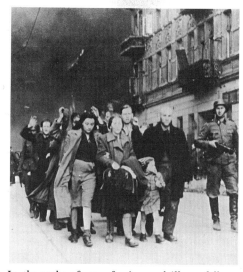

In the wake of war, famine and illness follow. When armies advance and floods of refugees enter new regions, infectious diseases arise. During the two world wars, people died by the hundred thousand, often as an indirect result of malnutrition and deficient hygiene.

from the sources of contagion to the kitchen. Even today, poor domestic hygiene and contaminated drinking water are still the major cause of epidemics.

As long as human existence in society is relatively isolated, there is an equilibrium between man and microbes in their normal habitat. Man's immune system builds up protective mechanisms against the surrounding bacteria and viruses. When people start to convene across village borders, the risk of epidemics increases. Not only do people barter goods; they also exchange disease-producing agents. A man's immunity to the bacteria in his local environment is no protection against new ones from outside. The immune system needs time to build up protection against them—during that time, one is ill.

Infectious matter spreads rapidly from one individual to the next in a densely populated area, and an assault by powerful bacteria or viruses can have disastrous consequences for society. History abounds with examples of resistance to a hostile army being broken down by the bacteria and viruses carried by soldiers, more than by their traditional weapons. And in our own time it is via modern transportation that infection spreads most rapidly: in a few hours, influenza can fly from Hong Kong to London or New York and beyond.

The transition from a nomadic hunter-gatherer's existence to agriculture and life in large, settled groups thus introduced contagious diseases as a grave threat to mankind. Never is this threat greater than when conflict erupts between societies: in the tracks of the armies come the scourges, from leprosy, plague, and smallpox to cholera, typhus, influenza, and other devastating infections.

Settlement also raises issues of ownership. Once a man has something to defend, another has something to seize—and what begin as small-scale skirmishes between neighbours and neighbouring communities grow, in time, into wars between tribes and peoples. War and its concomitant diseases are the primary forces of destruction in organised society.

Bacteria that normally occur in a limited area are conveyed by armies to new regions where people lack any resistance to them. Communities are wiped out, water is poisoned, and fields are laid waste. Starvation gains the upper hand, and epidemics break out.

There are many examples of how this double mechanism—war and disease—operates. One relates to *leprosy,* which until the decades preceding Christ's birth was confined to the eastern Mediterranean region; until that time, Europe had been spared. Caused by a bacterium, it has been the disease most feared throughout the ages. The tissues rot, and piece by piece the sufferer dies. Leprosy first came to Europe with Pompey's homebound legions and was spread by soldiers throughout the empire. The next time, a thousand years later, it was the Crusaders who brought it back from the East. During the fourteenth century, leprosy spread in Europe to such an extent that the Church and other authorities had to intervene—and they did so with a cruelty seldom witnessed before or since.

Another example is the *plague,* an infectious disease also of Asian origin. It was borne to Europe by warriors returning from the East. The first wave was during the reign of the Roman emperor Justinian, in the mid-sixth century A.D.; half the population of the Eastern Empire is said to have perished.

The plague is caused by a bacterium which, in origin, infects certain rodents, including rats. It spreads to humans via fleas that suck blood from the rats. The bacteria circulate in the blood, and when they kill the rat the fleas have to find a new host. Turning their attention to man, fleas transfer to him the plague bacteria that infest their intestines.

The second great plague, in the mid-fourteenth century, was the worst epidemic ever to strike mankind: the Black Death. It moved west in two stages. In the first, Crusaders sailing home from Jerusalem in the thirteenth and

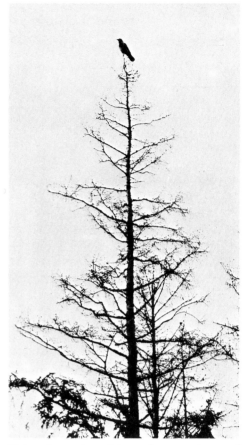

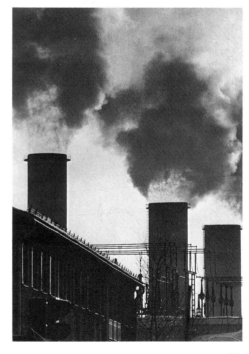

Today, destruction of the environment is one of the greatest threats to man's survival. Forests die when sulfurous ("acid") rain falls. The sulfur comes from the burning of fossil fuels in the major industrialized countries.

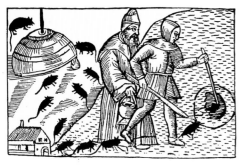

The black rat spread from Asia to Europe and was one of the main reasons for the rapid advance of the Black Death in the 14th century. The plague bacterium subsisted in fleas, which, in turn, infested the rats. When the rats died, the fleas had to find new hosts—and then it was the turn of man. Above, a ratcatcher luring rats from houses and leading them to water, in an effort to drown them. Illustration from Olaus Magnus, "History of the Nordic Peoples," 1555.

fourteenth centuries brought a hitherto unknown species of ship's rat with them, namely the black rat, *Rattus rattus.* This rat subsisted in the vicinity of man, and found conditions in medieval Europe—with its densely built, overpopulated, and unbelievably squalid towns—ideal. The black rat multiplied fast, and by the time the plague struck it had spread throughout the continent.

The year was 1347. In 1346, the Tartars had besieged the Italian mercantile base of Kaffa on the Crimean peninsula of Russia. The plague broke out among the besiegers; it had presumably arisen on the steppes between the Don and Volga rivers and had been transported south by rats. With giant catapults, the bodies of plague victims were hurled over the town walls—an early example of biological warfare. Rats gnawing on the corpses were infected, and the first cases of plague among the town's inhabitants soon occurred. The Italians, panic-stricken, sailed home. Most died on the way, but one ship made it to Genoa, thereby sealing the fate of 25 million Europeans. The epidemic raged for six years, killing around a quarter of Europe's population. No one knew what caused it, terror seized one and all, and the majority saw it as God's punishment.

Plague epidemics broke out again and again in the following centuries, but never on the scale of that pandemic, the world epidemic of the fourteenth century. Perhaps the most important reason for this was that another rat species—the brown rat, *Rattus norvegicus*—migrated from the East and outrivaled its black cousin. For a while the black rat took refuge on board ships, thereby causing plague outbreaks in ports, but in the eighteenth century it became extinct in Europe, as did the plague. We still use the word "quarantine," from the Italian *quarantina,* in turn from *quaranta,* meaning "forty": travelers had to remain in isolation for forty days before regaining their freedom.

Cramped living conditons, unhygienic surroundings, increased international traffic, war, poor diet, and lowered resistance to disease—these, together with ignorance of the nature and means of dispersion of contagious diseases, made epidemics the greatest threat to mankind right up to the beginning of the twentieth century.

Patterns of disease change through the centuries. Just as the fourteenth century was the age of the plague, so was the sixteenth century dominated by *syphilis,* a contagious venereal disease probably imported to Europe by returning New World explorers.

During the seventeenth century—an era of long and bitter religious wars—starvation, scurvy, spotted fever, dysentery, and bubonic plague killed millions. At this time, too, *smallpox* appeared, brought from Asia, and it made the eighteenth century its own. This virus disease came to a head in midcentury, killing around 60 million people in Europe alone. It was not until the British physician Edward Jenner, in the 1790s, discovered it was possible to vaccinate man against smallpox that the disease could be brought under control.

In 1812, Napoleon marched on Moscow with 600,000 men. Before crossing the Russian border, the army had already encountered an unforeseen enemy: *spotted fever.* It is caused by a rickettsia bacillus, a microorganism between a bacterium and a virus in size. Like a virus, it can reproduce only inside cells. It is spread by lice—and there were plenty of lice around. Within six months, more than half the Grand Army had fallen owing to pitched battle, typhus, spotted fever, and dysentery—not to mention the bitter cold of winter. During the retreat, the diseases also spread to civilians, who perished by the hundred thousand.

However, the greatest menace of the nineteenth century was *Asian cholera.* It swept across the continents in five major pandemics in the course of more than seven decades, killing around 100 million people. The culprit was a water-borne bacterium which can kill in a matter of hours. People who awoke healthy in the

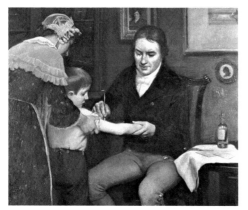

The British doctor Edward Jenner vaccinates a boy against smallpox. Jenner discovered that milkmaids never caught the disease: the reason was that they acquired immunity by catching the milder, bovine form. Painting by Ernest Board.

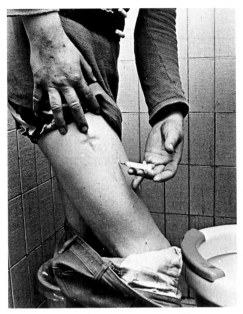

Drug abuse has become a severe problem among young people in certain industrialized countries. Below: Today, man is his own most fearsome and dangerous enemy. A nuclear war would cause genetic mutation, not only in man but in all forms of life.

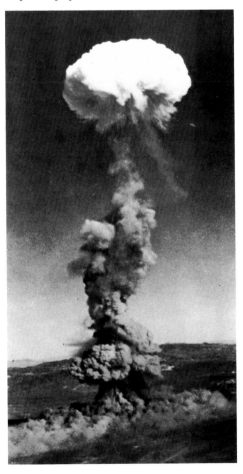

morning could be in their graves by the evening, struck down by circulatory collapse.

Until 1817, cholera was endemic in Hindustan. Thereafter it began to move westward through Persia and Russia. In 1830 it began to rampage in Europe. A complete lack of sanitation in the water supply meant that wells became the great source of infection. In urban areas, especially, death rates were so high that it was like the Black Death all over again. At night, carts bearing the dead rolled through the streets and the corpses were tossed into mass graves. Still no one knew how the disease arose or spread—until the British doctor John Snow in 1854 had the wells of Broad Street in London closed, and the German bacteriologist Robert Koch discovered the cholera bacillus in 1883.

It is difficult for anyone today to imagine the horror and sense of helplessness engendered in earlier generations by the great epidemic scourges. Death from contagious disease was ever present. Precautionary measures were in most cases ineffective since the art of medicine was almost entirely dominated by the ideas of the ancients until the eighteenth century. It was Pasteur, Koch, and other bacteriologists who, step by step, first disclosed the bacteria underlying infectious diseases and epidemics, and ushered in the era that would end their ascendance.

Most important of all, however, was improved hygiene in densely populated regions. Control of water supplies, drains, and refuse disposal; measures to reduce overcrowding; rules for the handling of foodstuffs; quarantine regulations; improved medical care; raised dietary standards—all these played their part in improving public health. In addition, laws were introduced for vaccination against smallpox and other diseases. Medicine became a natural science; the doctrines of Hippocrates and Galen, the physicians of antiquity, were replaced by the scientific study of physical functions and pathological mechanisms. The result was new, more effective methods of treatment and medicines, culminating in sulfa drugs, antibiotics, and vaccines. At last, man had the contagious diseases largely under control.

New threats, however, emerged. An accelerated pace of life subjected large groups of people to stress. Together with dietary deficiencies and work that is undemanding physically, stress has made *vascular disease*—arteriosclerosis and its complications, heart attack and cerebral hemorrhage—the gravest threat to man's life and health in modern times. Next comes *cancer*, caused by the mutation of genes and cells. This, too, is thought to be the product of environmental factors, notably dietary habits, toxins such as tobacco smoke and alcohol, radiation, air pollution, and water contaminants.

Modern man is poisoning himself and the natural environment. Alcohol and drugs damage vital organs and generate indescribable misery. The worldwide burning of fossil fuels, car exhaust fumes, and industrial wastes means an intake of substances that are difficult for our bodies to withstand. In addition, preservatives, colouring, and other additives and chemicals, whose long-term effects are unknown to us, are inserted into our foods. Increasing traffic congestion, in a more and more overpopulated world, claims millions of victims annually. Global warfare with radioactive weapons is a threat that looms ever closer.

Human life, then, has not become safer in the million-odd years our species has existed on this planet. True, many of the classic threats have disappeared. The risk of being attacked or devoured by wild animals is nowadays minimal (outside of a small number of reserves), and the great epidemic scourges of the past are unlikely to be repeated.

But our physiology retains from prehistoric times the seeds of our own destruction: on the individual level, the stress reaction; on the species level, aggression. Much has changed in his environment but, in essentials, man is still the same being who once fought for his life on the East African plains.

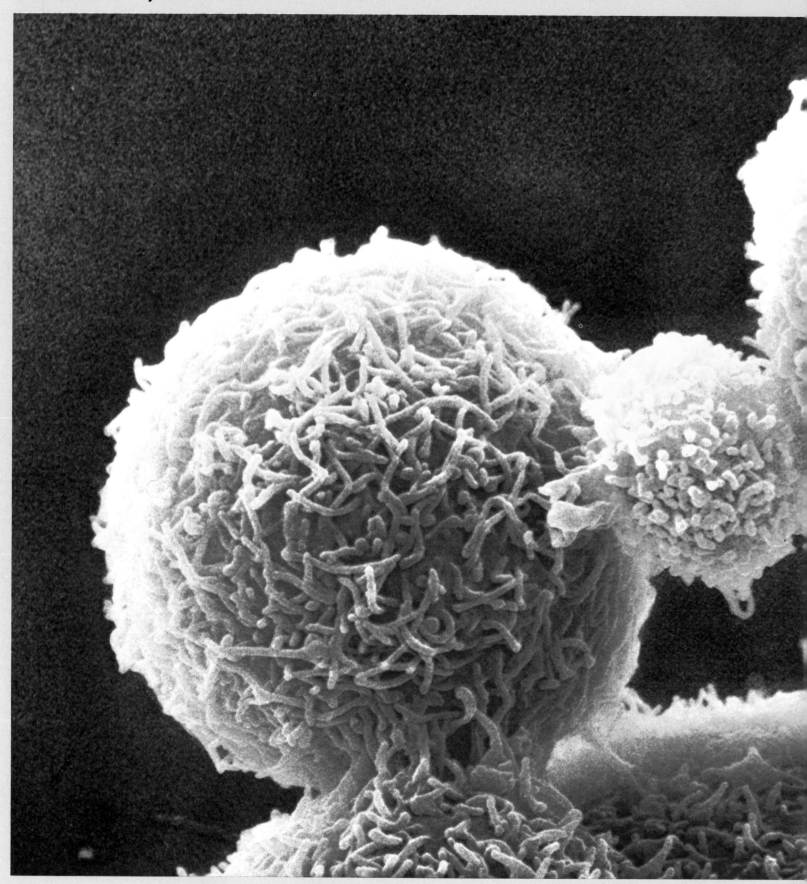

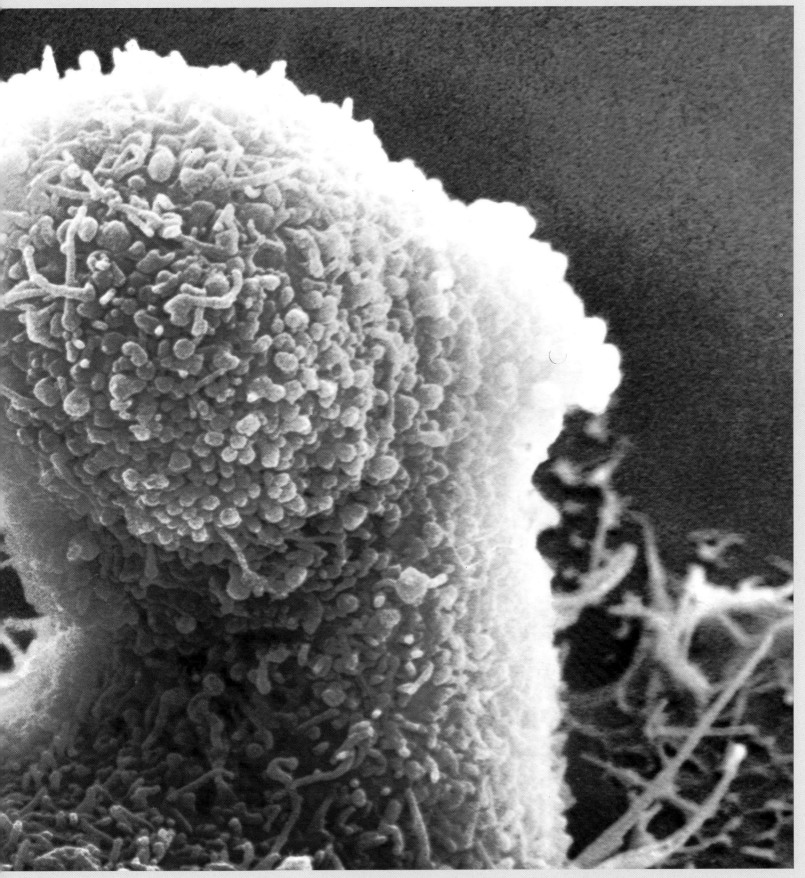

The immune system

Scratches on the skin, bacteria in the throat, and sore, infected sebaceous glands—all these are everyday occurrences and, as such, are entirely undramatic. After a few days, we are fit again and all is forgotten.

Visual and tactile sensations in these cases are superficial. The area around a skin wound reddens, seeps, smarts, and swells. The sore throat feels rough, the mucous membrane is red, and swallowing is painful. The pimple is a red bump which—if in a sensitive area, well supplied with nerves—constantly reminds us of its irritating existence. Then its head turns yellow, the tension diminishes, and in a few days the spot has vanished.

If, however, we could become as tiny as cells or bacteria, and visit the sites of these superficially undramatic events,

we would experience them as they really are—life-and-death struggles between attackers and defenders, waged with a ruthlessness found only in total war.

Suddenly the site of injury, previously so peaceful, is transformed into a battlefield on which the body's armed forces, hurling themselves repeatedly at the encroaching microorganisms, crush and annihilate them. No one is pardoned, no prisoners are taken—although fragments of the invading bacteria, viruses, rickettsias, parasites, and fungal microorganisms are conveyed to the lymph nodes for the rapid training of the defence system's true bloodhounds, the "killer cells." These cells learn in detail, molecule by molecule, how to recognise the adversary, whereupon they launch their offensive.

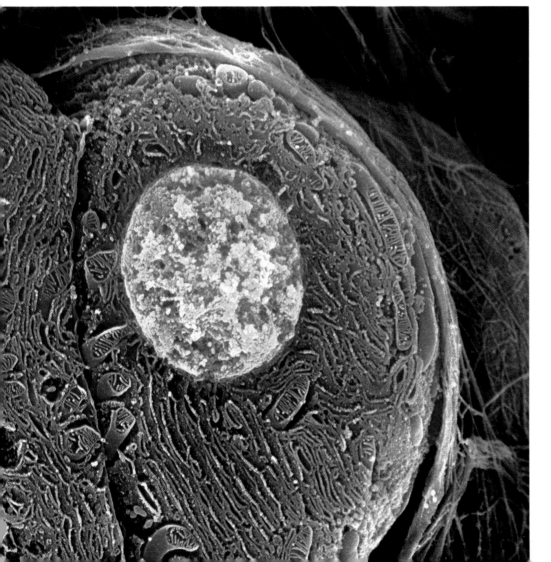

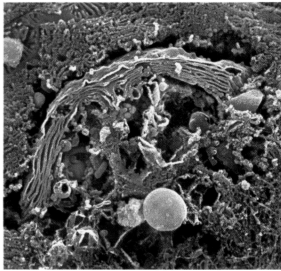

The Golgi body (above) *is particularly well developed in secreting cells. Proteins are collected there, wrapped up, and then sent off, in the form of spherical protein packages (yellow sphere in lower part of picture). (Magnification × 20,000)*

On the left, the cell's protective membrane (green) has been peeled off, and we see all the ingenious inner membrane structures that surround the light yellow nucleus and its chromosome contents. This glandular cell contains large quantities of mitochondria. (Magnification × 15,000)

The cell membrane: proof of identity

All these events take place in a microscopic world where nothing—neither the body's cells nor the microorganisms that assail them—measures more than a few thousandths of a millimetre across. Viruses are the smallest organisms of all: in relation to them, even the tiniest cell of the body is like a skyscraper to us. If we want to learn how the body defends itself against living invaders, toxins, and other menaces, we must descend to the cellular level. This is what bacteriologists, virologists, and immunologists have been doing for the past few decades. This scaling-down of perspective has yielded remarkable results—vaccines, antitoxins, antibiotics, and other pharmaceuticals which, together with improved hygiene, have to an astonishing degree made epidemics a thing of the past.

The photographs below show the principles of cell structure. In reality cells vary in size and shape, depending on their functions and the tissues to which they belong. The skin cell, for example, is flattened while the muscle cell is elongated, and the nerve cell has offshoots which transmit impulses to other cells.

Every one of the body's many billions of cells is equipped with "proof of identity"—a special arrangement of protein molecules on the exterior, the surface of the cell membrane. On the cells of all living creatures, the molecules form cell-specific structures. These constitute the cells' identity papers, protecting it against the body's own police force, the immune system.

A cell whose identification is faulty is immediately destroyed by the armed force which is constantly on patrol. Such a cell may be a bacterium which has penetrated the body or an ordinary body cell whose identification has been altered, for example by a virus. The human body's police corps is programmed to distinguish between bona fide residents and illegal aliens—an ability fundamental to the body's powers of self-defence.

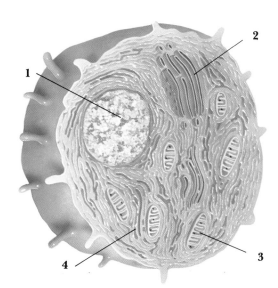

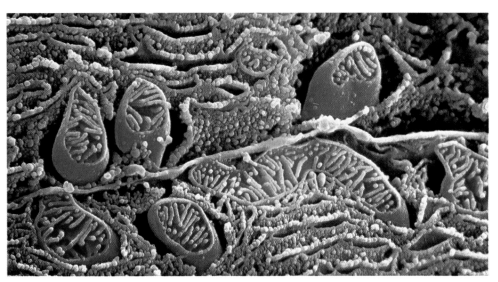

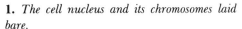

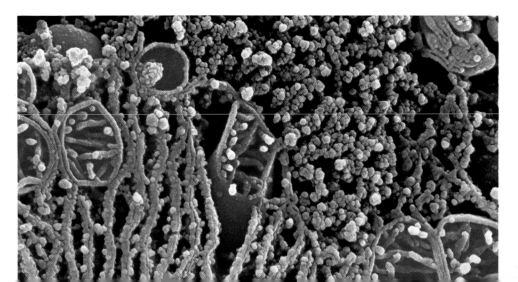

1. *The cell nucleus and its chromosomes laid bare.*
2. *The folded structure of the Golgi apparatus.*
3. *Mitochondria—the inner power plant of the cell. (× 30,000)*
4. *The endoplasmic reticulum. (× 60,000)*

The two pictures, right, show some of the cell's most important structures—the mitochondria and the reticulum. Ribosomes, like small light sacs, are visible on the reticulum walls; they are the site of protein synthesis. Mitochondria contain enzymes that convert the nutrients from food into energy.

Our immune system

The illustration on this page is a highly schematic and simplified picture of our immune system. *Top left,* the pale gray "house" symbolises the bone marrow, where all blood cells are born. *Bottom right,* a solitary bacterium (yellow) here represents the foreign invader that it is the task of the immune system to combat.

The light blue path represents the older defences, with various feeding cells that tackle all foreign substances and also function as a kind of cleaning system. They deal with all old, dead, and used-up material in the body.

The newer, special defence force, which develops later, follows the green path. Its cells are more specialised; they obtain their special training and reach maturity in organs such as the thymus gland and in the lymphoid tissue around the intestines and in the liver.

In the lymphoid tissue, the gray "half-way house" *(far right),* the B-lymphocytes are trained. These are the precursors of the large plasma cells—the pale green cells *(far right)* in the illustration—which produce the body's sniper ammunition, the antibodies (red and Y-shaped).

The three paths from the thymus are intended to show that there are different types of T-lymphocytes—among others, aggressive killer cells, helper cells, and suppressive cells. All of them have specialised tasks to perform when the immune system launches a counterattack.

The three blue paths of the older defences have three different kinds of feeding cells. First, the large and powerful macrophages (orange) advance on the enemy; then come the granulocytes (blue), smaller and faster moving, followed by the (pink) monocytes. The nuclei in the shimmering cell bodies are faintly discernible.

In addition, there is the important complement system *(middle),* symbolised here by a multicoloured range of small spheres flocking toward the foreign bacterium. These molecules play a large part in increasing the efficiency of both antibodies and feeding cells. In addition, they have the capacity to destroy bacteria by shooting holes in them. The complement factors are produced in many different cells in the body.

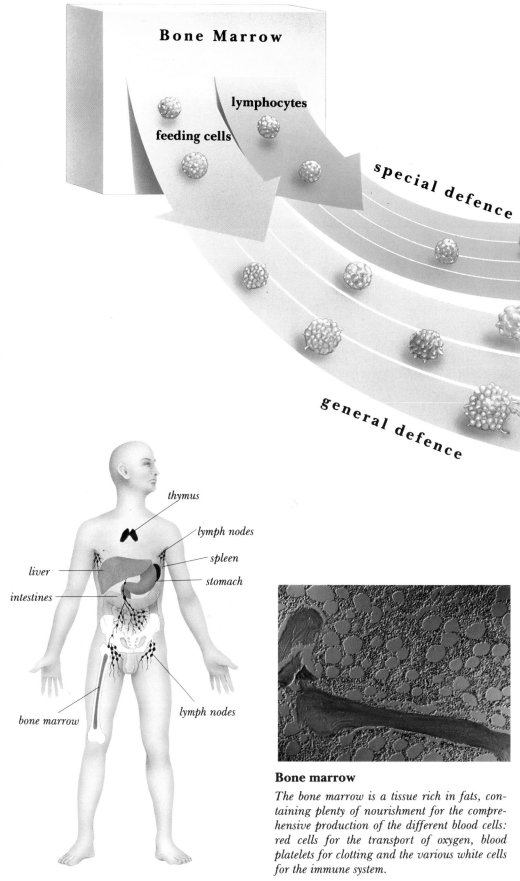

Bone marrow

The bone marrow is a tissue rich in fats, containing plenty of nourishment for the comprehensive production of the different blood cells: red cells for the transport of oxygen, blood platelets for clotting and the various white cells for the immune system.

Thymus

The thymus gland is perhaps the most important organ of the immune system. In it, the vital training of the different T-lymphocytes—such as killer, helper, and suppressor cells—takes place.

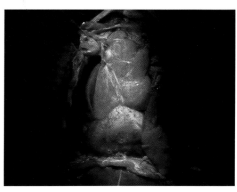

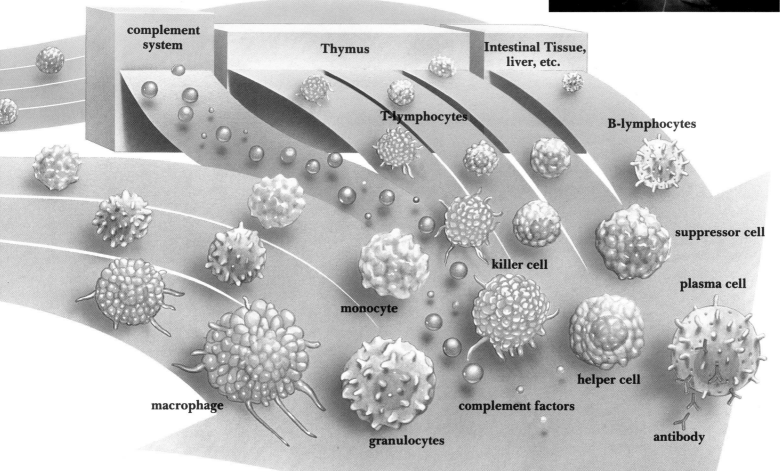

complement system

Thymus

Intestinal Tissue, liver, etc.

T-lymphocytes

B-lymphocytes

macrophage

monocyte

killer cell

suppressor cell

plasma cell

granulocytes

complement factors

helper cell

antibody

Bacterium

This bacterium represents the foreign invader, but it is only one of many invaders. Parasites, fungi, viruses, chemicals, parts of plants, mineral fragments, metal particles—these, and a great deal besides, set the immune system to work.

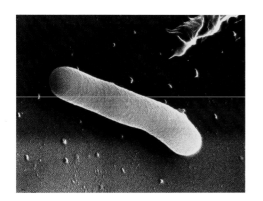

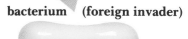

bacterium (foreign invader)

Mobile defences in the worm

The immune system is an extremely sophisticated array of mobile and stationary cells, killer cells, antibodies, and chemical substances, united in the purpose of destroying and removing everything that does not belong in the body. And their success rate must be 100 percent: 99, or even 99.9, is not enough. At a weak moment, the organism could be threatened by a single surviving bacterium.

The same applies to the tumour cell, another long-standing menace to the higher organisms. If a single tumour cell survives the assaults of the immune system, toxins, or radiation, it will soon create new cells to replace those which have been destroyed.

The need for defences against foreign organisms and toxins must have arisen early in the development of life. In a primitive form, defences exist even in unicellular organisms such as the amoeba. Insects attacked by bacteria produce substances that inactivate the invaders. Higher up the evolutionary ladder, in worms, we find not only this kind of antitoxin, general in action, but also specialised cells that can ingest the assailants. Sometimes the cells die from this unsuitable diet, but new ones appear, ensuring the worm's survival.

These mobile, bacteria-consuming cells, which constitute the worm's primitive immune system, also exist in the human body, in a more developed form. They occur in combination with a number of other defence components. Step by step, in the course of their development, organisms have been equipped with new weapons tested by an increasingly complex environment and found appropriate.

Vertebrate physiology displays the great leap forward from a simple to a more advanced immune system. The system is at its most advanced in primates, including man. Our lines of defence are ranked in order, with cells of many different types which remember, recognise, and eliminate noxious agents; with antibodies which adhere to bacteria, marking them so that they can be recognised by the body's police force; and with other substances which perforate hostile organisms so that their lives trickle to a halt.

Moreover, the whole of this (usually successful) struggle, waged from the cradle to the grave, is based on one simple fact, namely that the outer surfaces of foreign organisms or particles bear structures that do not occur in the body's own cells. The immune system identifies them as extraneous and thus to be eradicated. It is these alien structures, called *antigens* (a name based on the Greek word for "produce") which prompt the immune system to generate *antibodies*. The antibody fits the antigen in the way a key fits a lock, leading to the elimination of the foreign organism.

Standing army and special commandos

The organisation of the human immune system is reminiscent of military defence, with regard to both weapon technology and strategy. Our internal army has at its disposal swift, highly mobile regiments, shock troops, snipers, and tanks. We have soldier cells which, on contact with the enemy, at once start producing homing missiles whose accuracy is overwhelming. Our defence system also boasts ammunition which pierces and bursts bacteria, reconnaissance squads, an intelligence service, and a defence staff unit which determines the location and strength of troops to be deployed.

The backbone of the defence system is the white blood cells, transparent cells which circulate in the blood and lymph. There are several types, with different characteristics and defence roles (see pp. 22–23). Their total number is beyond belief: more than a billion in each human being, in other words about three hundred times the world's total population!

One type of white blood cell is the *granulocyte*. Granulocytes are small, fast-moving, and dynamic feeding cells in the blood, kept permanently at the ready for a blitzkrieg against microorganisms or foreign particles. They constitute the infantry of the immune system. Multitudes fall in battle, and together with their vanquished foes, they form the pus which collects in wounds.

Another type is the considerably larger *macrophage* (large feeding cell), the armoured unit of the defence system. These roll forth through the tissues, squeezing themselves through the tiny intercellular spaces and tracking down their victims, which are not only bacteria but also damaged cells and dead granulocytes. Macrophages keep the wound or injured tissue clean, devouring everything that has no useful role to play there. Their mode of operation is illustrated in the drawing on page 25.

The giant army of granulocytes and macrophages is, of course, a fearsome opponent for the invading microorganisms. Certain bacteria, however, are impervious to them, and viruses enjoy total impunity. Certain bacteria have, in the course of their development, learned to thwart both macrophages and granulocytes. Some, such as pneumococci (which cause pneumonia), use their cell walls to defend themselves. They cannot be ingested by the macrophages without the aid of antibodies. Other bacteria deceive killer cells into discharging their lethal shower of corrosive enzymes in the wrong place.

One refined method employed by many bacteria and all viruses is to hide inside the body's own cells. They disguise themselves, as it were, in a uniform which the immune system's soldiers have learned to overlook. In this situation, the defence system deploys its special commandos or frontline troops, the *B- and T-lymphocytes*.

Deadly embrace

The white blood cell—the feeding cell—moves in an amoeba-like fashion, that is, by dividing the cytoplasm within itself and pumping out "false feet," pseudopodia. Once it has reached its target (for example, a bacterium), it uses *phagocytosis*, a process which, quite simply, involves the defender eating the attacker.

Phagocytosis begins when the blood cell envelops the bacterium, isolating it in a cavity. Then it empties its enzymes into this cavity, covering its enemy and breaking it down into its constituent parts. The feeding cell is often poisoned by the bacterium, and dies, but is rapidly replaced by new granulocytes and monocytes (the largest kind of white blood cell). Most of the pus in a wound consists of bacterial remains and dead granulocytes.

In phagocytosis, the white blood cells not only attend to the elimination of invading microorganisms; another major task is keeping the tissues clean. They clear away cell fragments at the edge of the wound, so that new tissue can grow, and in the lungs special scavenger cells engulf particles of various kinds—dust, carbon, asbestos, silicon, and the like—which are capable of damaging the lung tissue. When organs are transplanted from unrelated donors, on the other hand, the action of the phagocytes is far from welcome: they set to work on the cells of the transplanted kidney or liver. With all their strength—and with the collaboration of other elements of the immune system—they try to eliminate the organ. The risk of rejection remains a major problem in organs transplants.

Phagocytic cells are classified into two groups, according to size: granulocytes are called *microphages* ("small feeding cells"), while histiocytes (the resting, connective-tissue forms) and monocytes are termed *macrophages* ("large feeding cells"). During an infection, when millions upon millions of granulocytes are lost in the struggle against the invaders, part of the macrophages' task is to ingest dead microphages—a phenomenon which might be described as a kind of small-scale cannibalism.

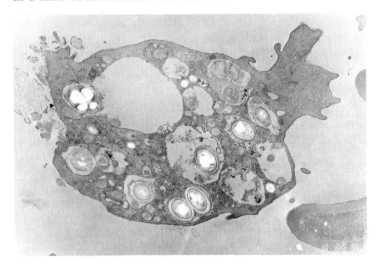

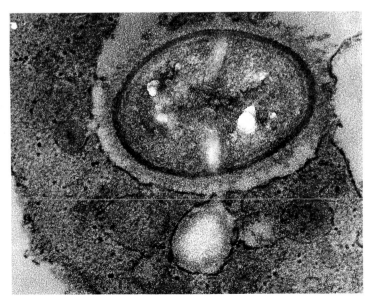

The feeding cell destroys its opponents—a process called phagocytosis, which consists of several stages. In (1) the feeding cell traps bacteria with its threads of cytoplasm. In the next stage (2) the deadly embrace begins: the feeding cell's membrane becomes concave around the bacterium. The bacterium is "swallowed": the hollow becomes a closed cavity around which digestive enzymes collect. Then they attack the bacterium. In (4) it is beginning to break down into its component parts, some of which can be metabolised by the feeding cell. The remainder—the waste—is transported (5) from the cell to the body's excretory organs.

The photographs on the right show, above, bacteria in a feeding cell during phagocytosis (× 5,000) and, below, magnified c. 40,000 times, the bacterium in its "death cell," surrounded by grains containing digestive enzymes.

The special defence forces rally

Lymphocytes are also white blood cells, but they are not feeding cells. They kill their opponents differently: by using homing projectiles (antibodies), and with some form of poisoning (killer cells). The ability to do so requires training. They attend the technical colleges of the immune system in order to acquire *immune competence.*

Like other white blood cells (and all red ones), lymphocytes are formed in the bone marrow. They are released in a constant stream from the stem cells and transported in the blood and lymph to their training sites.

About half of the unschooled lymphocytes go to the intestinal mucous membrane tissues, lymph nodes, and so on, which in man are called *bursa equivalents.* As the name indicates, these human tissues are the counterpart of a sac-like organ in birds, the bursa of Fabricius, which is definitely known to produce lymphocytes of a certain type, *B-lymphocytes* (the prefix B stands for "bursa"). The human body lacks the avian bursa, but has tissues which perform the same service.

When the round B-lymphocytes (or B-cells) muster in these tissues, they are like blank pages: they know nothing, and must learn from scratch. In the bursa-equivalent tissues, they acquire the capacity to react specifically against substances foreign to the body. A mature B-cell has on its surface *receptors* that can bind themselves to an irritant, an *antigen,* on the surface of the microorganisms. Every lymphocyte can, however, latch on to only *one* antigen: this is its specific property, its specificity. But since there are around a billion lymphocytes which, between them, are specific for about a million different antigens,

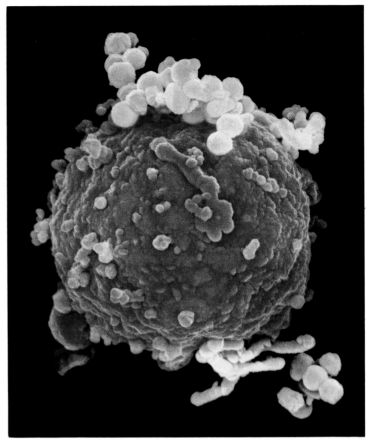

Every individual B-lymphocyte can make antibodies only against a specific foreign organism. The picture shows a B-lymphocyte, the large round body, with the ability to form antibodies against chlamydia bacteria, i.e., the clusters of small, round bodies. (× 14,000)

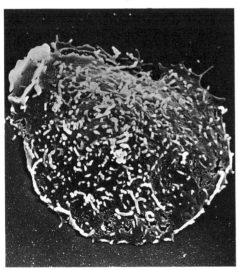

The artist here gives his vision of the smallest single weapon of the immune system—the Y-shaped antibody, so tiny that as yet no microscope has succeeded in revealing it in detail.

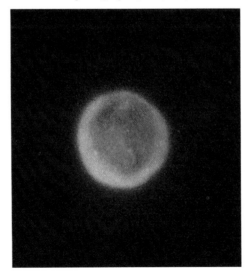

The B-lymphocyte matures and becomes a plasma cell, the factory where antibodies are made. Every cell makes only its own type of antibody. The antibodies are too small to be visible in this photograph. (× 5,000)

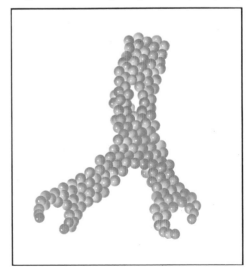

A technical trick makes the antibodies in the plasma cell visible: they are dyed with a substance which in certain kinds of lighting is fluorescent. Here, the antibodies are the light ring on the outer surface of the cell. (× 2,500)

the army of B-cells can together react against all foreign substances we meet in the course of our lives.

This is remarkable enough, but even more astounding is the fact that the lymphocytes develop these innumerable specificities at the fetal stage of human life. If we are born with a healthy immune system, it knows even at the moment of birth how to discover and neutralise foreign substances. Many of the billion B-cells are duplicated as regards specificity, but each one reacts against only one antigen.

The B-cells are dispersed in the body, and circulate in the blood or lie in wait for the enemy in the lymph nodes. When the invaders arrive—viruses, bacteria, fungi, parasites—every single one has on its surface antigens of some kind. Some of these are more important than others as recognition makers. The intruder moves in the blood and encounters B-cells, whose receptors are directed outward. When a particular antigen on the intruder hits the right receptor on a B-cell, the two are bound together and, at that moment, a signal is transmitted to the nucleus of the lymphocyte: "Produce antibodies against this antigen!"

The command is obeyed. First, the B-cell divides: one becomes two, two become four, and so on. Since all these cells, generation after generation, come from a single cell, they are called clones. The next step is for the clones' identical cells to undergo a change into *plasma cells*. This involves their transition into a phase of increased activity, higher metabolism, and greater resources.

Nothing goes to waste. The plasma cells' task is to manufacture, as rapidly as possible, *antibodies* directed against the antigens which issued the original signal. Every

plasma cell now discharges a couple of thousand antibodies a minute, 120,000 an hour. Since the clones of new plasma cells expand incessantly, it is not long before antibodies by the thousand million throng the blood. As soon as one meets the antigen for which it is custom-made, it attaches itself to it. When antibodies bind to the two or three "key antigens" of a virus, they thwart its ability to penetrate cells and cause disease. Cloning of plasma cells and mass production of antibodies continue until the bacteria or virus cells are wiped out and their antigens, which triggered off the whole process, have withdrawn from the tissues.

One important partner collaborating with the antibodies is the *complement system*. In its inactive form, it looks highly innocent: a set of special molecules, called *complement factors*, in the blood. But when antibodies have detected a bacterium and have become bound to its antigens, the complement factors are suddenly activated. One after another, they flock to the surface of the bacterium, and when the requisite nine factors are assembled, the complement perforates its membrane. The resulting inflow of liquid makes it burst.

The destination of half the lymphocytes leaving the bone marrow is a gland behind the breastbone called the thymus. It grows during childhood, reaching maximum size at puberty; thereafter, it diminishes. The lymphocytes which attend the technical college of the thymus are the *helper, suppressor,* and *killer cells* called T-lymphocytes (or T-cells). They are among the most indispensable armed forces of the immune system.

Helper cells constitute the defence staff unit, directing

The complement—biological dynamite which blows up bacteria

1. *The Y-shaped antibody latches onto the antigen on the bacterium's surface.*

2. *Another antibody attaches itself, and now chemical signals are transmitted, to be received by substances in the blood.*

3. *These substances are complement factors, digestive enzymes at their preliminary stage in the blood.*

4. *Step by step, the activated complement factors gather on the bacterium's surface, which starts to dissolve.*

5. *When the ninth factor is in place, the complement turns into biological dynamite and . . .*

6. *. . . perforates the bacterium, which explodes when fluid rushes in, and is then disposed of by the feeding cell.*

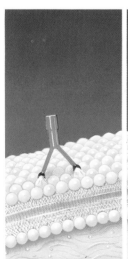 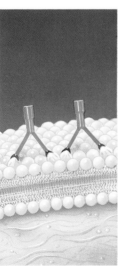 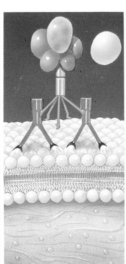 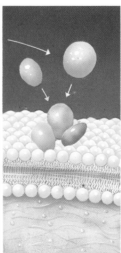 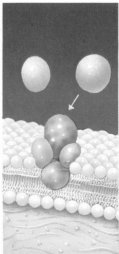 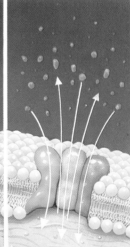

troop operations. They communicate with B-cells and feeding cells via hormone-like chemical signals which they transmit throughout the body, rousing the defence forces to battle. When required, they also affect the *suppressor cells,* which curb the aggression of other lymphocytes.

Killer cells are formed in the thymus to kill those of the body's own cells which contain foreign antigens. This situation may arise, for example, when a virus invades the cells, or when bacteria or parasites hide in them. Tissue cells that have become tumour cells are another target of the killer cells.

The killers subsist in the lymph nodes, to which feeding cells come with their ingested fragments of antigens. The killer cell needs only to brush against an antigen, and at once it starts to divide. Swelling hordes of killing cells depart in search of the specific antigen. On finding it and the antigens of the body's own cells, it makes short work of the diseased cell.

Every episode of this kind generates T-cells with a particular task: to *remember* for decades to come—perhaps for life—the disease-producing substances which then invaded the body. The intruders' descriptions are stored in the vast criminal records of the immune system. When a substance matching one of the stored descriptions makes a new appearance, the memory cells see to the swift manufacture of antibodies to combat it. The invasion is defeated before it can make us ill. We are *immune.*

In the spleen—the dark red part of the picture below—the majority of blood-borne intruders are put out of action.

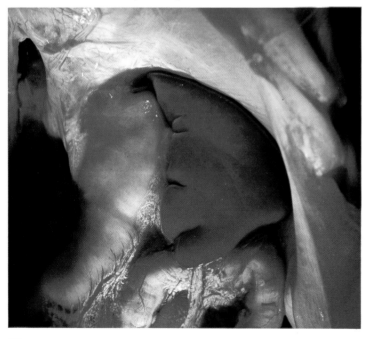

Meeting the enemy: inflammation

White blood cells of various kinds, lymphocytes , antibodies, killer cells, complement factors—these are the fundamental components of the immune system. How they combine and successfully counterattack invaders is shown in the *inflammation* which results from a skin wound.

Inflammation is the body's way of responding to a localised attack. It may be caused by bumps and blows, a prick on the finger, too much sun, burns or frostbite, radiation, or corrosive acids and alkali. Bacteria and other microorganisms are thus not essential causes of inflammation, although they are the most common. Inflammation follows a pattern which is in all respects classic—doctors in ancient times first described its four stages: namely, heat, swelling, reddening, and pain. Each of these steps has its medical justification, and hastens the healing process.

The *first line of defence* of the immune system consists of the skin, the membranes, and the stomach. If they are intact, the skin and membrane tissues constitute *good mechanical protection* against most microorganisms. In the respiratory tract, this protection is reinforced by dense cells with millimetre-long flagella (cilia) forming a web with mucus. The cilia flutter like a cornfield in the wind, constantly shifting mucus with inhaled material upward for us to expel, by clearing our throats or coughing.

The first line of defence also includes *chemical warfare.* The skin's sweat and sebum (sebum is the glandular secretion that lubricates the skin) contain bacteria inhibitors such as *lactic acid* and *oleic acid.* The membranes of the eye and respiratory organs, the intestines and the sexual organs are covered with secretions containing the substance *lysozyme.* This is an enzyme that can dissolve and break down the bacteria's protein sheaths, denuding the bacteria and making normal life impossible for them. Bacteria in food entering the stomach meet another fate: They are annihiliated by the high concentration of hydrogen ions in the acid gastric juice.

Airborne microorganisms are constantly landing on the skin and in the respiratory tract, or being swallowed with food. But the respective local defences hold them at bay, as long as the person is healthy and the membranes intact. Thus we live in equilibrium with the world of microbes.

This equilibrium may, however, be disturbed. If we are simultaneously attacked by large quantities of vigorous—or *virulent*—microorganisms, or if our defences have been weakened by starvation, illness, mental disturbance, or advanced age, our powers of resistance may fail. The assailants then break through the first line of defence and into the organism. This also happens when our skin is scratched or punctured. Suddenly, a promised land of nourishing substances is opened to the microorganisms which until now have been languishing on the poor soil of our skin. They flood in through the wound, and with their rapid proliferation they can quickly seize the advantage.

Infection causes the formation of substances that activate the feeding cells. Before combat, they gather and prepare to attack: they change their appearance, becoming more like heads of lettuce than fluffy balls. Here, three are ready to attack, while the fourth has not yet been activated. (× 3,000)

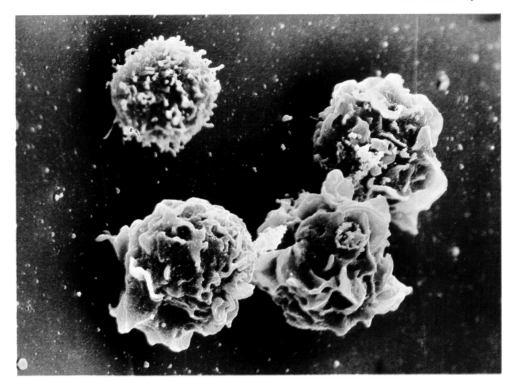

What inflammation means

The bacteria (yellow) stream from the scratch on the skin into the body tissues, like enemy soldiers on the warpath, through a gap in a defence line. They confront antibodies (red), which adhere to them. Then the complement system (blue) starts its complex defence reaction, whereby chemical "scents" are formed. These make a path guiding the feeding cells to the battlefield. Feeding cells squeeze through the blood vessel wall and move toward the enemy, with amoebalike movements. The antibodies stimulate their appetites and, on contact with the bacteria, the feeding cells immediately start to swallow them. The battle is in full swing.

The aggregation of white blood cells causes swelling and pain. Increased blood flow engenders redness and a sensation of heat. These are the symptoms of an ongoing inflammation process, when the immune system is combating an infectious enemy organism.

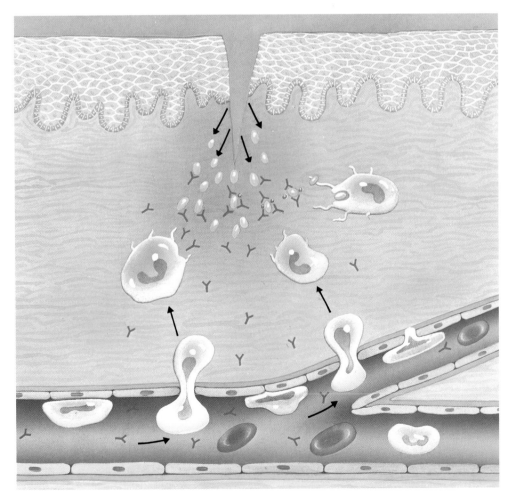

War on the second front

The wound is a bridgehead for invading bacteria, and events in the tissues closely parallel those of a military engagement. The enemy attacks; the alarm sounds; the defence forces strike back; the area is barricaded; reinforcements are summoned; the enemy is wiped out and order is reestablished. The story does not always have a happy ending, but luckily this is usually the case.

All the above-mentioned phases have their counterparts in the body's fight against infection. Bacteria rush in over the border, crossing one barrier after another and attacking the exposed, nutrient-rich cells beneath the skin. This is the signal to the body to open a second front.

The alarm sounds. When cells are torn in a skin injury, they release substances that enter the blood and lymph. At once, these substances are borne out into the surrounding tissues, paving the way to the invasion area for white blood cells such as granulocytes and monocytes. Some also affect the blood vessel walls, which first contract and then expand, at the same time becoming more permeable to blood plasma and white blood cells.

Reddening: the circulation increases and the body broadens the immune system's access routes. The area is immersed in blood, which the eye perceives as redness.

Heat: more blood coming from the interior of the body, where the temperature is 37°C (98.6° Fahrenheit), to the skin, which is 5° to 10° cooler, raises the temperature of the wound area. This is an advantage for the enzymes, the substances involved in the body's biochemical processes. Certain enzymes function best at high temperatures—39° to 40°C (approximately 102°–104° Fahrenheit)—and this means that a generally elevated body temperature (fever) undoubtedly makes a positive contribution.

Swelling: in the initial stage, the spaces between cells in the blood vessel walls enlarge. This means that a large quantity of blood plasma—the fluid in which blood cells are suspended—leaks out into the wound area. The area contains proteins, including antibodies targeted on the microorganisms which have previously infected the body. If the antibodies come into contact with the infectious matter, they latch on to the antigens, making the cells easier for the phagocytic white blood cells to identify. The outflow of fluid causes local swelling and at the same time dilutes the bacterial toxins. Fibrin is produced and forms a web in the wound, trapping blood cells and bacteria. Torn blood vessels are sealed, and the infection is contained.

Pain: the skin possesses an abundance of nerve endings that respond to the growing pressure caused by the congestion of blood and fluid. The pressure may rise further when the blood—because of plasma loss—becomes so sluggish that stasis arises. The pain increases. The pain of a skin wound activates hundreds of sensory nerve cells, which frenetically send progress reports to the brain.

The reinforcements arrive

The wound is a scene of devastation. In the fragments of torn tissues, the invading microorganisms are bathed in a warm, nourishing solution of blood and fluid. Perhaps they count themselves lucky. But right from the start the fluid contains millions of poisonous granulocytes, poised to attack. Antibodies and complement stand by, ready to shoot holes in the bacteria as soon as the antibodies have pointed them out.

The granulocytes are drawn to the spot by chemical signals from damaged cells, and they follow the "scent" to the battlefield. They are not confined to the blood vessels: they can move straight across the terrain, slipping between cells. On reaching their destination, they immediately start feeding on the enemy.

In due course, reinforcements—the large feeding cells (macrophages)—arrive. The battle rages; the slain pile up in the wound. Dead bacteria and granulocytes cover the area, appearing to the naked eye as pus. The gradual disappearance of pus as the wound heals is due to the macrophages, those voracious eaters which clear the battlefield of debris.

While the giant army of unspecific defence forces tries to hold its positions, information arrives from the rear guard, the specific immune system. A stream of B-lymphocytes arrives on the scene. With their "receptors," they test the antigens they meet, and if there is something that fits the fork of a receptor, in little or no time the first custom-made antibodies are on the spot. This is because an antigen that fits is a signal to the lymphocytes to start dividing and producing antibodies against the antigen.

The macrophage is the most efficient feeding cell. It combats invaders of all kinds with strength and stamina. (× 2,500)

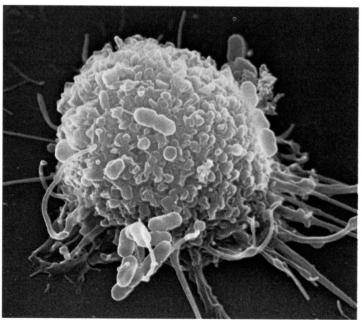

The lymph nodes, too, are a hive of activity. Large feeding cells, loaded with antigens from the vanquished enemy cells, are conveyed there in the lymph. As they pass through the lymph nodes, they introduce the antigens to the T-lymphocytes. Here, too, the encounter with an antigen functions as a starting signal for cell division: killer cells stream out of the lymph node and into the blood, where they search for adversaries with the right antigens.

Now the body has mobilised all its defence forces. If the bacteria break through and manage to spread, they meet the migrant macrophages in the tissues. If they nonetheless intrude farther, they are usually absorbed by the lymph and taken to the lymph nodes. These are the fortresses of the immune system, manned by macrophages and lymphocytes. Now the specific defence forces are in position: antibodies and killer cells throng the blood and deliver the coup de grace to all microorganisms they find. This is the third line of defence.

The final phase of the battle is the healing of the wound. This is an automatic process in which there are thirteen coagulation factors involved. Their activity ceases with the formation of a crust, or scab—nature's own bandage. Beneath the scab, macrophages clear away the debris and new tissue grows in from the edges of the wound.

The immune system versus the body

The immune system, with its microbe-tracking cells, its complement factors and its antibodies, its interlocking systems, is a remarkable phenomenon. Dispersed throughout the body, it conducts a permanent search for microorganisms, poisons, foreign particles, and diseased cells. It has an amazing ability to recognise minute details in the construction of foreign substances. There are millions of different details—or antigens—and it is extremely rare for the immune system to confuse them with those of the body's own cells, despite the similarities. And since some portions of the system—for example, the complement—are biological dynamite, nature has been careful to install safety valves and brakes.

The activation of the complement factors parallels the blood-clotting process which, if it errs in one way or another, may lead either to undesirable blood clots or to unchecked bleeding. Blood clotting, or coagulation, is based on numerous steps which must occur in a certain sequence if the process is to succeed.

Complement activation follows a similar pattern. On their own, suspended in the blood, they are inactive and harmless; once they are activated, it is another story.

The process starts with an antibody attaching itself to, say, a bacterium and thereby obtaining an address label to pass on to the execution patrol. Now complement factor 1 can bind to the bacterium surface, followed by factor 2, and so on. When the ninth factor joins, the process is complete. The complement factors have perforated the cell, causing an inrush of fluid, whereupon it bursts.

In spite of all the precautions, the immune processes sometimes err, turning on the body's own cells. Allergies, such as eczema, hay fever, and asthma, are one result and autoimmune disease another, often more serious, one.

There are many theories of how this faulty functioning in the immune system arises, but no one knows for certain. Since an immune attack against the body's own cells is prompted by some kind of surface alteration that provokes the immune system, there is reason to suspect external factors. For example, viruses and certain medicines have been inculpated in many cases, since a profusion of antibodies destructive to the body can be demonstrated after viral infections and medical treatment.

Autoimmune disease may affect whole organs, or parts of them. Chronic inflammation of the thyroid gland (Hashimoto's syndrome) is an example of how antibodies attack a vital organ. Another is insulin-dependent juvenile diabetes, in which antibodies are directed against the insulin-producing cell islands in the pancreas. This destructive process may have been initiated by a virus infection.

Several diseases of the connective tissue, such as systemic lupus erythematosus and rheumatoid arthritis, are also thought to have an autoimmune background. Perhaps the most common cause of kidney inflammation (glomerulonephritis) is damage to the small glomeruli (bunches of capillaries in the kidney) that act as blood filters, caused in various ways by the immune system.

For the unfortunate few, the system designed to combat disease *causes* illness. Nothing is perfect in this world, not even our exquisitely sensitive immune system.

When the immune system becomes autoimmune, as in rheumatoid arthritis, cartilage may be destroyed and the surfaces of the joints impaired. (× 12)

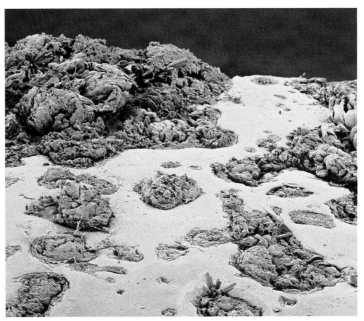

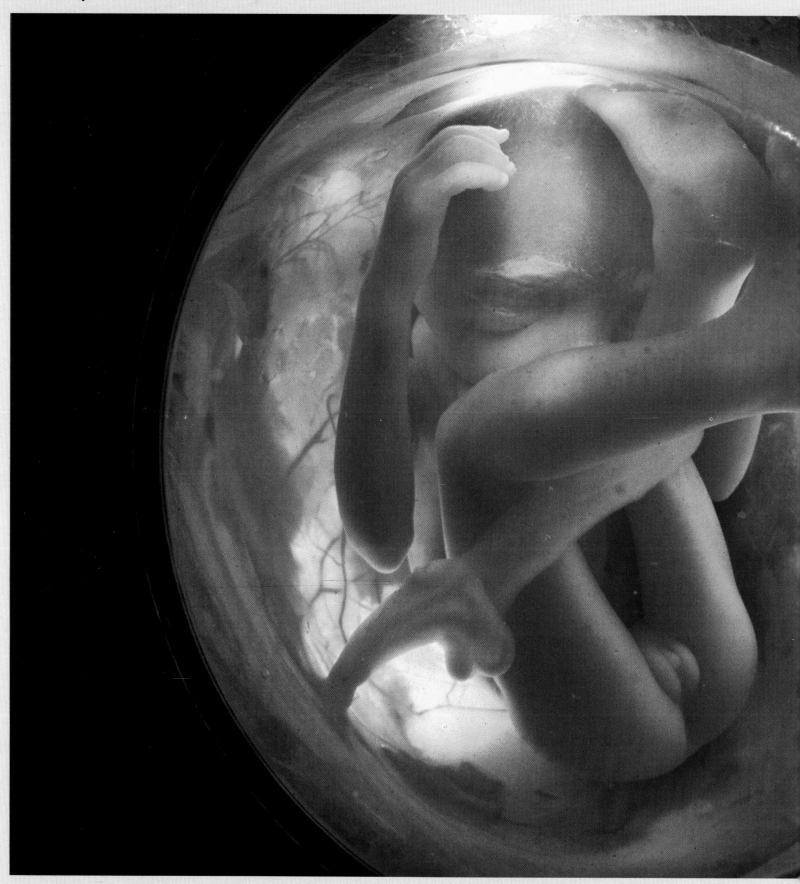

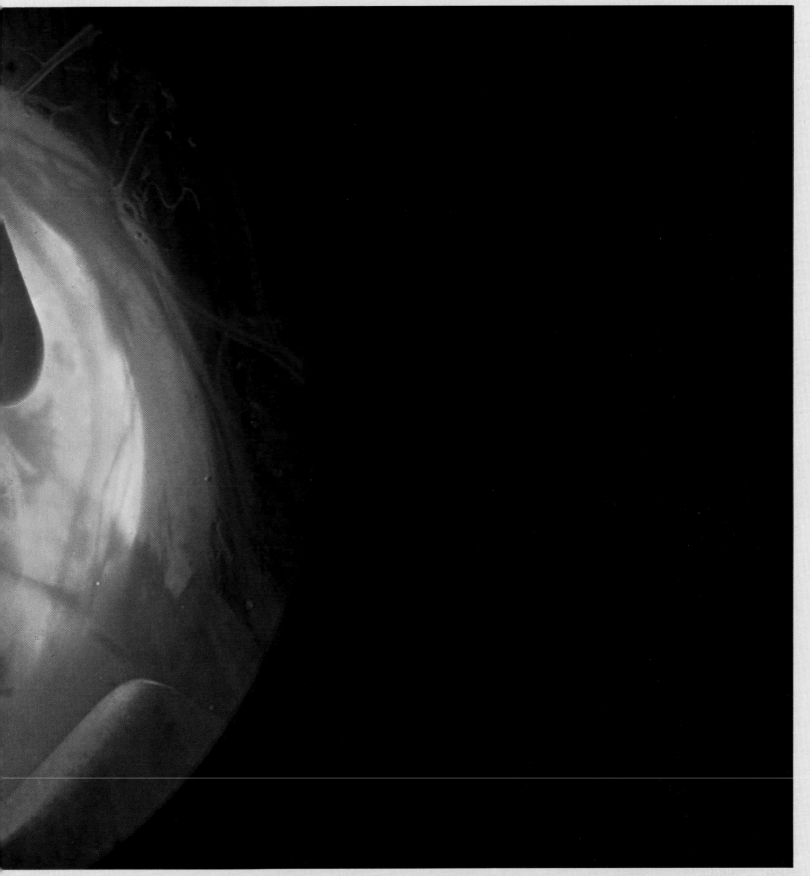

Slightly over five months old, the fetus is suspended in the fluid of the amniotic sac.

Immunity in the newborn child

At the moment of birth, a baby is exposed to the massive onslaught of ubiquitous microorganisms. They land on the skin and in the lungs; via the mouth, they rapidly enter the alimentary canal. Life has begun: from now to his last breath, the new human being will combat bacteria, viruses, parasites, and fungi. By the moment of birth, however, the child's immune system is in place. Teeming antibodies circulate in the infant's blood; feeding cells have already penetrated the tissues.

It is a remarkable phenomenon. But what is even more remarkable is that there can be a fetus at all. For a fetus is, in a sense, a transplant, comparable with organs transposed from one individual to another. Both the fetus and its portion of the placenta are composed of cells with hereditary traits differing from the mother's.

The normal reaction when tissues from one individual come into contact with those of another (unless it is an identical twin) is that the transplant is rejected. The recipient's immune system fights back, destroying the new tissue.

The growing fetus has, of course, inherited certain characteristics from the mother; but the father has also contributed, and if, for example, a piece of the newborn baby's skin were to be grafted onto the mother's body, her immune system would immediately attack the graft.

However, for one or more reasons not yet entirely clarified by research, the rejection response does not take place between a mother and the child in her womb.

Is it the placenta which makes peace between irreconcilable tissues? Does the mother produce special hormones, or other substances, which suppress the immune system during her pregnancy? Alpha-fetoprotein is one substance capable of having this effect. Or does she develop specific suppressive lymphocytes and antibodies to prevent immune reactions that could pose a threat to the life and well-being of the fetus? We do not know; it is an enigma.

But the child is born, not rejected. Moreover, the mother's body takes great pains to ensure that the child gets a good immunological start in life.

The immune inheritance passes from mother to child in two phases, first during the fetal stage, in the blood, and second, during breast-feeding, in the milk. When microbes assail the mother, her immune system develops antibodies against the intruders. The antibodies, which vary in size from IgG (immunoglobulin G) upward, circulate in her blood.

During pregnancy, the mother's blood conveys numerous important substances to the placenta, the major building site adjacent to the growing fetus itself. The placenta functions as a sophisticated filter, preventing the entry of molecules exceeding a certain size. Blood cells cannot pass through, and neither can bacteria or hormones. Larger antibodies, too, are turned away—but IgG sprints past the checkpost, becoming a constituent of the fetal blood. When the child is born, its blood contains antibodies in an even higher concentration than that of the mother herself. And it receives a booster dose of antibodies immediately before birth.

The child's existence and powers of self-defence are entirely dependent on the mother's (genetically determined) generosity. Even though its own production of IgG antibodies begins toward the end of the fetal stage, the process is a slow one. And when the inherited antibodies have served their purpose, after a few months, the level of IgG antibodies in the child's blood declines. By that time, however, it has long since raided another immunological weapon arsenal: breast milk.

Fetal immune mechanisms develop in stages.
• The first stage is the *yolk sac*, a short-lived embryonic appendage (it disappears as early as the eleventh week of life, when its blood-forming functions are assumed by other organs). In the walls of the yolk sac, stem cells—shortly to migrate to the fetal bone marrow for the production of lymphocytes—are formed. Later, in lymphoid organs, they are fashioned into weapons (i.e., they acquire "immune competence").
• Alongside the massive transfer of IgG antibodies from the mother's blood, the fetus begins producing its own type IgG and IgA antibodies in the fifth month. Normally, the fetus is not exposed to infections, since neither bacteria (except for syphilis spirochetes) nor most viruses can pass through the placental filter. Occasionally, however, it happens, and the fetus can then, in fact, defend itself by the generation of antibodies. For example, if the mother is infected by a measles virus, a five-month-old fetus can begin to produce antibodies against measles. This takes place in its first plasma cells (lymphocytes).
• The portion of the immune system termed the *complement* is made by the fetus, not provided by the mother. At birth, however, it has not attained its full powers.
• Feeder cells—macrophages and granulocytes—have al-

ready at the time of birth been delivered by the bone marrow, and are ready to protect the newborn baby against bacterial invasion.

The foundations of the immune system have thus been laid before birth, but the ultimately decisive firepower is still provided by antibodies acquired from the mother.

Breast-feeding initiates a new phase in immune system development. With the breast milk, the infant sucks in large quantities of antibodies, including IgA, which is too large to pass through the placental filter. The first few days' breast milk, *colostrum,* is particularly rich in antibodies. They line the membranes of the alimentary canal and—in close collaboration with the complement factors—can immediately counterattack assailants.

The newborn baby is a satellite state, heavily dependent on its superpower mother. This fact is underlined by a comparison with bottle-fed infants, who suffer infections of the nose, ear, and throat more often than breast-fed babies do. The disadvantage of products designed to replace maternal milk in the early neonatal period is particularly pronounced in developing countries when hygiene is neglected. Whereas the breast provides sterile, antibody-laden nourishment, bottle-fed babies succumb more readily to infections, and, as a result, their mortality is higher. In developing countries neither bottles nor water used in making up a formula are usually sterilised.

For animals that suckle, such as calves, foals, and piglets, the mother's milk is absolutely crucial for their survival when they are newborn. This is because they receive no antibodies from the mother's blood: everything must come from the milk. It is vital for the young to latch on to the mother's teat as soon as they possibly can.

For human young, the important thing is to be capable of responding to a microbial assault by the age of two or three months. By then, weapon manufacturers in the red bone marrow and thymus are working flat out. When the child is ten years old, the human immune system is at its strongest, armed to the teeth. Thereafter, its powers gradually deteriorate.

A world swarming with viruses, bacteria, and fungi confronts the new-born child. Now it is vital that everything has gone as it should—that the infant's body is well provided with antibodies from the mother, and that its own immune system is ready for the starting signal. Soon, the new individual must be capable of withstanding attack without external help.

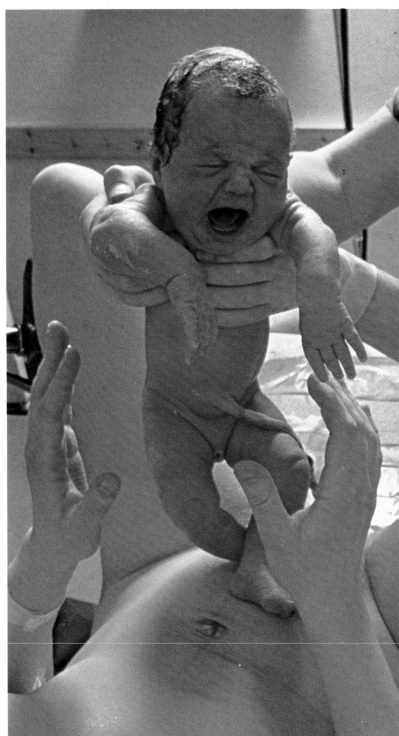

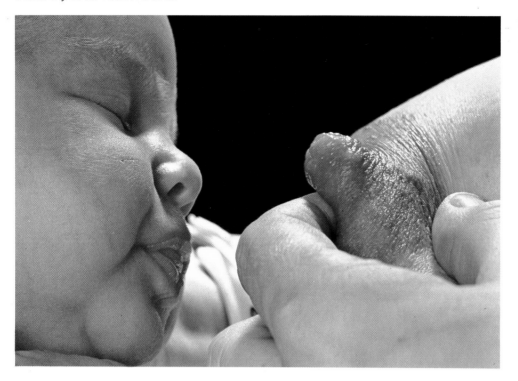

Immunity comes with breast milk

In all mammals, including man, the first milk brings a rich supply of antibodies. Termed "colostrum," it is more watery in consistency than maternal milk in general. *Below,* we see a millimetre-wide drop of colostrum on the heavily pigmented skin around the nipple.

Colostrum contains antibodies of various kinds. They line the newborn baby's intestinal membrane and give local protection against infections of the stomach and intestines.

During the fetal stage, the child has acquired IgG-antibodies from its mother's blood. During breast-feeding, it assimilates other types of antibodies with the milk. After a few months, however, the infant's own immune system starts to produce the various kinds of cells involved in an immune response. The child is no longer dependent on the protection it received from the mother.

The mother often has to squeeze the breast *(left)* to express enough colostrum.

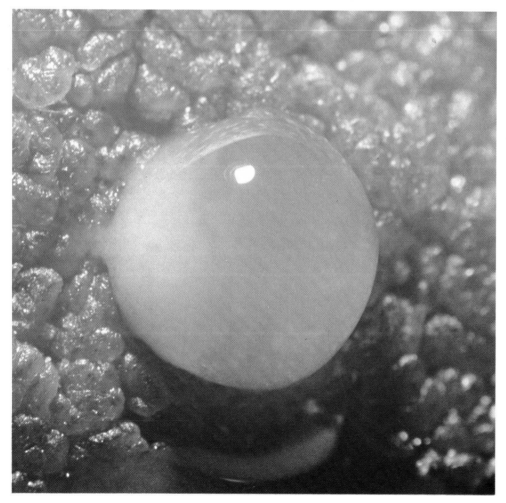

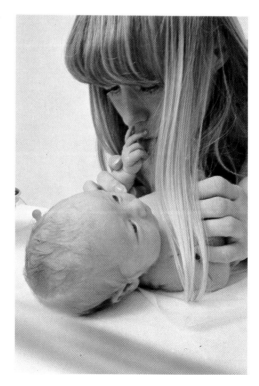

and food comes with security

Below, we see colostrum trickling out of the nipple. The first milk has a different composition from that of ordinary maternal milk. Above all, colostrum contains immunoglobulins and antibodies which protect the newborn child against infections during its early weeks. If the mother catches cold, her immune system produces antibodies against the infectious substance, and some of them are transferred to her baby in the milk. The same happens in other mammals.

The advantage of maternal milk is that it is of the correct composition with regard to nutrients and substances needed for growth, at the right temperature, and in a hygienic package. Another advantage is its accessibility.

But suckling is not merely a question of the right food at the right time. It also satisfies the infant's strong sucking and security needs. Breast-feeding consolidates the mother-child relationship.

Physiologically, a diet with the composition of maternal milk is all a newborn baby's intestinal canal and excretory system can cope with. Its kidneys, for example, are immature and inefficient in the first few months of life. Maternal milk is perfectly adapted, and makes no demands.

The composition of maternal milk varies considerably among different mammal species. In man, it is richer in carbohydrates than in other species; in the cow there are more proteins; and in the dog, more proteins and fat. One-third of the milk imbibed by whale calves is fat.

A drop of colostrum, full of ingredients which help to build up the child's resistance to infection, trickles out of the nipple.

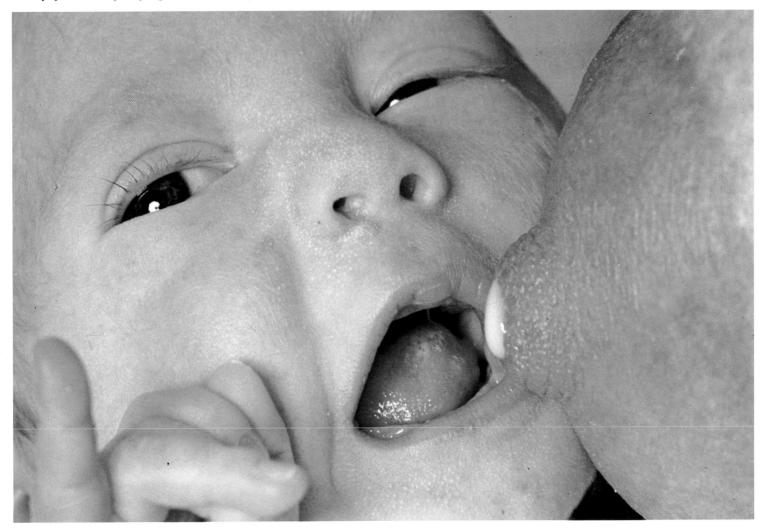

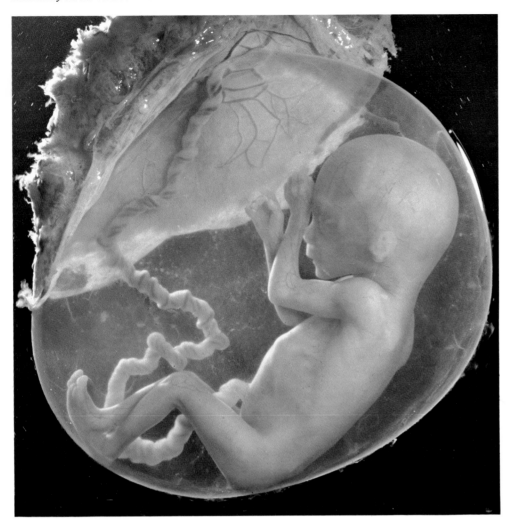

Immunity in the newborn child

We do not enter the world defenceless. Even a fetus (*left,* in the fourth month) is laden with antibodies from the mother, and the milk a newborn child receives at the beginning of breast-feeding is particularly rich in those antibodies which cannot pass the "placental barrier," i.e., are too large to flow through the placenta.

The protection afforded by breast milk is, however, short-lived. To survive, the newborn baby must be capable of rapidly mobilising its own immune system—and this is exactly what happens. Even before birth, the stem cells of the bone marrow produce lymphocytes (white blood cells) which travel to either the thymus or lymphoid tissue (e.g., the intestinal membrane and lymph nodes) for further training. In the infant's blood, therefore, there are lymphocytes which can react against practically all the substances with which one comes into contact in a lifetime. These "B-lymphocytes" have specific molecules (receptors) on their surfaces, structured in such a way that they exactly fit particular antigens on the surfaces of foreign substances, such as bacteria and viruses. It is the B-lymphocytes' tremendous range of specificities that enables the baby to become independent, from the point of view of immunity, after only a few months.

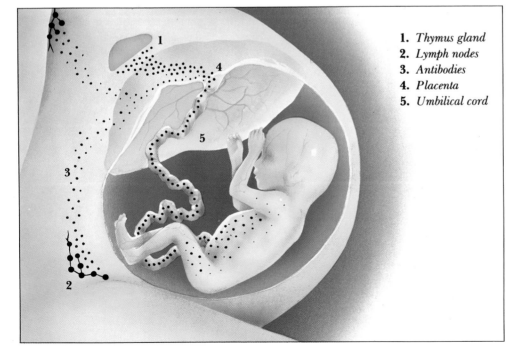

1. *Thymus gland*
2. *Lymph nodes*
3. *Antibodies*
4. *Placenta*
5. *Umbilical cord*

The drawing to the left *elucidates what is happening to the fetus in the illustration above. Antibodies originating in the mother's bone marrow receive their "further education" in (1) the thymus gland and (2) lymph nodes or other lymphoid tissue. Figure (3) represents the stream of antibodies carried by the mother's blood to (4) the placenta. This is where the mother provides the fetus with nourishment and collects its wastes in return. The small outgrowths (villi) of the placenta, immersed in the mother's blood, filter out all molecules over a certain size. Thus only the smallest antibodies can be transferred to the fetus via the umbilical cord (5).*

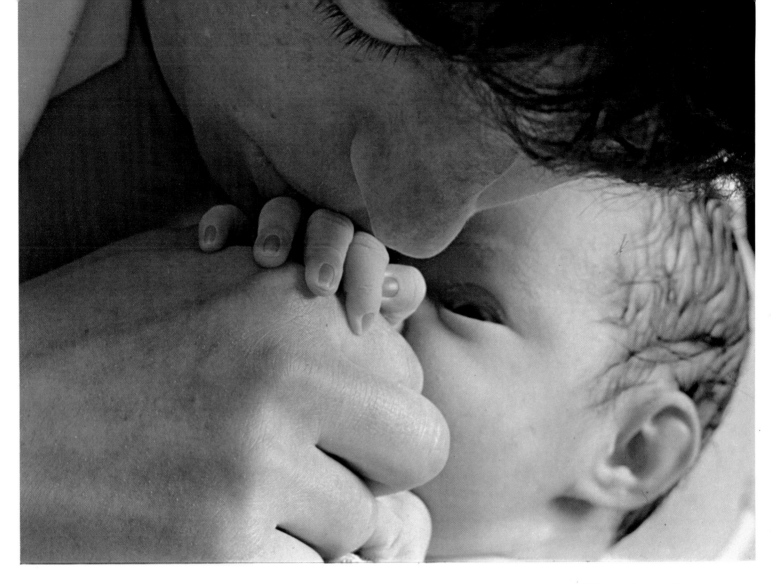

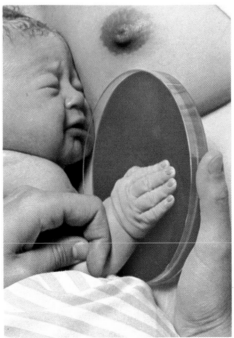

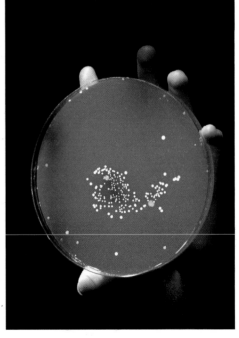

Right, a plate containing nutrients for bacteria. The child's hand was pressed against the plate and, within 24 hours, the bacteria that adhered have multiplied, forming several visible colonies, with millions of bacteria in each.

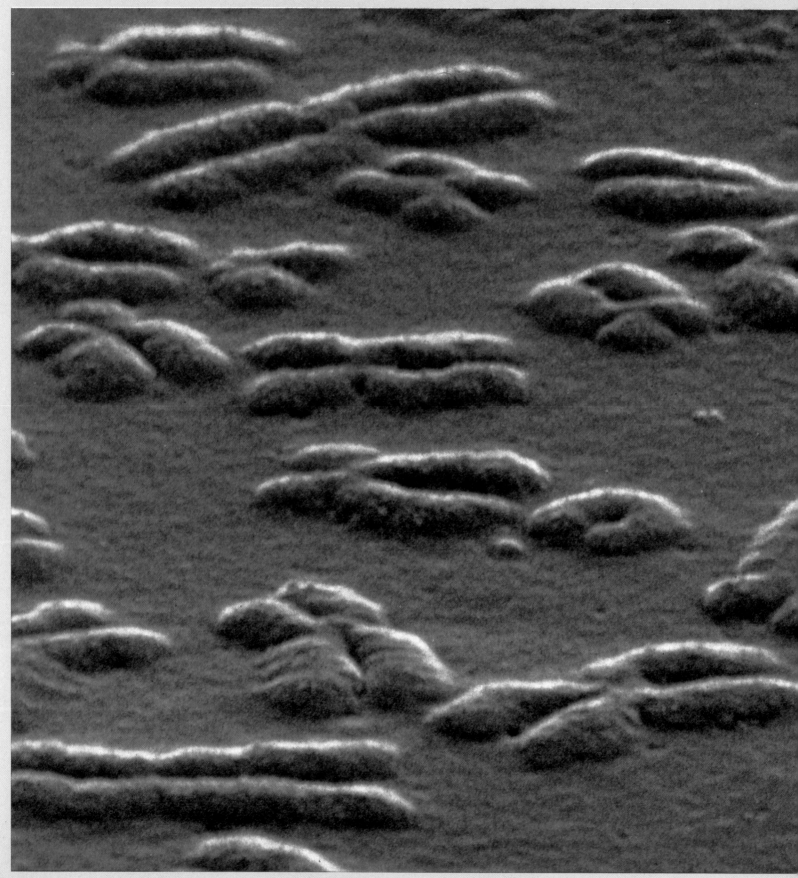

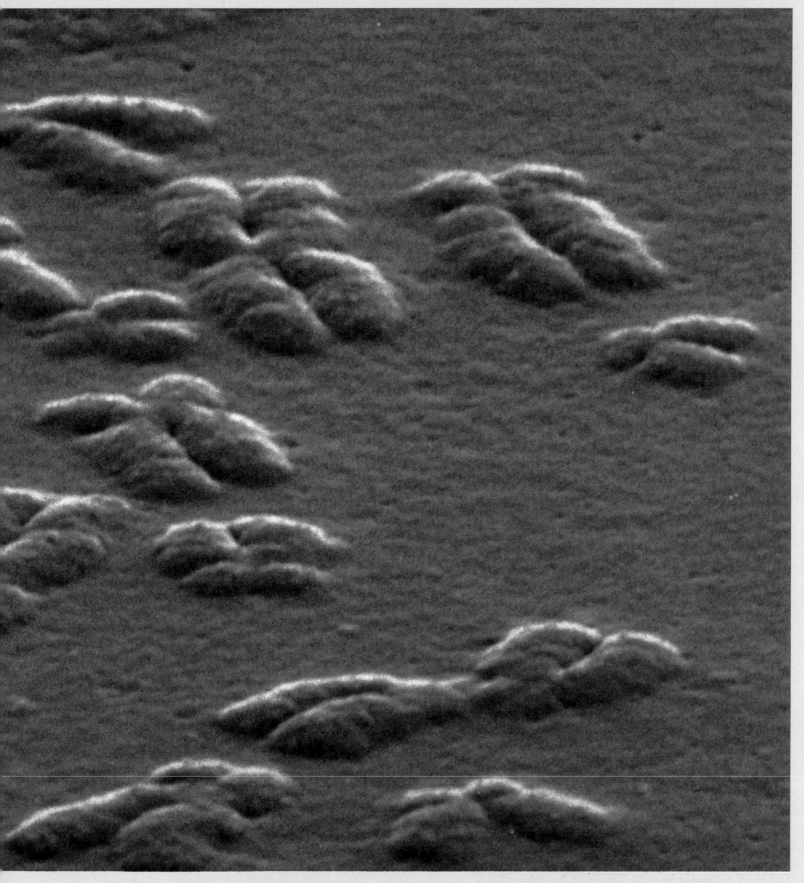

Chromosomes

Right inside the cell, in its microscopically small nucleus, the body's most valuable material is kept—the genetic blueprint. In man, it is organised into forty-six suggestively shaped bodies called chromosomes, which resemble the mysterious script of some forgotten civilisation.

The chemistry of chromosomes is dominated by nucleic acid, which at life's earlier beginnings joined with fat, carbohydrates, and protein to make a substance called chromatin, thereby paving the way for the unparalleled development of organisms. Chromatin has a good memory—it is the stuff of memory itself. And if there is one thing the genetic blueprint needs, it is a memory that never fails. In chromatin, in fact, all information required for life and development is stored.

If we penetrate the microanatomy of the chromosomes, we find that they are constructed of infinitely fine and extremely long strands of nucleic acid, DNA (short for deoxyribonucleic acid). The DNA strands in the inherited material of a single cell are all together about 150 centimetres long. If it were possible to lay all the DNA in the body's many billions of cells end to end, making one long thread, it would stretch from the earth to the moon.

It is these strands which bear, inscribed in code-like chemical formulae, the genetic information. The genes, the material of inheritance, are like entries in a giant chemical dictionary. If their information were written out in the form of letters, it would fill 1,000 thousand-page books with three thousand characters on each page—and that is just the hereditary blueprint in one cell.

Without this blueprint, we would never have come into existence, nor could we live. It controls all the functions of the cell, and its division, down to the tiniest detail. Today, we are (rightly) impressed by the tremendous memory capacity and speed of computers; but the performance of the DNA molecule is an even greater wonder.

Our hundred thousand–odd genetic traits provide careful instructions as to how the cell is to deliver the products for which it is programmed—everything from a hormone, a few enzymes, mucus, sebum, and the weapons of the immune system to spark-like impulses in the brain's network of nerve cells.

One may well ask how the encoded information is deciphered, and how this abstract script is converted into concrete molecules of protein and other substances. The process in our cells is an unceasing one—it is life itself—and it takes place on an inconceivably small scale, in cells only a few hundredths of a millimetre in diameter.

It works as follows: Special messengers—chemical cousins of DNA, called messenger RNA—seek out a particular piece of information, or gene, and make a copy of it. They transport this copy from the control centre in the cell nucleus, where the ribosomes are. Ribosomes are tiny granules attached to the cell's nourishing plasma. They function as protein synthesisers: the messengers come here with their sketches of what is to be done and, from the building blocks of protein—the twenty amino acids—the protein molecule is constructed along the lines of a brick house. The protein molecule is then sent out to serve in the process of life.

In reality, this buildup of molecules to form increasingly large molecule chains is not as simple as it might appear. Most remarkable are the vast effects of the genetic code and molecule construction. They underlie everything that makes us as we are. They mean that we become people, not animals; they determine sex, body size, and the colour of skin, hair, and eyes. They control intelligence, health, and even disease—among the genes, there are certain defective ones that make us liable to be struck by hereditary diseases sooner or later in our lives.

And all these traits are established at the moment when the genes in the male sperm fuse with the genes in the female ovum.

The instant of fertilisation, with its uncontrollable amalgamation of genes from two individuals, is the draw in life's great lottery. It is then that our offspring draw prizes or blanks; it is that moment which, once and for all, decides whether defective genes occupy sites in the DNA where they can do mischief, or whether good genes are dominant. The immune system is one example: every so often, the parents' genes combine in such a way that the child receives a weak immune system. It is destined to be harassed by infections and, perhaps, to die a premature death.

The most important chromosome as far as the immune system is concerned is the one geneticists call number 6. It contains most of the genes which control the body's defences. First and foremost, it regulates what are called the T-lymphocytes, which are important for the whole immune system. They function as a kind of command unit for the great army of defence cells. Some of them stimulate, others suppress and balance; a third type works in conjunction with the antibody-producing B-lymphocytes.

People who are unfortunate enough to be born with some damage to the sixth chromosome often become what might be called immunological invalids. They suffer ever-recurring infections, and not infrequently die in childhood or early adulthood. Much contemporary research into the body's defences is therefore concentrated on this chromosome. Researchers hope to be able to unravel its secrets in order to alleviate the suffering caused by immune system deficiency. Their efforts include the current struggle against AIDS (acquired immune deficiency syndrome), a lethal disease correlated with male homosexuality, also spread by means of blood transfusions. It is characterised by a severe reduction in the activity of the vital T-cells.

The material of inheritance is extremely conservative by nature. This is evident from the fact that human beings today differ very little from those who lived a hundred thousand years ago. Nonetheless, the genetic blueprint can be altered at various points. Over the long term, these changes have generally been beneficial to the species. However, in the short term, individual perspective, gene modification may do more harm than good. Radiation, vibrations, chemical effects, and other environmental factors can lead to genetic mutation, as it is called. If changes of this kind occur at the fetal stage, miscarriage is often the result. Nature has its own protective mechanisms.

Improved medical care, however, means that certain hereditary defects that formerly killed the individual before he or she became reproductively mature are now becoming more widespread. Diabetes of the juvenile type is one example; allergic diseases are another. Their victims now attain a normal age and have children, who also carry the seeds of the disease in their genes.

Whether modern genetic engineering—the ability to manipulate genes—will in the future counteract this new tendency for defective genes to spread remains to be seen. In any case, genetic manipulation opens up a whole new research front whose concrete results could include new medicines, vaccinations, and methods of treatment.

Suddenly, man holds some of the keys of life in his hand.

It is the genes which determine skin colour, hair type, skull configuration, and certain facial features, such as the shape of nose, mouth, and eyelids.

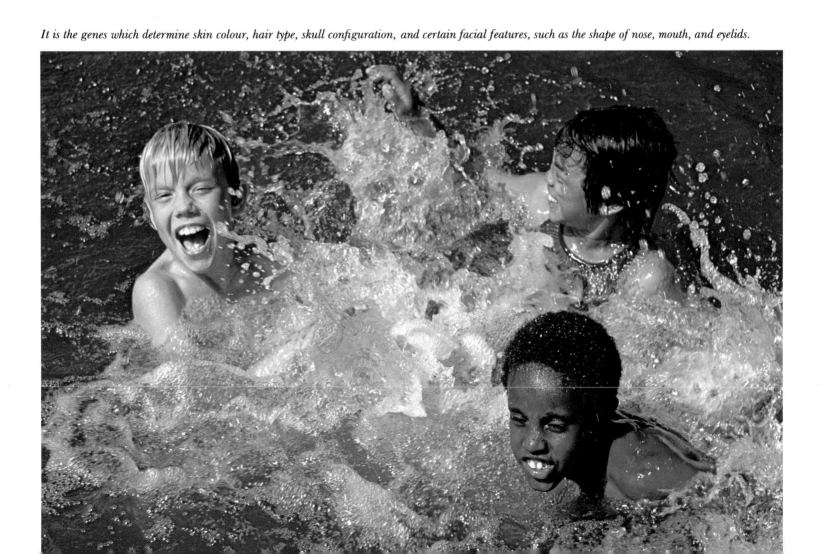

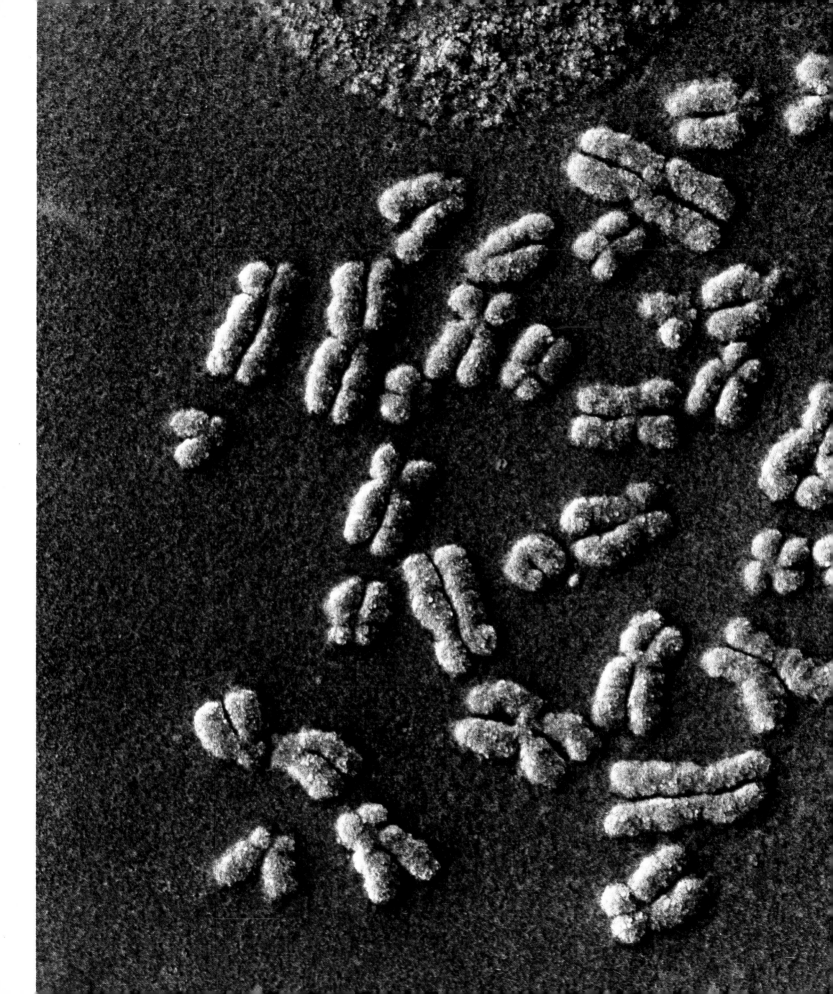

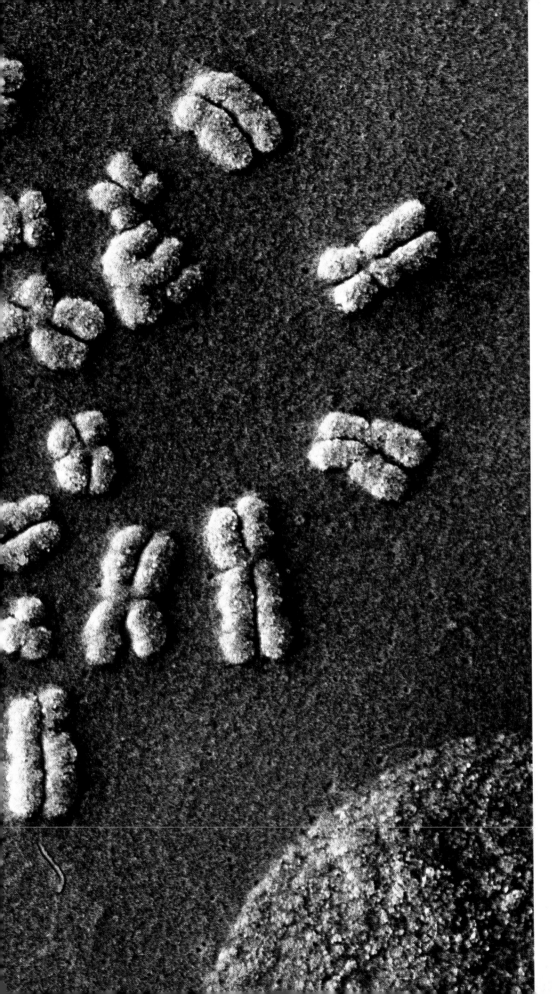

The cells' chemical punch cards

Human cells contain 23 pairs of human chromosomes. The variation in size between chromosome pairs is considerable: the longest is about ten times larger than the smallest. The chromosomes contain genes, half of which come from the father and half from the mother. The combination is determined at the moment the genetic blueprint of the sperm fuses with that of the egg. Some scope remains for the genes, however—the phenomenon of crossing-over, as it is called, between genes. This creates variation and is one of the mechanisms behind genetic modification to adapt the species to changed environmental conditions.

The genes may be likened to chemical punch cards. Stored on them is all the information the cell requires to perform its tasks. The information consists of four kinds of amino acids—thymine, adenine, cytosine, and guanine—arranged serially in such a way as to form a code, the genetic code. There are an infinite number of ways of arranging the varied sequences of the four amino acids. Cell messengers, as they are called, read the code for a protein—for example, an enzyme—and transfer the information to the cell units, which assemble the enzyme according to the design. The procedure is the same for all the proteins in the body: the genes on the long chromosome ribbons contain the genes, and production takes place in the cell factories.

In man, there are about 100,000 genes—and they are to be found in the nucleus of every single one of the body's many billions of cells! However, the cell utilises only a few thousand genes; the rest constitute dormant, or mute, information. How the cell "turns on and off" different genes is still not fully known.

The dominant chemical substance in the chromosomes is DNA, deoxyribonucleic acid. It contains the material of inheritance in all living things, both plants and animals, and has passed it on from one generation to the next since life began, around 4,000 million years ago. It is hard to find any chemical compound whose potential exceeds DNA.

Human chromosomes. The rounded formations in the lower and upper sections of the picture are cells. (x 40,000)

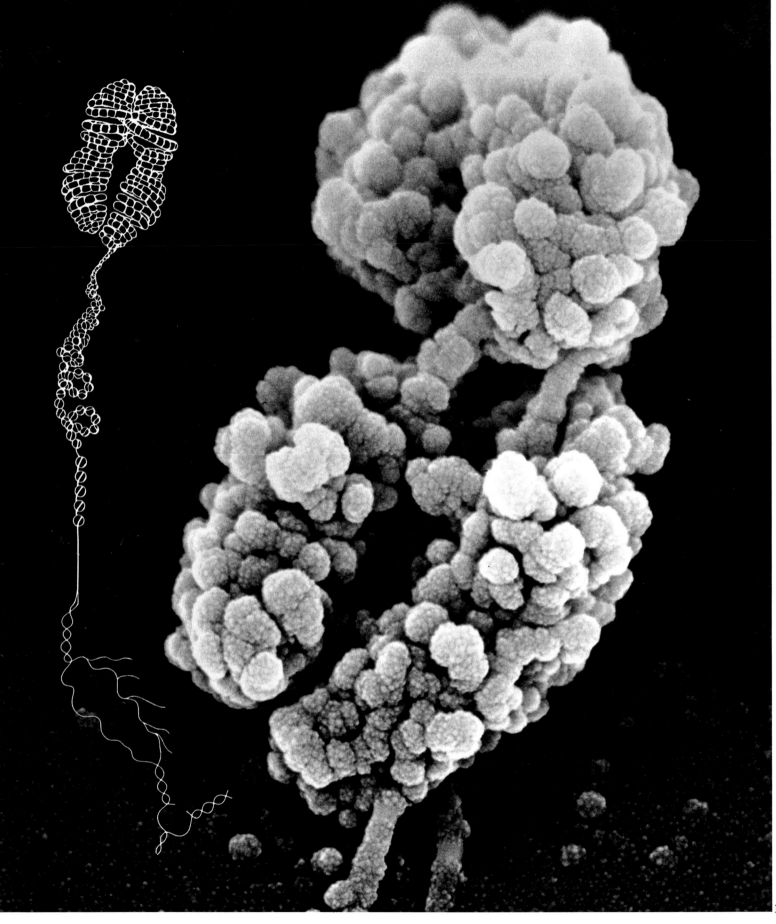

Opposite, we see a pair of chromosomes magnified about 125,000 times in the scanning electron microscope. The adjacent illustration is a diagram of chromosome construction. Chromosomes consist of extremely fine DNA strands, more than a metre long, spun around a protein nucleus. Returning to the large picture, we see the cluster of DNA strands on the chromosome. When the cell divides, each strand is split into two exact copies. Thus from one cell two genetically identical cells are created—a precondition for the correct functioning of cells, tissues and organs.

Below, single and sometimes double strands of DNA, represented as dotted lines and rosettes. The grainy substance surrounding them is proteins. This remarkable picture was taken by means of a transmission electron microscope.

How, then, is the information distributed between the 46 chromosomes? DNA hybrid technology has enhanced man's ability to map the genes in our chromosomes. Today, we know the exact construction of several hundred genes; in the future, perhaps, we shall have access to all the entries in the vast gene library of the cell nucleus.

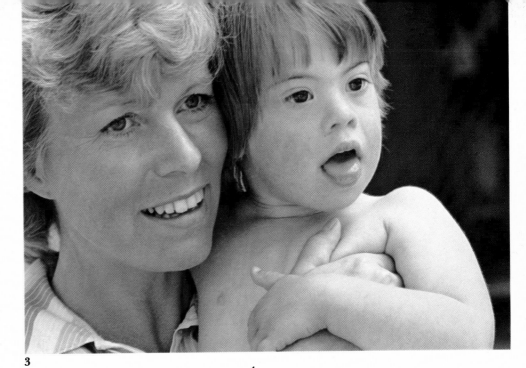

3

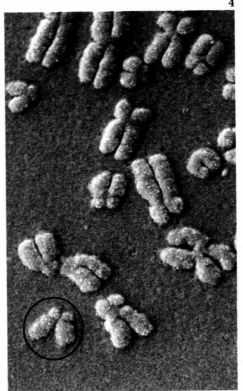

4

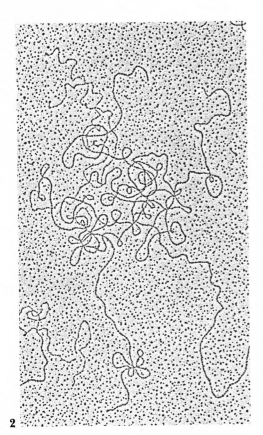

2

1. *Human chromosomes, magnified about 125,000 times, with a diagram showing the construction of DNA strands.*
2. *DNA strands.*
3. *Mother and Down's syndrome child.*
4. *Detail of a human being's normal chromosomes, with a ring around the 21st. In mongoloids, the 21st chromosome consists of three sections instead of two.*

Down's syndrome

Chromosomes and their genes contain the design for all cells and tissues. Barely visible defects in the chromosomes can have devastating consequences. One example is Down's syndrome, also called mongolism. This malformation produces congenital heart defects, malformation of the intestines, severe brain disorder resulting in retardation, extreme susceptibility to infection, and the risk of leukemia, to mention only a few characteristics. Its cause is an excess of chromosomes: the child has 47 instead of 46. Chromosome number 21 (with a ring round it in the photograph) has three, instead of two, sections.

When the excessive genes in chromosome 21 dictate how the body is to develop, countermands and misunderstandings arise. Superficial characteristics include slanting eyes and malformed outer ears, but the internal damage is more serious. One child in 600 to 700 is affected by Down's syndrome. The risk increases with the age of the mother: For the 40-year-old mother, one in a hundred; for the 45-year-old, one in sixteen. Surgical correction of internal malformations, together with other medical treatment, means that mongoloids now have an approximately normal life expectancy. In days gone by, they died young. Today, Down's syndrome can be detected by means of amniocentesis (extracting and testing a sample of amniotic fluid) while there is still time to terminate the pregnancy.

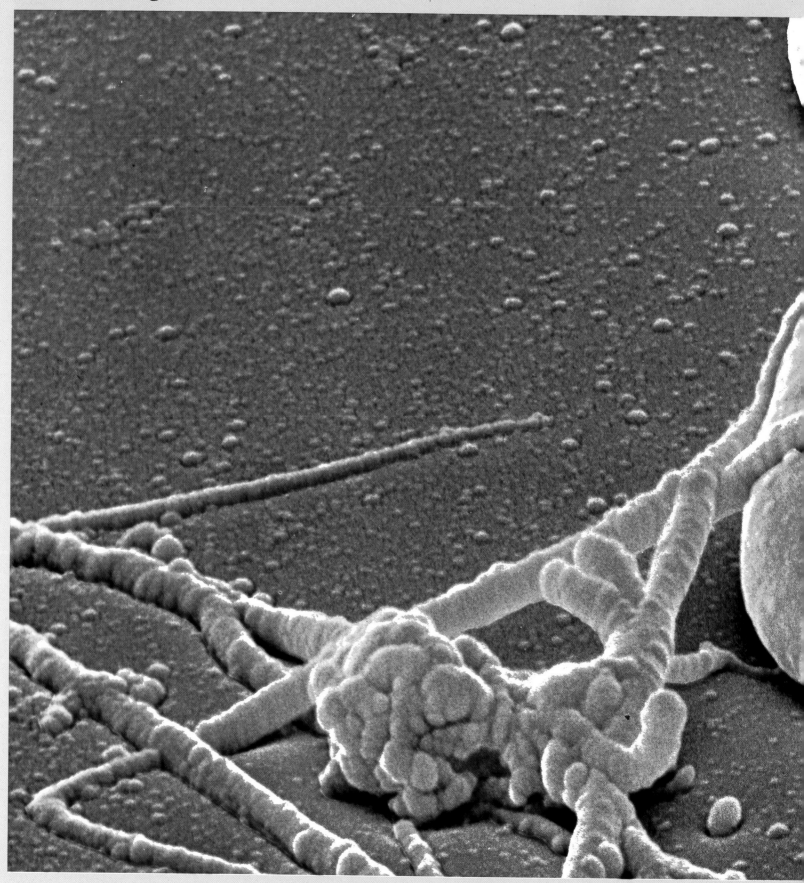

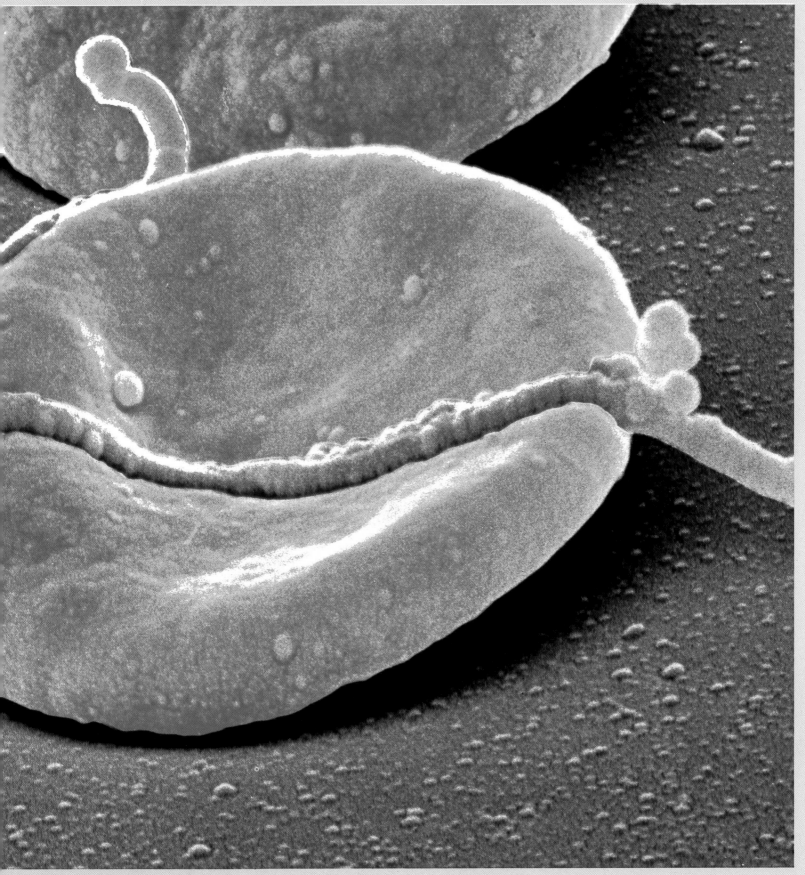

Blood clotting

A blood clot in an artery of the heart may be no more than two millimetres thick and weigh only a fraction of a gram.

Yet it kills a human being within about half an hour.

The misplaced blood clot (or thrombus) is a biological deviation in one direction; persistent bleeding, or hemorrhage, is a deviation in the other. In each case the body is manifesting a disturbance in one of its most intricate chain reactions: clotting, or coagulation, of the blood.

It is easier to understand that an unchecked hemorrhage causes life, literally, to ebb away than it is to see how an insignificant lump of clotted blood can quench the flame of life. The explanation lies in the fact that it blocks the life-sustaining network in a vital area, cutting off the blood supply and choking the cells. Large portions of heart muscle suddenly stop working, and the remainder are unable to maintain the circulation. In the case of a clot affecting the brain, essential centres are incapacitated and the flow of spark-like impulses between nerve cells ceases.

Prolonged hemorrhage and the formation of thrombi are pathological extremes in a system that normally functions with unremitting precision, and that is essential to life. If the coagulation process did not automatically seal leaks arising in the smallest blood vessels, the capillaries, or in surface wounds, life would be rendered impossible. If the clotting system were not equipped with safety mechanisms to prevent coagulation taking place at the wrong site in a blood vessel, clots could develop anywhere.

The ability or inability of blood to clot is thus a good example of how, by a finely tuned balancing act, the body has learned to make use of biological dynamite. Its successful use is based on the fact that blood clotting is a step-by-step process. In other words, the body has no blood clots stored ready for use; everything is done on the spot. All the tools and ingredients needed for this process circulate in the blood. When a blood vessel is damaged, an alarm signal is transmitted, setting off a clotting process comprising no fewer than fifteen stages.

The first stage consists of an instantaneous change in the nature of the blood platelets (thrombocytes) when they come into contact with the site of injury. Normally, they move freely in the blood without adhering either to each other or to the blood vessel walls. But when tissue is damaged, substances in the connective tissue alter the characteristics of the passing platelets: suddenly they become very sticky and start fusing both with the damaged blood vessel wall and with each other. They rapidly build a preliminary dam, at the same time producing substances which initiate the actual clotting.

Step by step, various substances in the blood are thus activated, and at the final stage two substances are crucial. One is an enzyme called *thrombin,* the other a protein called *fibrin.* The thrombin's role is to promote the process, and that of the fibrin is to supply the clot with a network of fine threads which trap blood cells.

The strong, tough fibrin threads are produced by a method chemists call polymerisation. It is the same as that employed by a spider when it spins its web and, in the plastics industry, in the making of nylon thread. Rubber is another example of the many natural polymers—that is, chain-like molecules—which have arisen from the coupling of simple molecules. Our own body processes thus paved the path now followed by high technology. By means of the enzyme thrombin, a soluble substance called fibrinogen is converted into a solid called fibrin.

If, however, the thrombin were to activate the fibrinogen and build a network of fibrin threads at the wrong site in the circulatory system, disaster would result: It would lead to blood clots which might be fatal. To inhibit their formation, nature has therefore developed a number of safety mechanisms; several chemical stages must be undergone before the thrombin is ready to function.

For a blood clot to form, it is essential for the coagulation factors to act in a particular sequence. Some individuals lack one or several of these factors, and as a result their blood does not clot normally. The hardest hit are *hemophiliacs,* who on being injured must receive treatment in order not to bleed to death.

In addition to blood clotting, which is a *chemical* process in the blood, the body also has *mechanical* methods at its disposal to reduce blood loss. These come into play when a blood vessel is cut or torn: it tightens at the site of injury, and the blood which has seeped out into surrounding tissue exerts pressure on the vessel from without. Defence measures of this kind are important since the loss of as little as half a litre of blood can bring about a state of shock, which is a serious condition.

There are, then, substances in the blood which in the course of a complex series of events make a blood clot form. But there are also substances that can counteract clotting, "dilute" the blood, and act directly to dissolve the fibrin in a clot. The clotting system on the one hand and the dissolving system on the other must function in equilibrium, so that neither outweighs the other. If a clot were to be dissolved prematurely, blood would start leaking out again. And if it remains too long in one artery, it can cause tissue damage, since not enough blood then gets to the cells.

The great, and growing, problem in our society is that coagulation so often takes place at the wrong site in the blood vessels. The cause is damage to the vessel walls, leading to fatty degeneration or atherosclerosis: the diseased, rough walls easily give rise to blood clots, and vessel constriction increases the risk that loosened clots will join together and form thrombi. Nowadays, the initial stages of atherosclerosis may be observed in young people between twenty and twenty-five. Although hereditary factors also play a part, faulty nutrition and living habits are dominant: excessive consumption of animal fat and carbohydrates, insufficient exercise, too much stress, and smoking. Vascular diseases increasingly often affect younger men, and nowadays also women in growing numbers.

The dramatic final phase need not necessarily be the lodging of a blood clot in the coronary vessels. Much autopsy evidence indicates that the cause of sudden death is much more often a spasm—a sudden tightening of the coronary arteries—and that no clot is formed in the majority of cases. However, underlying this phenomenon is the occurrence of pathological changes in the heart's coronary vessels, namely, their becoming increasingly blocked.

Red blood cells, seven-thousandths of a millimetre in diameter, on their way through the body's tiniest blood vessels, the capillaries. Capillaries easily break as a result of blows or cuts, but leakages are rapidly sealed in a person whose blood clots normally. (×1,200)

A hemophiliac boy, equipped with helmet and protective pads for the joints, which reduce the risk of dangerous bleeding. In hemophiliacs even small leakages in minor blood vessels can have consequences that are hard to deal with, and preventive measures such as these are therefore essential.

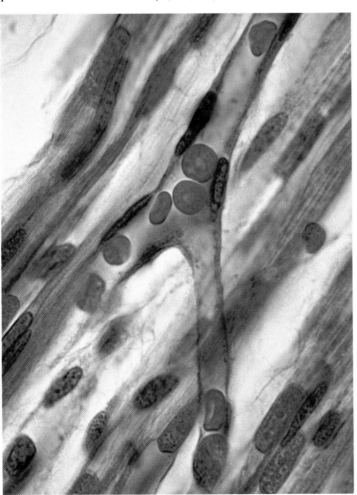

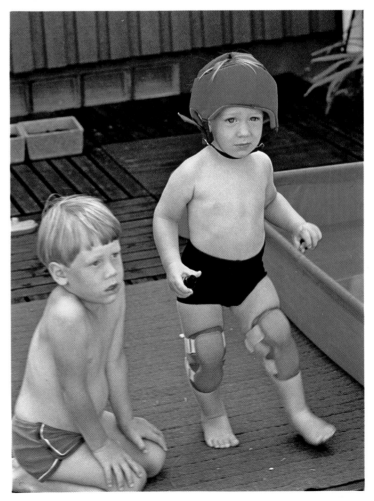

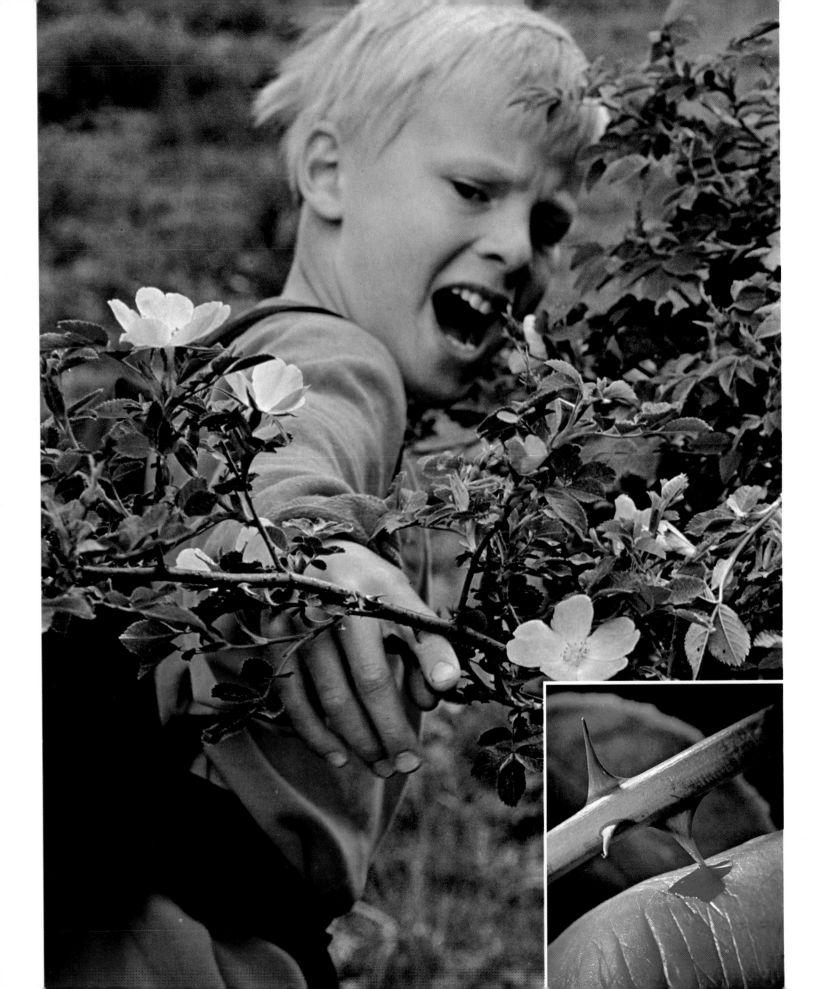

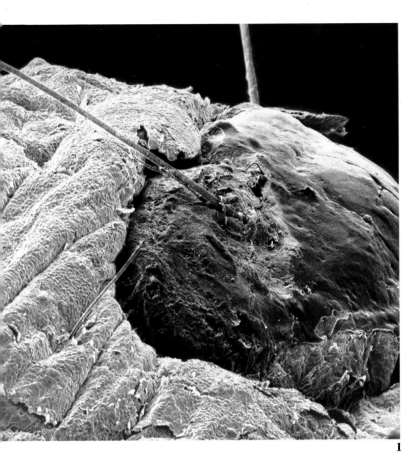

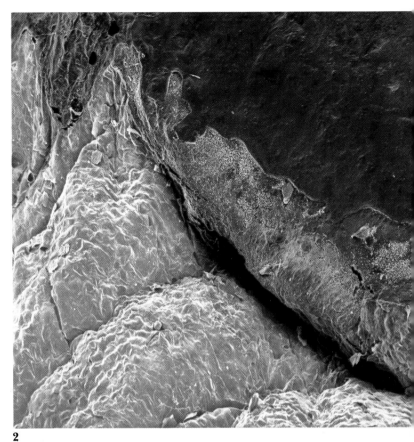

1   2

An everyday drama: the healing of a wound

Breaking the skin is easy—a scratch from the thorn of a wild rose is enough. When it happens, the body's first line of defence collapses. Bacteria living permanently on the skin are now able to enter the underlying tissues, an environment rich in nourishment.

Even a small, superficial wound poses two problems for the body: to stop the bacterial invasion and to inhibit bleeding. If the immune system is defective, even normally harmless skin bacteria may become a threat. And if blood clotting does not function properly, a tiny wound also leads to a large loss of blood.

In the healthy body, however, the correct reactions are triggered immediately and automatically. The tissue injury prompts the release of substances which make the thrombocytes in the blood adhere to each other and start forming a clot. At the same time, the various frontline troops of the immune system rally to the wound, where they attack the intruders and remove debris from the damaged cell tissue.

Above, magnified about 40 times, we see how a crust, or scab, has formed over a wound (*1*). There is a clear line of demarcation between the scab (the smoother surface) and the undamaged skin epithelium. Strands of hair stick up through the scab. The picture on the *right, above (2)* shows the demarcation line between undamaged skin and scab, magnified about 80 times.

Of the two illustrations nearest to the *right*, the one *above (3)* shows the appearance of the scab after a few days. It is nature's own first-aid bandage, a web of fibrin threads packed with red blood cells and thrombocytes. In the picture *below (4)*, we see how the scab has become detached: new skin has formed beneath it. The everyday drama of healing is almost complete.

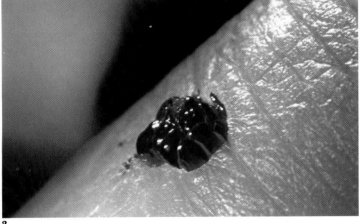

3

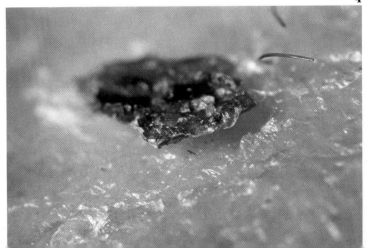

4

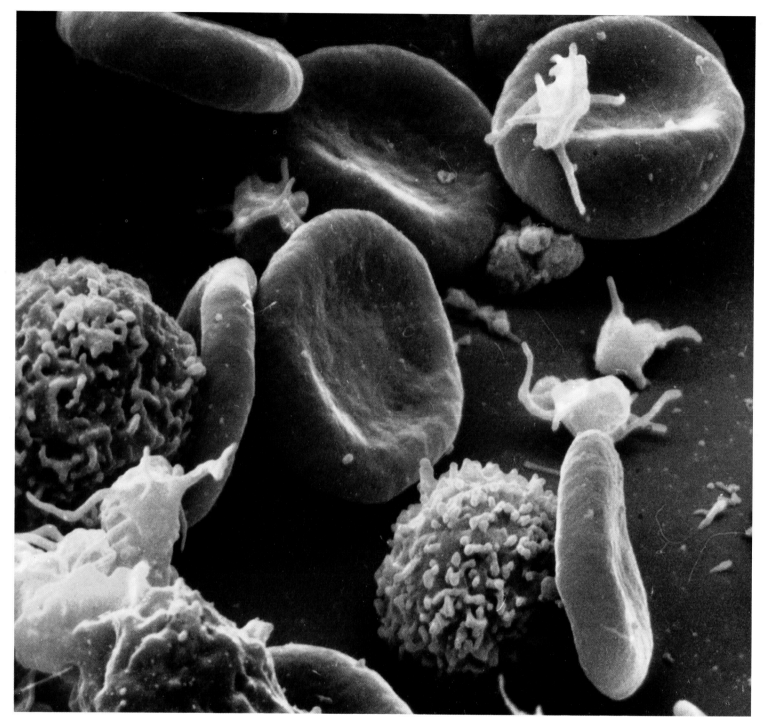

Blood—our liquid organ

Blood is a liquid tissue with many important tasks to perform. It consists half of yellowish, watery plasma and half of red and white cells and thrombocytes (also called platelets).

Left, we see biconcave red cells, spiky white cells (granulocytes) and irregularly shaped, tiny thrombocytes which have been activated. (×10,000) The red blood cells are elastic, in order to squeeze through the often narrow capillaries. Their task is to convey oxygen from the lungs to the cells of the body, and to transport the waste-product dioxide from the cells to the lungs.

In an adult there are around 25 thousand million red blood cells, with a total surface area of 3,000 square metres—thus, our oxygen absorption resources are enormous!

Granulocytes are white blood cells that are part of the immune system. They circulate in the blood and attack foreign substances such as bacteria. They are small feeding (phagocytic) cells, differing in both size and combative endurance from the hardier, larger phagocytes, the macrophages.

Thrombocytes are cell fragments that become detached from

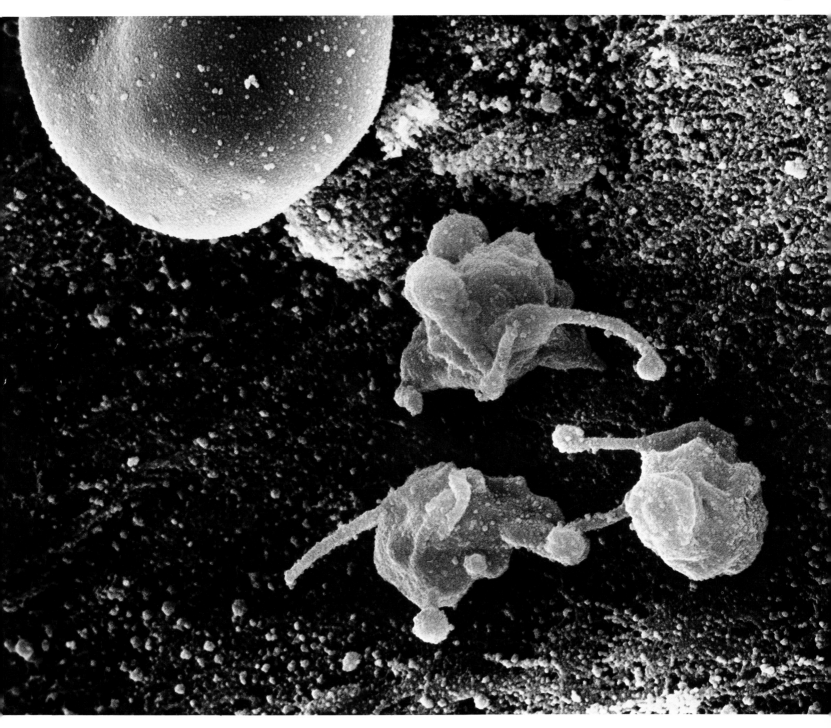

megakaryocytes, giant cells with several nuclei stationed in the bone marrow. In one cubic millimetre of blood there are between 200,000 and 500,000 thrombocytes. Thrombocytes may be described as the key that unlocks blood coagulation. They circulate constantly in the blood without adhering to each other or the blood vessel walls. But if a tissue injury arises in a blood vessel, they immediately change character. Under the influence of substances released from the site of injury, they adhere to each other, forming a preliminary dam, stopping the leakage,

then issuing the chemical signals that initiate the blood-clotting process.

The picture to the *right,* magnified about 15,000 times, shows a red blood cell *(top left)* and the wounded region of a blood vessel. The endothelial cells, which normally constitute a barrier between the blood and the vessel wall, have been torn off. Three thrombocytes adhere to the exposed tissue and have started to release their contents, some of which promote the coagulation of the blood. Others stimulate the growth of cells that repair the wound.

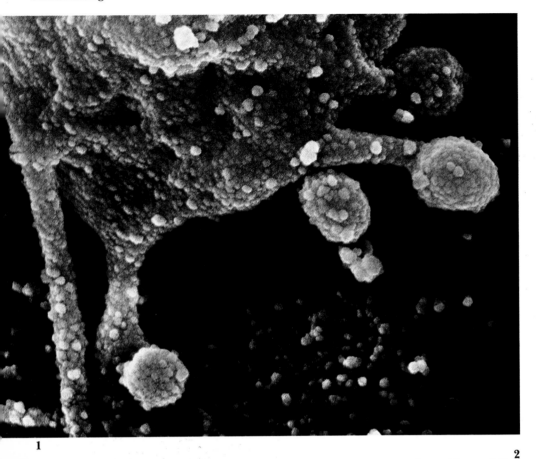

1

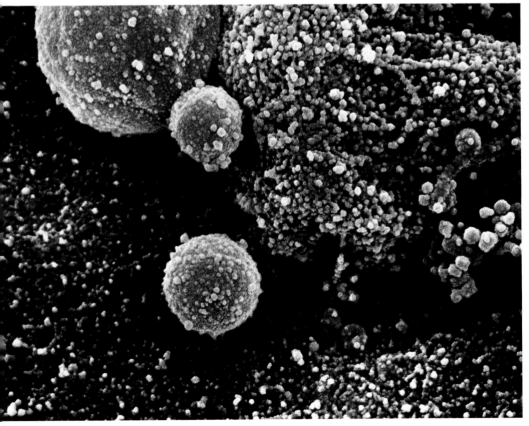

2

The body makes its own bandage

Further magnification of a thrombocyte shows how grains are secreted from its offshoots. These grains contain substances that are important for the coagulation process. The thrombocyte collects on its surface biologically active substances from the blood plasma. Finally, the coagulating enzyme thrombin is formed.

The task of the thrombin is to activate a substance in the blood plasma, fibrinogen, which is rapidly transformed into fibrin. This fibrin forms a mesh of threads, which becomes the shell of the blood clot. The *upper* picture *(far right, opposite)* shows how the formation of threads has started, and the picture *below* shows part of the mesh in the complete fibrin web, enclosing trapped red blood cells.

Blood clotting is a complex process that must undergo fifteen stages before it is completed. These stages must follow each other in the correct sequence, otherwise no blood clot will be formed.

The clot is a temporary first-aid bandage providing a protective cover beneath which the real repair work is done. For this reason there is a dissolving system based on the enzyme plasmin, which causes the disintegration of the clot when it has completed its task.

Fibrin is produced by the same method as that used in the plastics industry for making nylon thread: polymerisation. Here, simple fibrinogen molecules are being linked together, forming fibrin chains. *Opposite, upper left,* we see the thread growing out of the thrombocyte in the foreground. It is this thread that starts the process, at the moment when it comes into contact with damaged tissue. The whole area around the wound immediately changes character. The thrombocytes stick together, fibrinogen (hitherto an invisible component of blood plasma) is shed and, under the influence of the enzyme thrombin, becomes fibrin. The fibrin forms threads which are spun into a net. Finally, thrombocytes and blood cells are trapped and a dam is formed.

1-2. *Details of thrombocytes adhering within an injured blood vessel. The grains from the thrombocyte are ejected as small balls and leave craterlike openings on the cell's surface. Magnifications: 1. X 40,000, 2. X 60,000.*

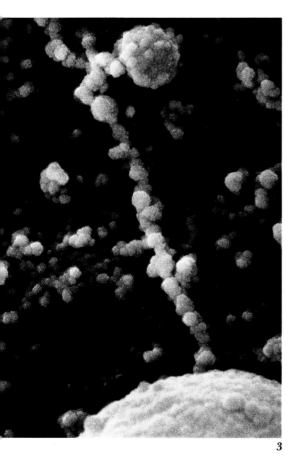

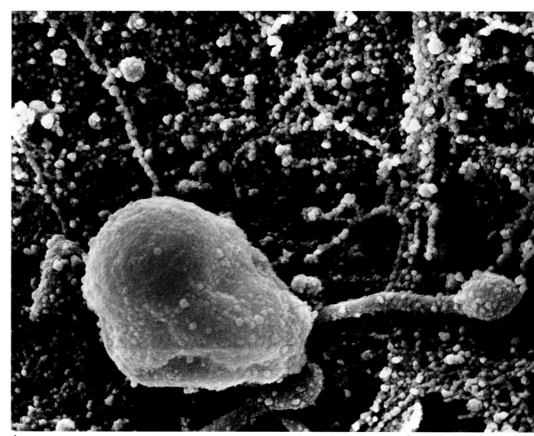

3

4

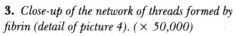

3. *Close-up of the network of threads formed by fibrin (detail of picture 4). (× 50,000)*
4. *Thrombocyte and threads during formation. (× 20,000)*
5. *Fibrinogen molecule. (× 235,000)*
6. *Red blood cells, trapped in the finished fibrin network. (× 7,500)*

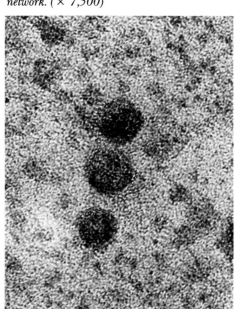

5

6

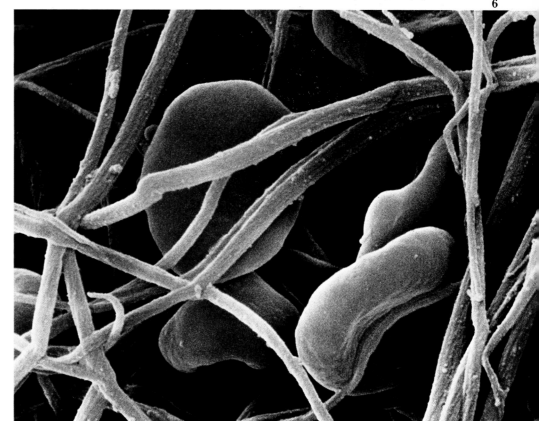

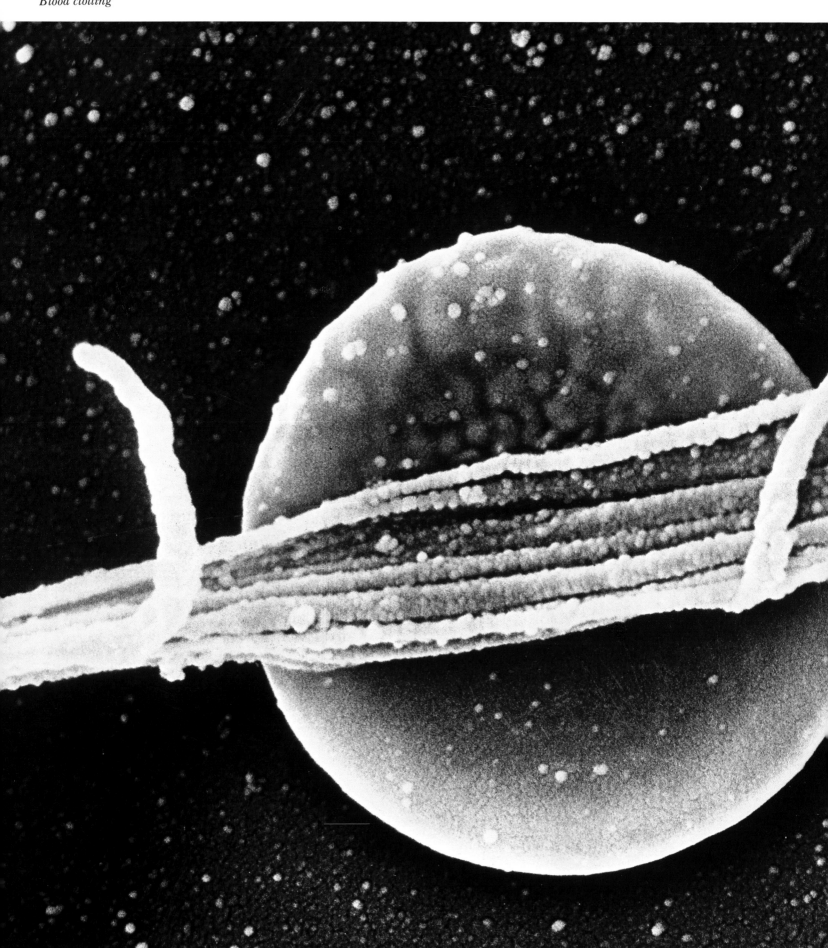

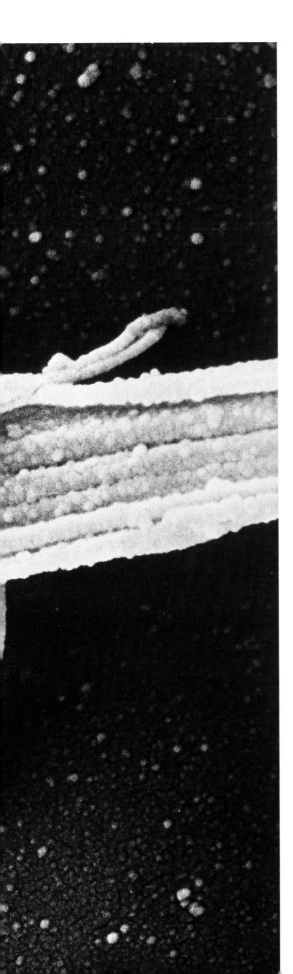

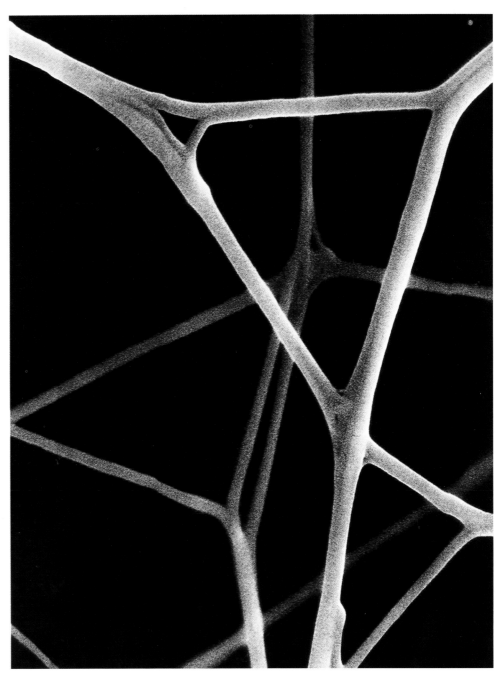

Nature as designer

This could be a picture of the planet Saturn, with its rings, but it is a red blood cell trapped in a bunch of fibrin threads. The blood cell's diameter is in reality no more than about seven-thousandths of a millimetre: the magnification is thus 25,000 times.

Nature's skill as a designer is also evident in the illustration, *above*, showing (magnified 75,000 times) some threads in the fragile fibrin web—the elegant initial phase of blood clotting. These threads trap blood cells and platelets; together, they form a clot that seals leaks in the blood vessels. Fibrin threads are to a blood clot what reinforcing bars are to reinforced concrete.

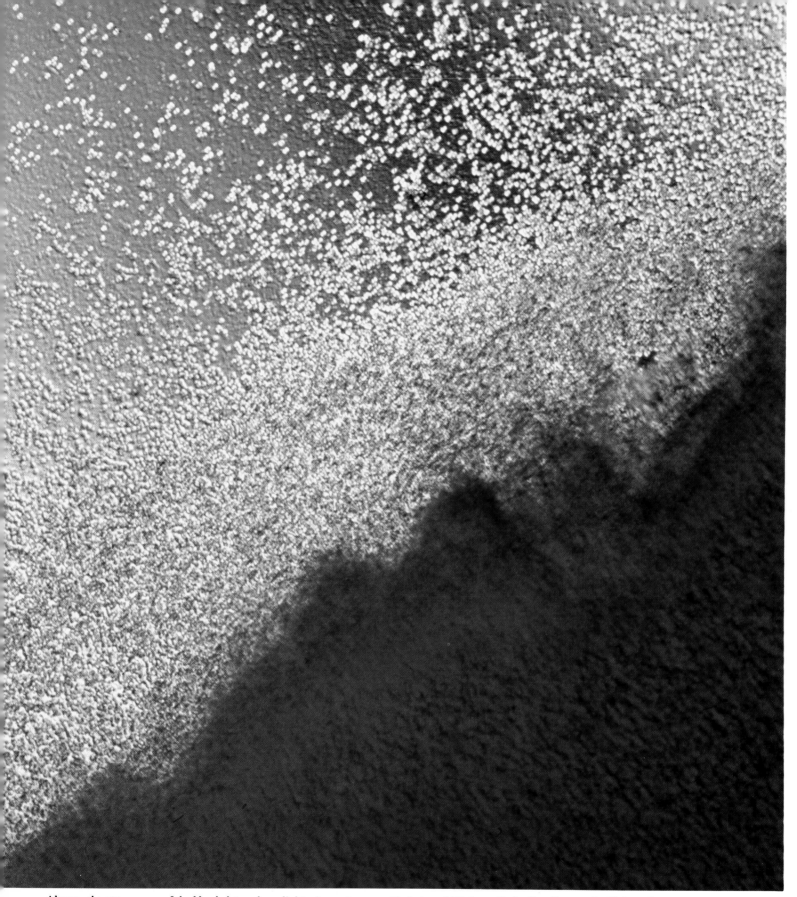

Above, *the appearance of the blood clot under a light microscope, magnified about 200 times. Red cells adhere to the fibrin web.*
Right, *fibrin net magnified about 2,100 times—but still under the light microscope. We see the fibrin web is filling up with trapped blood cells.*

60

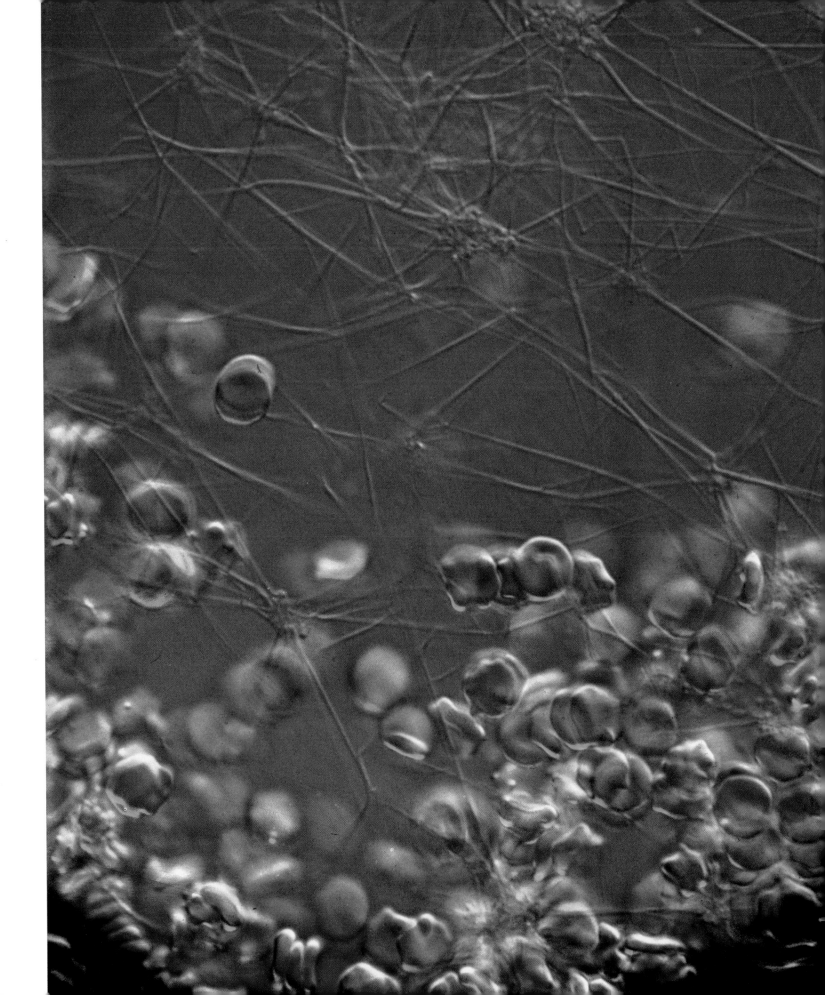

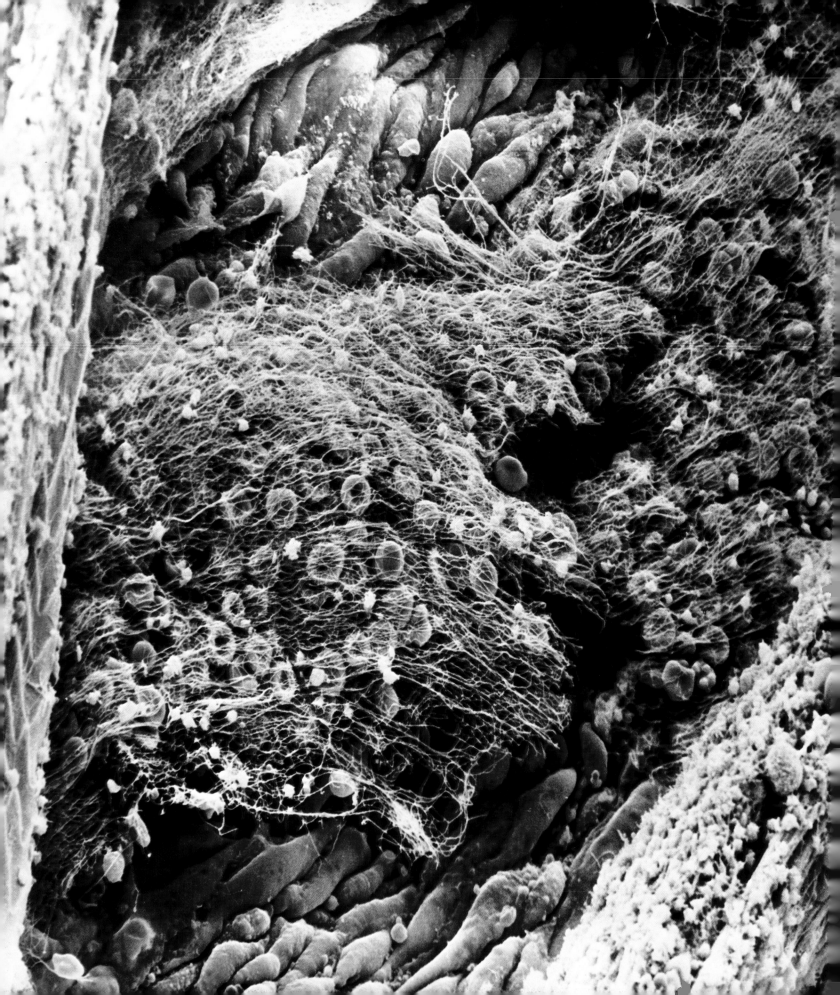

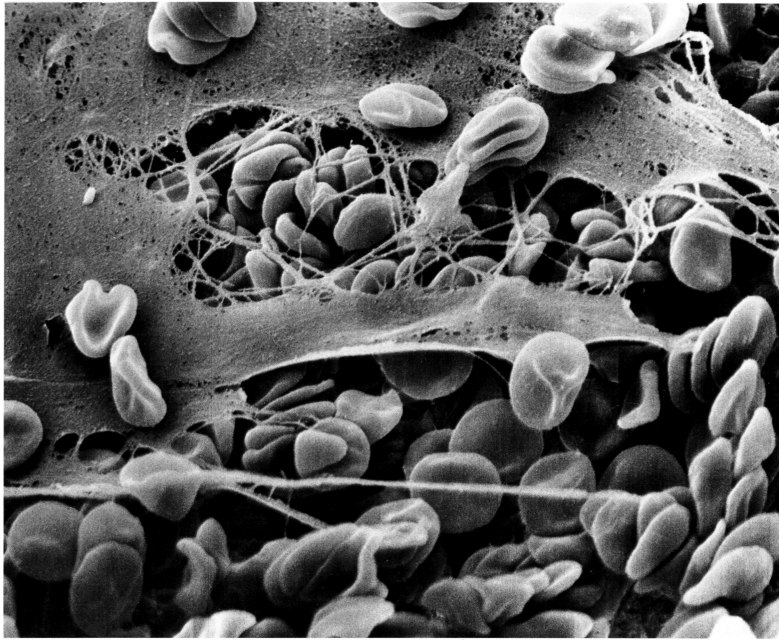

Above: *blood clot, under a scanning electron microscope. (× 3,400)*

Left: *birth of a blood clot in a blood vessel. Red blood cells are trapped in the fibrin web. (× 1,300)*

An increasingly fine mesh

Once the thrombocytes have given the starting signal, the blood clot grows fast. There is no lack of material for it to utilise: each cubic millimetre of blood contains about 5 million red blood cells and between 200,000 and 400,000 thrombocytes. They are trapped in the increasingly fine mesh of the fibrin web, eventually forming a tight plug at the site of bleeding.

The pictures on this page show the genesis and growth of the blood clot, under a scanning electron microscope.

Left, we witness the dramatic moment when a blood clot has just been born in a blood vessel. In the middle of the picture, we see how the red blood cells have been trapped in the fibrin web like fish in a net.

Opposite, magnified further, we see the blood clot several minutes later. The coagulation process is already much more advanced and the fibrin web has taken on an almost textile appearance. Passing blood cells are packed in ever more tightly.

The life-threatening blood clot

The greatest pestilence of our time is vascular disease, with cerebral hemorrhage, stroke, and heart attack as its most dramatic manifestations. When arteries become clogged—which may happen in various organs—part of the organ dies. The cause is an insufficient supply of oxygenated blood. In some cases, a blood clot has formed in a vessel and arrested the blood flow; in other cases, a clot formed elsewhere in the body has traveled to the vessel and adhered there. Third, the cause may be a vessel severely clogged by atherosclerosis, through which the flow of oxygenated blood is inadequate.

Atherosclerosis in the blood vessels is considered to have many causes: hereditary disposition, a diet rich in fat and cholesterol, overweight, high blood pressure, stress, cigarette smoking, and insufficient exercise. The inside of the blood vessel becomes damaged. Cholesterol crystals are deposited at the site of damage, the wall in due course becomes rough, and thrombocytes, with misdirected zeal, initiate a coagulation process. The vessels become steadily narrower and stiffer.

Below, a blood clot blocking the descending branch of the left coronary artery (often called the artery of sudden death) in a 48-year-old, overweight man.

Right, a blood clot in the left ventricle of the heart. The darker streaks are ligaments in the ventricle wall, while the lighter areas are thin parts of the wall. The blood clot in the picture is not dangerous if it stays put. Fragments of it may, however, loosen and block arteries elsewhere, which can be fatal.

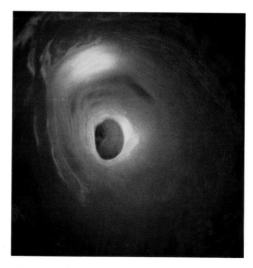

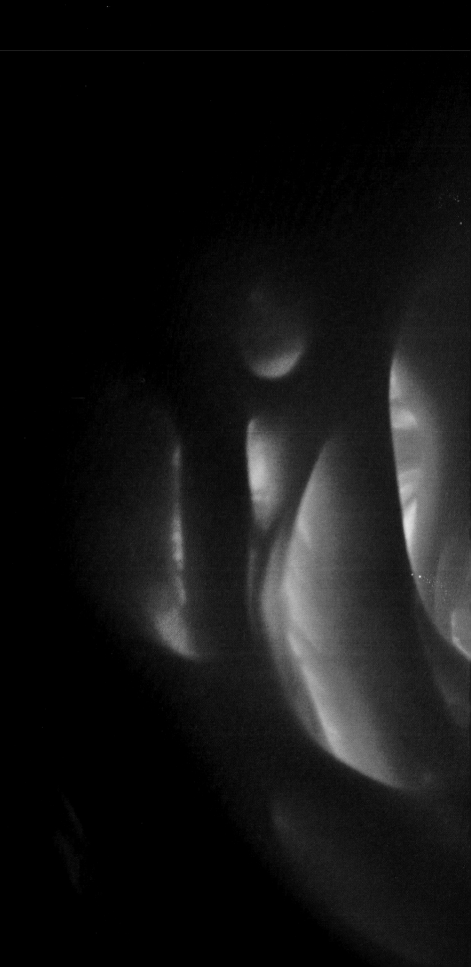

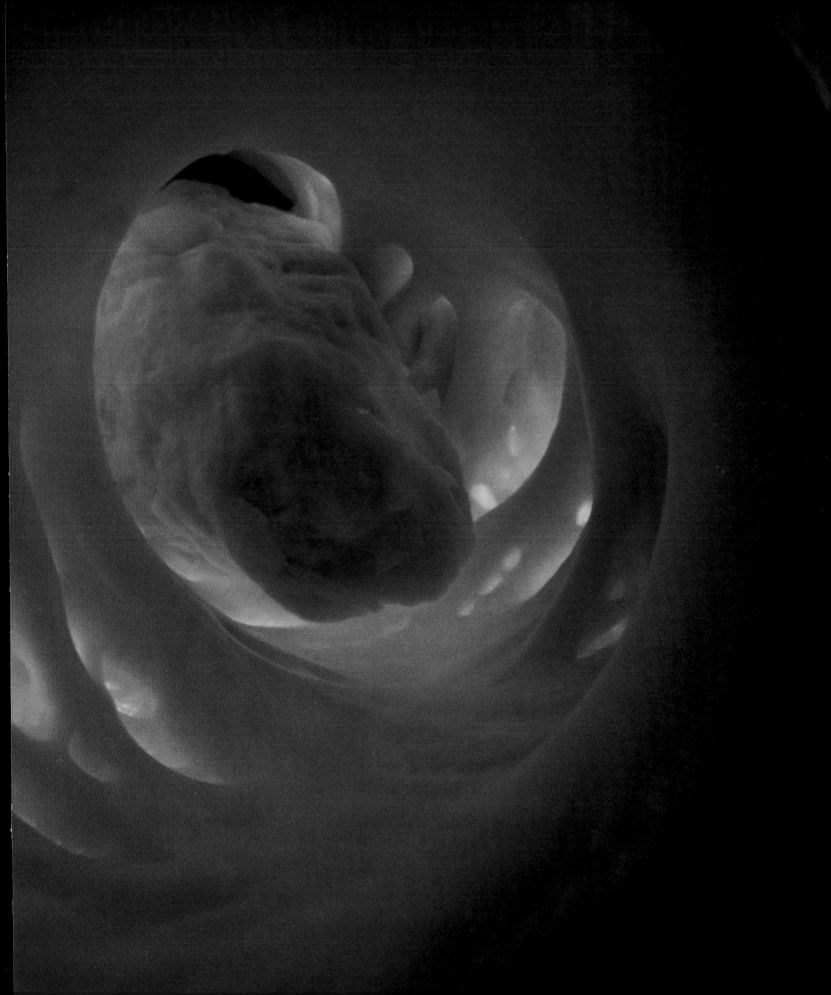

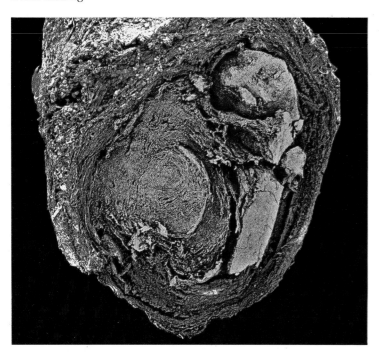

Atherosclerosis can lead to a heart attack

In a young person, the blood vessels of the heart have a diameter of about 3 mm. Their inner walls are smooth and polished, enabling the blood to flow unimpeded. However, the inner layer of the wall may change: The surface may become uneven, and the wall itself may thicken and lose its elasticity. The result is a deterioration in blood throughout, sometimes culminating in a complete blockage.

Not all the causes of atherosclerosis have yet been ascertained. Important risk factors where the heart is concerned include excess cholesterol in the blood and high blood pressure. Smoking is another major culprit.

Left, the coronary vessel of a middle-aged man—overweight and a heavy smoker—is totally clogged up. In this picture, taken with the aid of a scanning electron microscope, the blood vessel wall is thickened and brownish red. The yellow portions are the calcified material which has plugged the vessel completely.

The picture *below* shows the heart infarction (attack) resulting from atherosclerosis in the coronary vessels. (× 3,500) The yellow cells advancing over the muscle cells are white blood cells, whose task is to deal with dead and dying muscle cells, paving the way for the healing process.

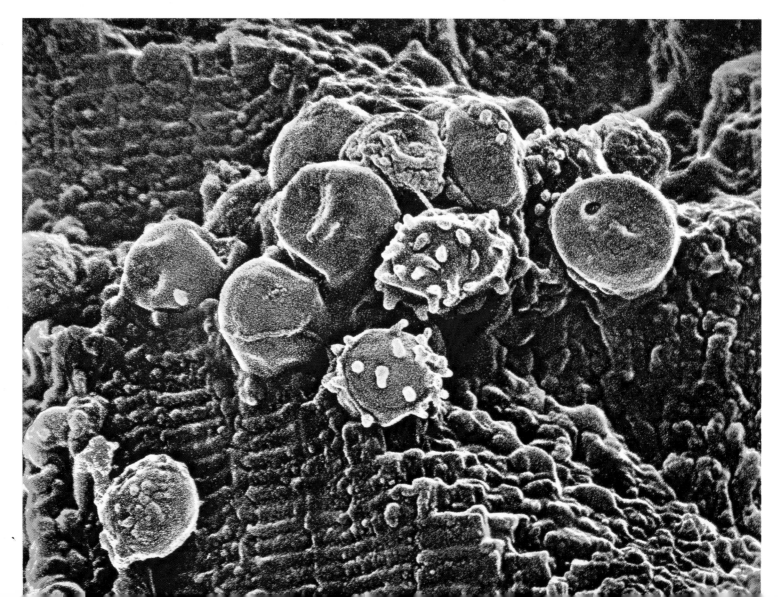

Exercise increases the "good" cholesterol

Cholesterol occurs in the body in many different forms. It is also an important raw material for the production of vitamins and hormones. Some cholesterols are good for the blood vessels, while others can harm them. With regular exercise it is possible to increase the "good" cholesterol in one's body and reduce the "bad." As a result, the risk of the blood vessel walls being damaged, or affected by the beginnings of atherosclerosis, declines.

Apart from taking exercise, wise precautions include cutting down the sources of stress and the amount of animal fat in the diet, giving up smoking, and keeping blood pressure under control.

Near right, particles of the "good" cholesterol, HDL (high-density lipoprotein); *far right*, the "bad," LDL (low-density lipoprotein).

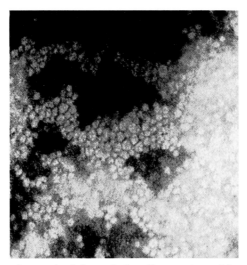

The "good" cholesterol, the yellow portions of the picture above, functions as a cleansing agent. Women normally have more than men, and this is thought to be one of the reasons why they suffer from heart and vascular diseases less frequently.

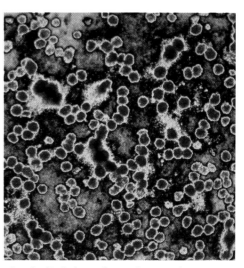

The "bad" cholesterol can, in excessive concentrations, be harmful and contribute to atherosclerosis.

Both pictures were produced by a special computer system for colour simulation of electron microscope photographs. (× 100,000)

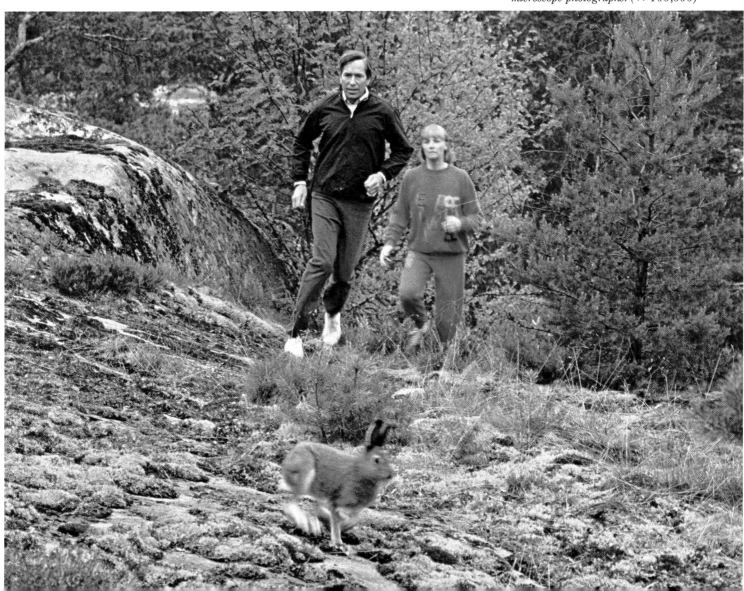

What is life-threatening to the hemophiliac . . .

For the blood to clot normally, fifteen coagulation factors must be activated in sequence. If only *one* factor is missing, the whole process is disturbed, and if it is the eighth factor, the result is *hemophilia.*

Blood from a healthy individual clots *in vitro* in three to six minutes. A hemophiliac's blood can take anything from half an hour to several hours. The prolonged coagulation time means that even tiny wounds and capillary breakages can be life-threatening.

The disease is hereditary, and the gene that causes it is carried on the female sex chromosome. Classic hemophilia strikes only men—it is transmitted from a hemophiliac man to half of his grandsons through the female line. Although his daughters do not suffer from the disease, they pass it on to their sons.

Hemophilia was described in Jewish writings from as early as the fifth century A.D., in connection with fatal circumcision. But it remained an enigma well into the nineteenth century, when it acquired the status of a royal disease. Britain's Queen Victoria bore the gene and passed it on through her daughters to the Spanish and Russian royal families. No fewer than ten of her male progeny of the first and second generations suffered from the disease.

It was not until 1947 that research was able to establish that hemophiliacs lack a certain substance, antihemophilic factor (AHF) in their blood, and that it is this lack which causes the disease. Approximately 85 percent of all hemophiliacs lack this very factor, which is the eighth in the coagulation schedule.

Further research showed that there were various types of hemophilia and that one form, von Willebrand's disease, affects both sexes. It was also found that lack of factor 9 occurred in certain types of hemophilia.

The symptoms vary according to the degree of severity of the disease. In some cases, the quantity of the critical factor in the blood is only slightly below par, and sufferers can cope with everyday life without any trouble. In other cases, where the lack is more marked, internal bleeding occurs spontaneously, particularly in the joints and beneath the skin. For such individuals the most minor operation, such as a tooth extraction, is impossible without preventive treatment.

This treatment nowadays consists mainly of injections of AHF. Large quantities are given, for example, before an operation. Hemophiliacs can lead a relatively normal life provided they receive a dose of AHF every few months. However, they may not take medicine without consulting a doctor, since many common medicines, including pain relievers derived from salicylic acid, affect blood-clotting ability.

In about 10 percent of hemophiliacs, the immune system launches an attack against the AHF. This creates problems, which may, however, be solved in some cases by the use of chemotherapy.

Since the gene causing the disease is carried by the hemophiliac's daughters, early abortion of female fetuses is offered to hemophiliacs in some countries. Sex can be determined by amniocentesis and other newer tests.

Nowadays, the hemophiliac can keep his disease under control by taking the coagulation factor VIII, i.e., antihemophilic factor (AHF), he lacks.

A 100 ml ampoule once a week may be sufficient. When bleeding is acute, several ampoules a day are needed. Sterile equipment is essential.

The hemophiliac is surrounded daily by serious threats—for instance, a broken glass bottle. Even small hemorrhages can be life-threatening and must be counteracted with AHF.

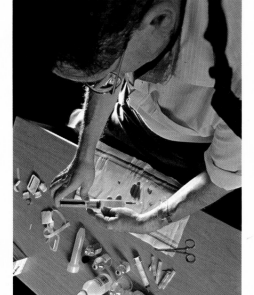
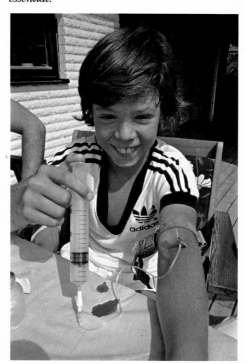
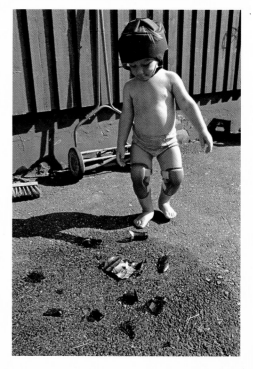

. . . is vital to the female mosquito

Our blood normally starts to clot as soon as a vessel wall ruptures and the thromboyctes respond to the injury. The coagulation process then begins and the leakage is sealed. However, there are exceptions, one of which is constituted by the blood-sucking female mosquito. To survive, she has evolved a method of thinning the victim's blood and preventing it from coagulating.

When the mosquito carves her way down into the blood vessels of the dermis with her bunch of seven knife- and saw-like instruments, the vessel walls are damaged. Normally, this would lead to coagulation. But the mosquito simultaneously injects saliva that contains a blood-thinning substance. Thus she has long known what to do, whereas man's discovery of how to prevent coagulation by means of anticoagulants is only forty to fifty years old.

The mosquito's saliva pumped into the microscopic wound also contains single-celled fungi, which irritate the tissue, drawing blood to the site. It is only the female that sucks blood: she needs the blood protein for the eggs in her abdomen to develop. Subsequently, she lays the eggs in small pools of water.

It is the saliva that causes itching and allergic reactions to a mosquito bite. Most of us, however, develop a certain immunity to the sting at the beginning of the mosquito season. Surveys carried out in mosquito-infested regions have shown that a rate of three hundred mosquito bites a minute on a naked forearm is not unusual. If the whole body were exposed, it would mean nine thousand mosquito bites a minute and a swift death from loss of blood. But humans are able to protect themselves to a tolerable extent with clothes and insect repellent. Not so for penned-in livestock: indeed, it is not unknown for cattle and horses to die after massive attacks by mosquitoes and blackflies.

These red blood cells do not coagulate, since the mosquito injects an anticoagulant, heparin, into the dermis. Otherwise, its "drinking straw" would get blocked.

It is only the female mosquito that sucks blood from animals and man. The male contents itself with plant juices. The female digs her venom bristle in through the skin, injects the gland secretion that prevents coagulation, and sucks her fill.

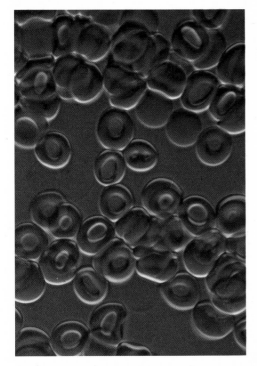

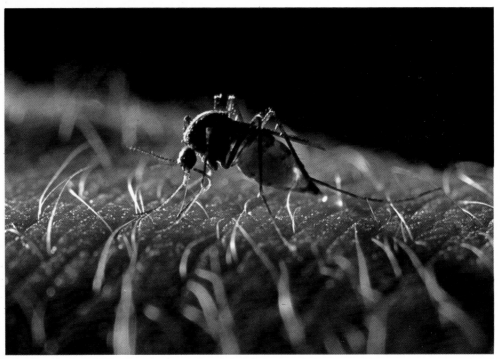

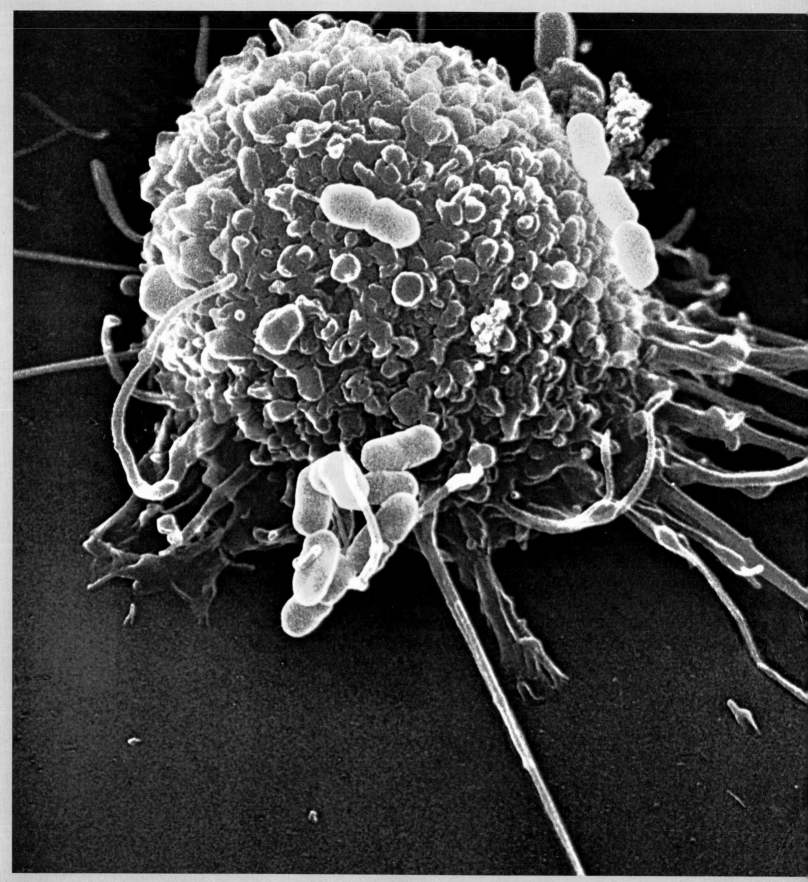

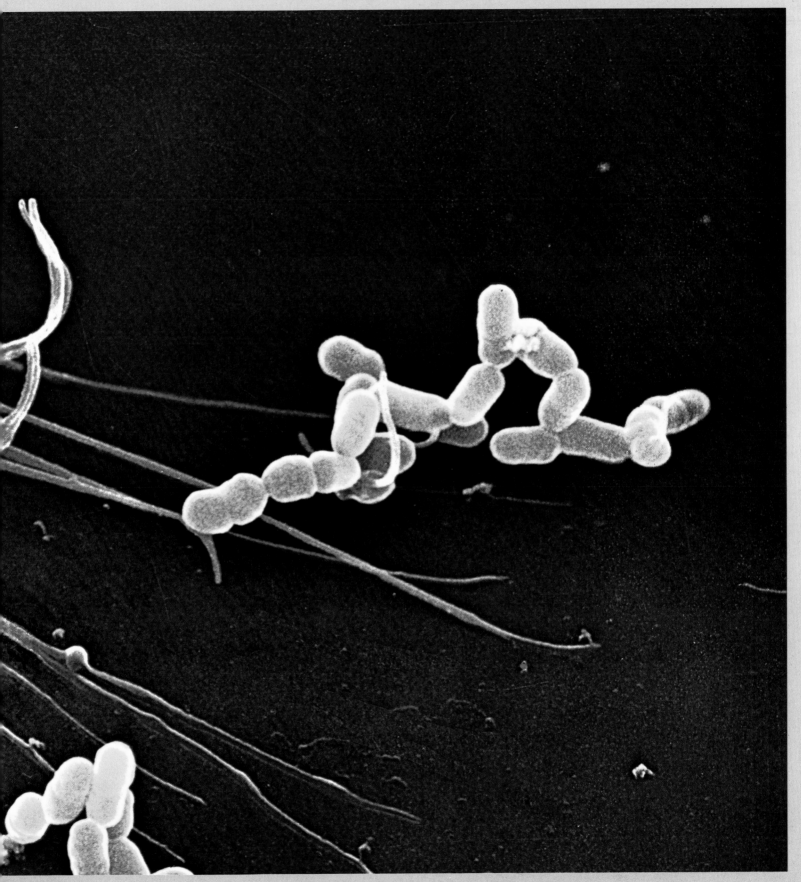

Bacteria, trapped in the cytoplasm "lasso" arms of the macrophage.

Bacteria

Throughout his development, man has coexisted with bacteria. These one-celled organisms—shaped like spheres, rods, commas, or spirals, and a few thousandths of a millimetre in size—are found in profusion in air, soil, and water. The biomass of bacteria in the decimetre-thick topmost layer of a single acre of farming soil may amount to over one thousand pounds.

Most bacteria living on our skin or in the alimentary canal are either harmless or positively beneficial to us. They help us to break down nutrients and build up vitamins, for example, vitamin K, which is necessary for blood clotting. The large intestine is host to at least a hundred types of bacteria that do no harm whatsoever, and dead bacteria compose about half of human feces.

Both parties, man and bacterium, benefit from this symbiosis (coexistence)—as long as the balance is not disturbed. If illness strikes, lowering our powers of resistance, even otherwise friendly bacteria may go to the attack. The balance may also tip the other way, for example, if we take antibiotics: then intestinal bacteria perish en masse and we get "a funny feeling" in the stomach.

A completely different situation, however, arises when we are assailed by disease-producing (pathogenic) bacteria. They may be in the air we inhale or the food we eat; they may penetrate through skin wounds. Bacteria are also adapted to living inside the human body. Many are so specialised that they cannot develop in tissues other than those of man, and cause only human diseases.

Our first lines of defence against bacteria are mechanical and chemical. Undamaged skin is almost impenetrable to bacteria, and the sebum that lubricates the skin contains antibodies. The same applies to the liquid bathing the eyes, the wax in our ears, and saliva. Intact membranes are in small danger of a bacterial attack, and the hydrochloric acid of gastric juice is strongly bactericidal.

The female vagina contains a special defence mechanism, the Döderleins bacteria, which produce lactic acid and thereby create an acid environment in the vagina which other bacteria entering the vagina find lethal. The acidity also makes it more difficult for spermatozoa to move, so most of the man's semen goes toward neutralising the environment.

But the body's specialised weapon against bacteria that penetrate the barrier of skin or membrane is of a totally different kind: feeding cells, or phagocytes. These are white blood cells that capture their opponents, lock them into a stomach-like cavity, submerge them in digestive enzymes, and destroy them. The feeder cells register the substances exuded from damaged bacteria and tissue cells, and can in this way "track" their prey (a process known as chemotaxis). They also have the capacity to penetrate cells in tissues, and to move outside the circulatory and lymph systems.

In his many millennia of contact with bacteria, man and his predecessors have developed several different kinds of feeding cells. Granulocytes—the small, nimble but not particularly tough type called neutrophile—are one kind. They mobilise rapidly, attack, and suffer major losses, but help confine a bacterial invasion. If the bacteria, instead of being localised, stormed their way into the blood and lymph, they could be quickly dispersed throughout the body.

From the battlefield, the substances from disintegrating cells spread in the blood, calling for reinforcement troops. One may refer to a kind of "scent" leading soldiers along a well-defined path to the field of battle. Along it come the armoured tanks of the immune system, the macrophages. They are slower but have considerably greater stamina than the granulocytes. They fight with more perseverance, and each individual consumes more bacteria.

Other parts of the immune system also have a role to play, namely the antibodies and the proteins of the complement system. These adhere to bacteria, marking them and making them more appetising for the feeding cells. This process is called opsonising, and antibodies called opsonins are the "aperitif."

As soon as the feeding cell begins to approach the bacterium, it extends its lasso-like cytoplasm arms, binds the bacterium, and encloses it in a cavity in its cytoplasm, called a phagosome, exposing it to a salvo of powerful enzymes and corrosive hydrogen peroxide. The bacterium's fate is usually to be broken down into its component parts. Some of them will be reused, others discarded.

The complement factors function, broadly speaking, as "magnetic mines." They are sucked toward the bacterium and perforate it, causing it to explode. The complement system has a formidable chemical arsenal—one of its constituents is identical with cobra poison!

However, it is not always the bacteria that fare the worst in the battle with the feeding cells. Just as man has become adapted to them, so have bacteria adapted themselves to us. Some of them have a cell surface on which it is difficult for the feeding cells to get a grip. They slide out of the way. Others have such a resistant cell surface that they can withstand the shower of enzymes in the phagosome. They hibernate, later emerging to cause infection. Infections that flare up once more after appearing to have been vanquished may be the result of these undefeated pockets of resistance inside the feeding cells. In extreme cases, the spread of infection to different parts of the body can give rise to sepsis, general blood poisoning. This state, once so feared, is nowadays treated—usually with success—by means of antibiotics. The drug gives the immune system time to mobilise its own forces and launch a full-scale attack.

One advanced example of the art of deceiving the immune system is the "hospital germ," *Staphylococcus aureus*. If it is enclosed in a feeding cell's "stomach," it excretes a substance which makes the digestive enzymes empty themselves *outside* the stomach! The bacterium has, in addition, developed a resistance to antibiotics, and it thereby leads to intractable problems. Hospitals reserve certain antibiotics exclusively for cases of this "hospital disease."

Sulfa drugs and antibiotics, which came into general use following World War II, laid the foundation for the greatest revolution in the history of medicine. Bacterial infections, a scourge for millennia, vanished from the top ten causes of mortality list—and gave way to more modern pestilences, namely vascular diseases and cancer.

Bacteria and, above all, viruses are globe-trotters. Within a few hours, an influenza virus can fly from Hong Kong to Los Angeles or London. Within days it is traveling by train, bus, and Underground. Every cough, every sneeze, propels hundreds of millions of virus particles into the air—invisible passengers in unseen droplets of water and particles of dust. Those who have already had the disease are immune, but those who lack antibodies against the virus fall ill.

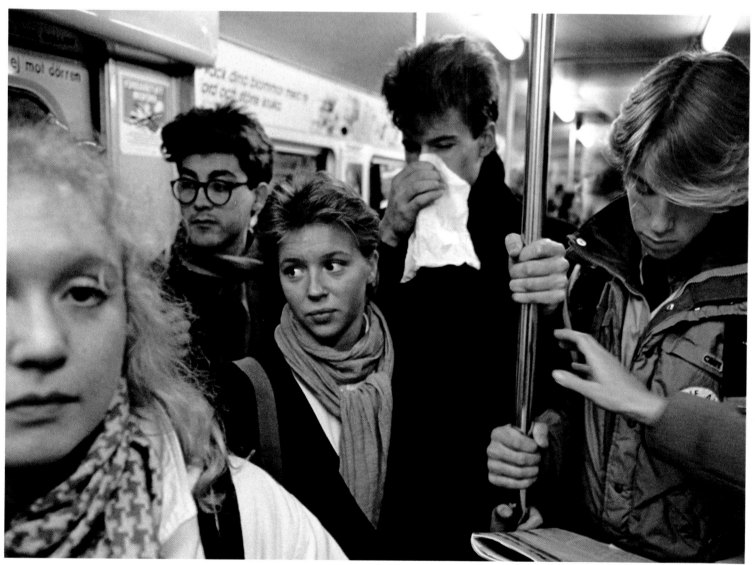

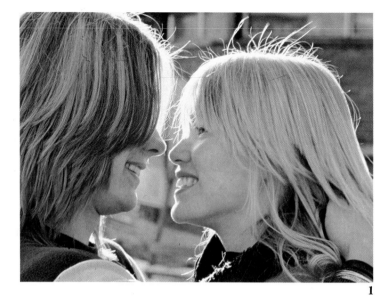

1

The spread of infection

Bacteria and viruses are travelers in the microscopic drops of water we constantly breathe in and out. When people gather, it is virtually impossible to prevent the transfer of infectious matter between individuals. The urban environment favours the spread of infection.

The large picture, *right,* shows mucus and bacteria from a normal cough. The bacteria in the bottom right of the picture look like acorns on the outer edge of a ragged "textile weave" of mucus. Some bacteria are particularly fluffy: they are equipped with a sticky sheath that makes it easier for them to adhere to most substances. *Above right,* in close-up, we see some bacteria of both kinds, and the picture below shows how two bacteria have attached themselves to the epithelial cells of the nasal membrane. The bottom close-up shows, greatly magnified, a bacterium in the act of sticking onto the smooth cell surface, using its special adhesion organ.

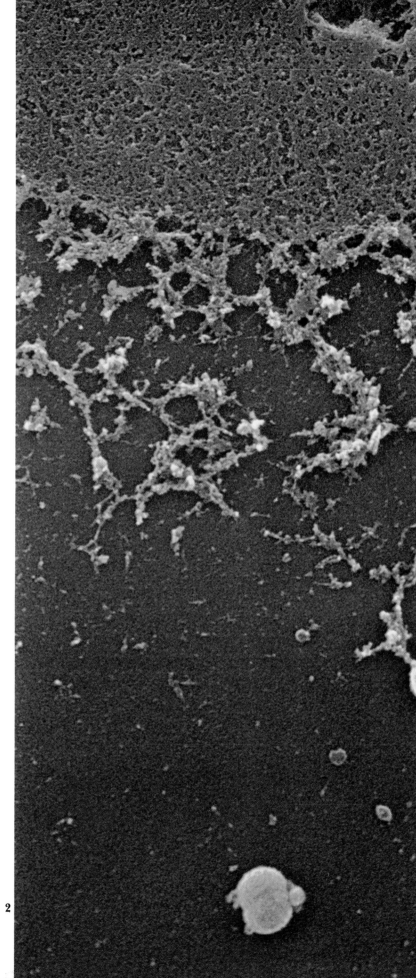

1. *A loving encounter—also for bacterial populations!*
2. *Bacteria* (below) *and mucus* (above) *ejected in coughing. (× 4,000)*
3. *Close-up of some bacteria. (× 25,000)*
4. *Two bacteria adhering to the epithelial cells of the nasal membrane.* *(× 35,000)*
5. *Detail of a bacterium's sticky adhesion organ. (× 90,000)*

2

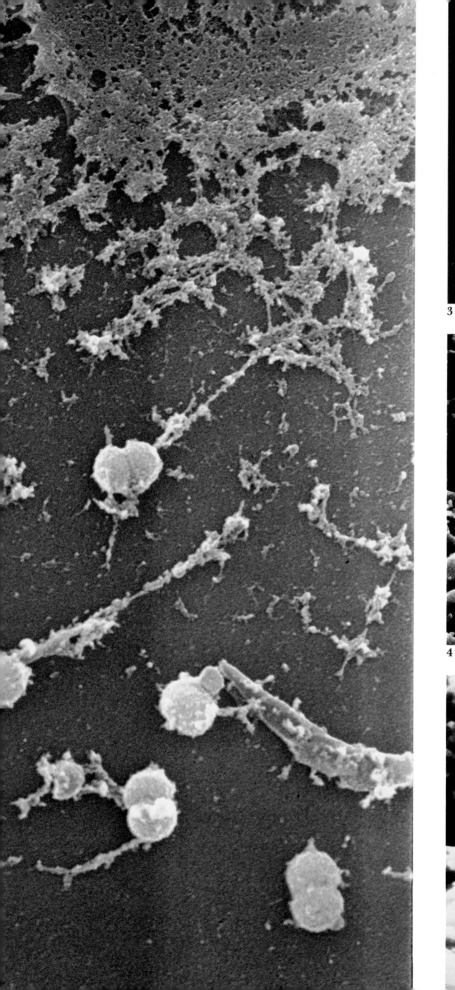

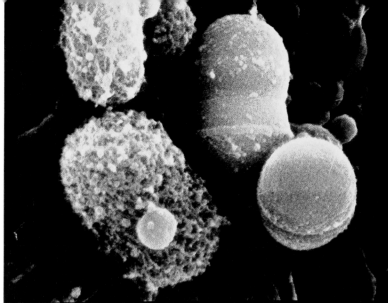

3

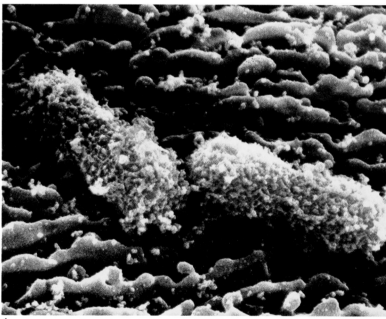

4

5

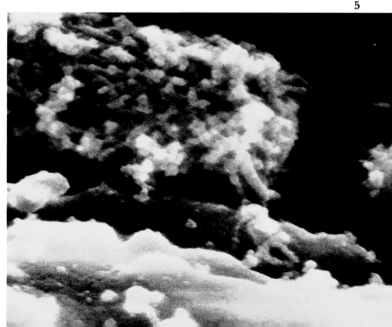

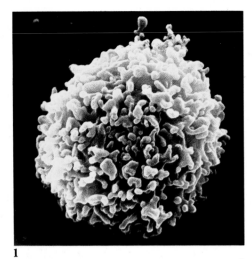

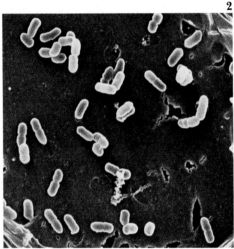

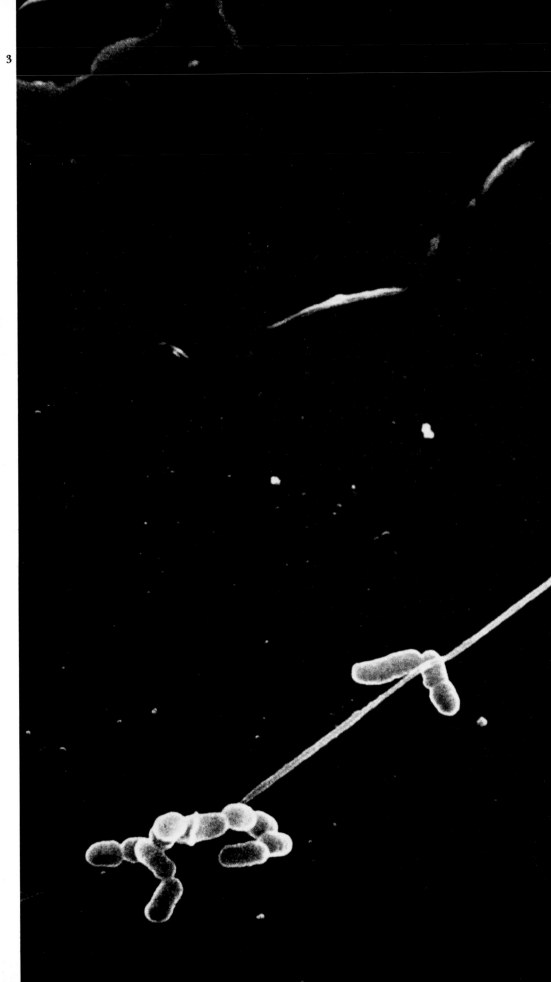

The macrophage traps bacteria

A macrophage, a large feeding cell, has begun close combat with *E. coli* bacteria in the intestine. It shoots out a kind of "flypaper," a sticky cytoplasm outgrowth to which the bacteria adhere. The macrophage then pulls in its prey, or moves in its direction. The result is that the bacteria are shut into a cavity, a vacuole, in the macrophage's body. This cavity is none other than a "death cell": here, the imprisoned bacteria are showered with enzymes that make protein dissolve. They disintegrate and are discarded as useless debris.

The macrophages have a considerably greater bactericidal capacity than the smaller granulocytes.

1. *A macrophage, magnified about 5,000 times.*
2. *Bacteria magnified 3,000 times.*
3. *The macrophage in combat with small, sausage-shaped* E. coli *bacteria.*

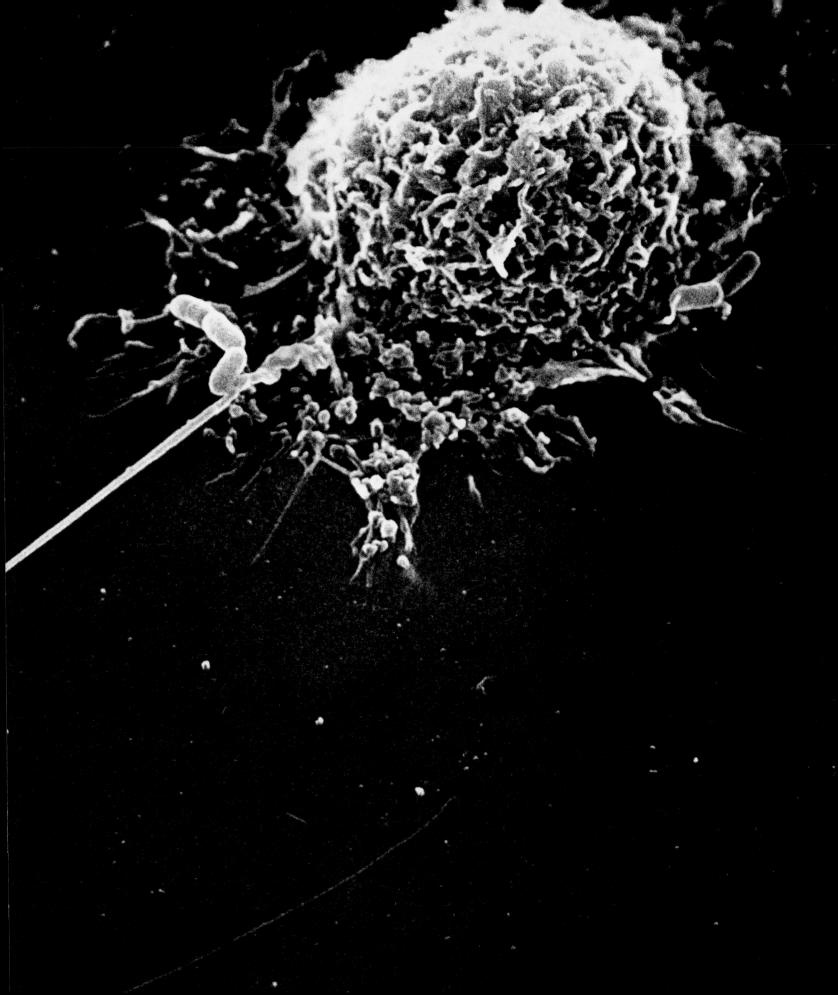

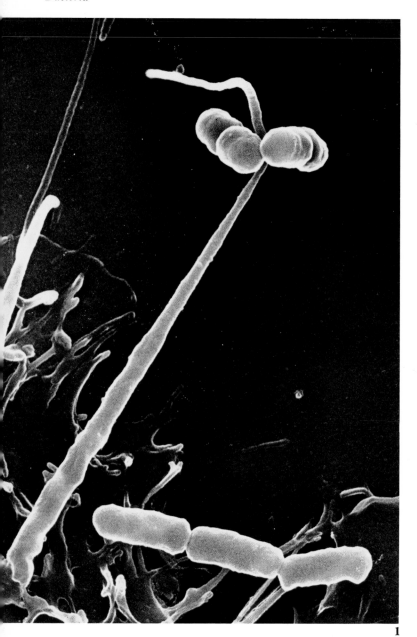

1

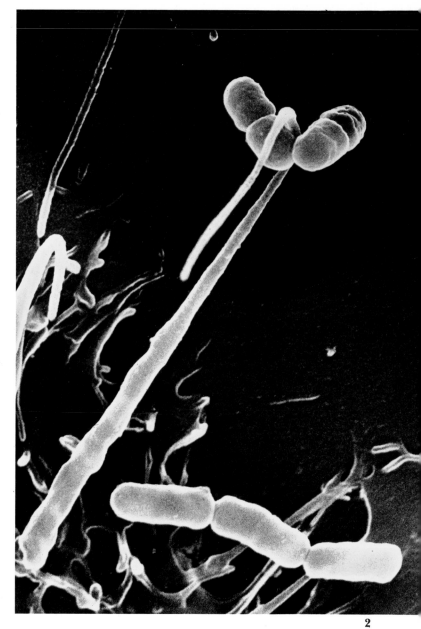

2

Macrophage meets bacterium

Here, a series of remarkable photographs, taken using the electron microscope, show the different stages of a macrophage's onslaught on bacteria. *Above left* (*1*): rod-shaped *E. coli* bacteria, which are common in the intestine, have been snared by the cytoplasm outgrowth, the macrophage's "flypaper." In the following picture (*2*), the snares are being tightened and the prisoners drawn in toward the macrophage's body.

The large picture, *right* (*3*), shows the conclusion of the battle: The macrophage pulls the bacteria inward to deliver the coup de grace. Antibodies and complement factors play an important role in the capture of bacteria. They position themselves on the bacteria, serving as appetisers (opsonins). The macrophage then locates the enemy more easily in the wound's disordered medley of blood and cell fragments.

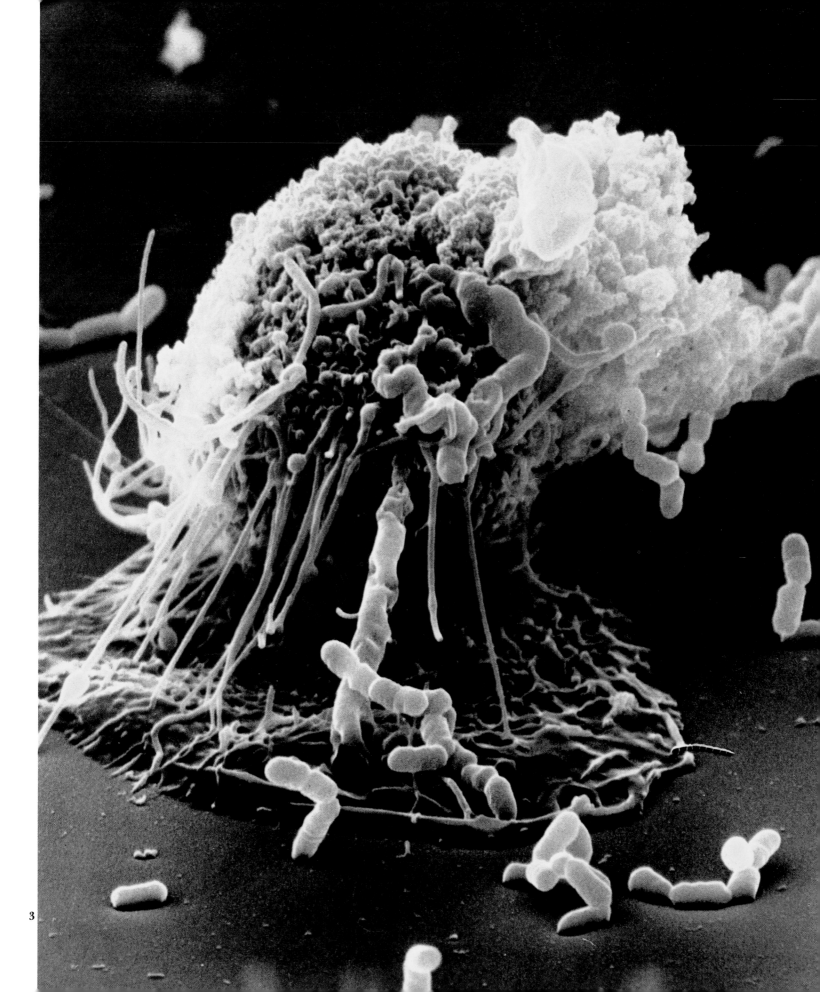

3

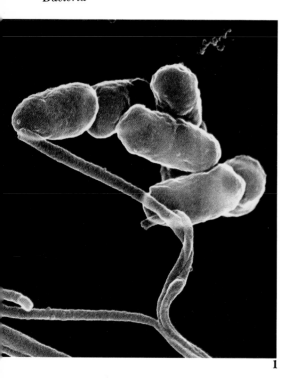

1

The feeding cell lassoes the bacteria

When the feeding cell has homed in on the invading bacteria, it pushes out cytoplasm threads that infiltrate them. The antibodies have made them more appetising. The feeding cell's way of capturing its enemies resembles the use of a lasso.

The body's methods of disarming invasive microorganisms developed many hundred million years ago. Even worms have feeding cells circulating in their blood. In the higher animals and man, the methods have evolved further and been refined.

The pictures were taken under a scanning electron microscope, and the degree of magnification in the large picture is about 45,000.

1. E. coli *bacteria, caught in the feeding cell's cytoplasm threads.*
2. *The bacteria are pulled nearer and nearer to the feeding cell.*
3. *A* Staphylococcus bacterium *is about to be enclosed in the feeding cell.*

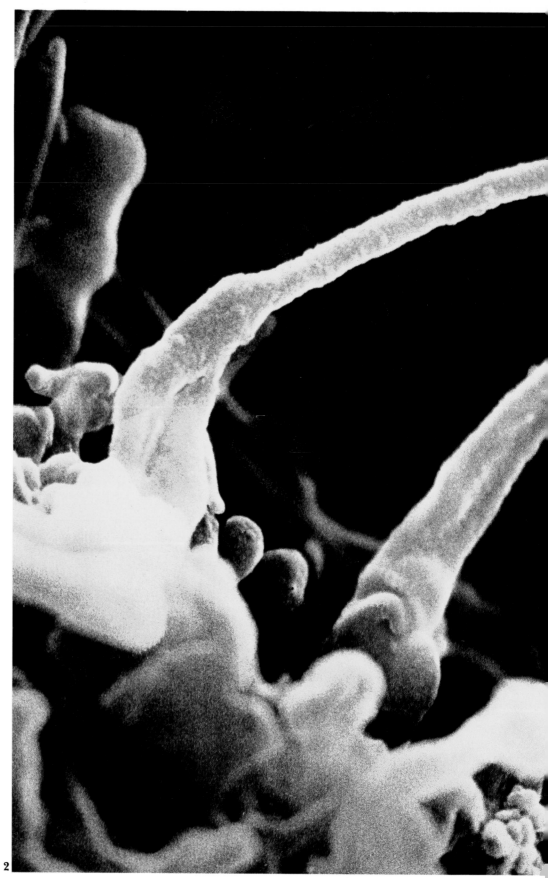

2

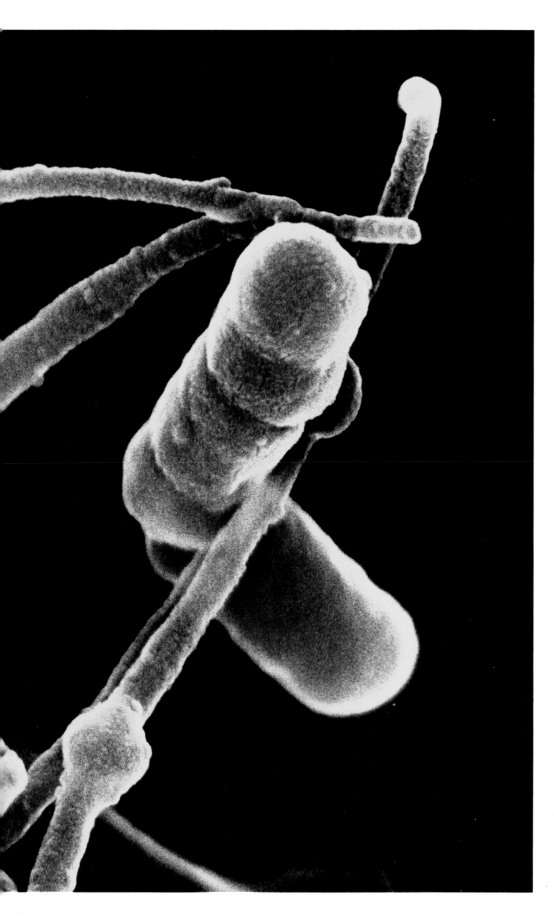

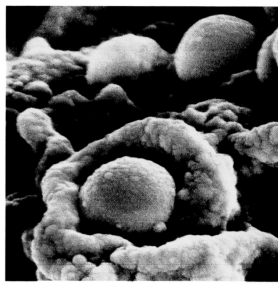

3

How does the feeding cell swallow the bacterium?

The war between bacteria and macrophages is in reality waged between cells measuring only a few thousandths of a millimetre across. In these photographs, they are magnified 10,000 to 45,000 times. Above, the staphylococcus resembles the egg in a bird's nest. It is in the embrace of the macrophage, inside a hollow which gradually closes, becoming a "death cell."

One of the remarkable properties of the macrophage is that it can suddenly increase its surface area, enclosing an enemy sometimes many times larger than itself—for example, an asbestos fibre, a grain of pollen, or some other material inhaled into the lungs. Bacteria, however, as shown in the photographs above, are considerably smaller than the macrophage.

When the walls have closed around the enemy, the execution—phagocytosis—takes place. The prisoner is showered with hydrogen peroxide or other deadly toxins. Digestive enzymes are sent into the death chamber to dissolve the bacterium.

The disintegration of foreign proteins that occurs during phagocytosis is one of the most important aspects of the immune system. The effect of antibodies and complement factors is to make the process more efficient. This is particularly conspicuous in the immune individual at the onset of a bacterial attack. Ready-made antibodies then immediately bind to the invasive bacteria, marking them for the feeding cells, which rapidly incapacitate them by phagocytosis.

Antibiotics in action

The advent of penicillin in the mid-1940s meant that man could exploit one of nature's own bactericides. The raw material is produced by a species of mould fungus, *Penicillium notatum,* which subsists in the soil and elsewhere and uses its "penicillin" to protect itself against attacking bacteria. As early as 1928, the microbiologist Alexander Fleming observed the effect of penicillin fungus on a bacteria culture, but it was not until more than a decade later that conclusions were drawn and one of the greatest medicinal discoveries of the age was made.

Below, we see how penicillin attacks a colony of spherical bacteria, staphylococci. Penicillin makes its presence felt when the bacterium has divided and begun to construct walls, or membranes, around its own cytoplasm. This is a multistage process, and penicillin obstructs the final stage. As a result, the cell wall becomes mechanically defective—tight, in places torn, incapable of withstanding the rising mechanical and osmotic pressure in the growing cell plasma. The bacterium explodes.

Near right, a colony of pus bacteria (staphylococci), the middle one in the process of division. The colony is under attack by penicillin, and the picture beneath shows the empty shell of a staphylococcus after the explosion. It is then the feeding cells' task to clear away the debris. *Far right,* a rod-shaped bacterium divides and, *below,* destruction is complete: the penicillin has synthesised with the cell wall, causing the bacterium to split immediately.

Penicillin attacks a colony of staphylococci. Above left, *we see a greatly diminished and dying bacterium and, in the middle, the penicillin.*

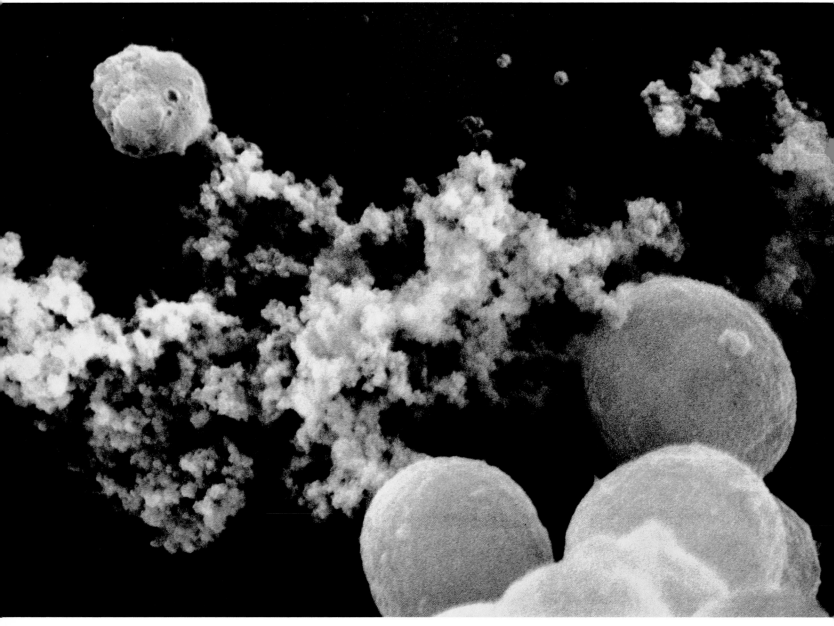

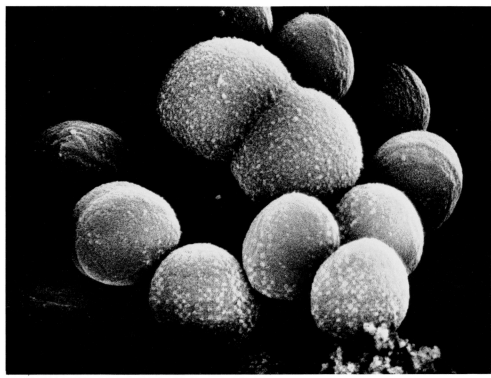

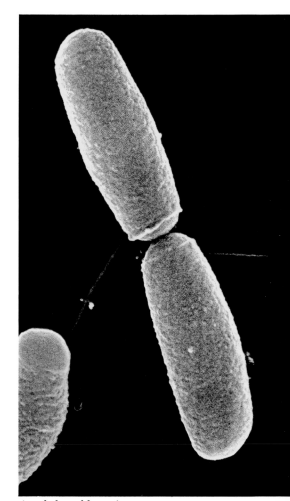

Staphylococci. The large one is in the process of division.
A dead staphylococcus looks like a skull. (× 75,000)

A rod-shaped bacterium.
The same bacterium after an attack by penicillin.

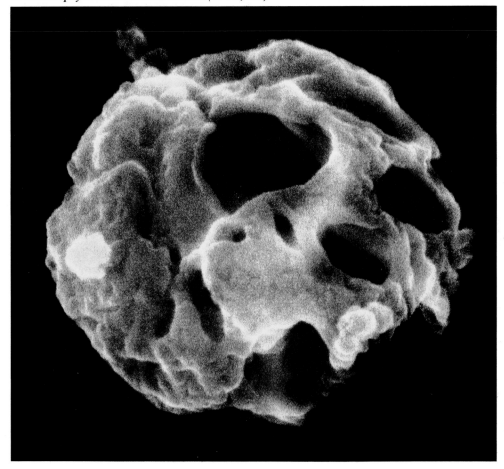

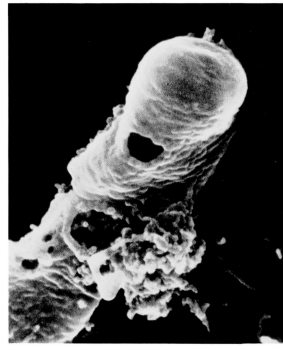

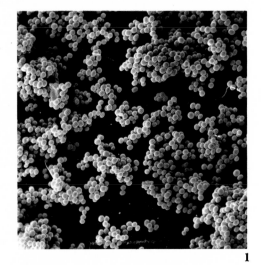

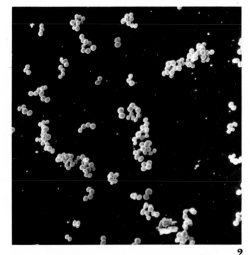

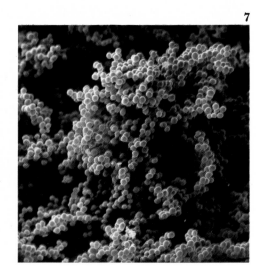

1

2

3

Resistant bacteria

In the early years, penicillin was used indiscriminately to treat both severe infections and the common cold. People were negligent of dosages, and a problem suddenly arose: bacteria developed resistance against penicillin. By natural selection, species which make an enzyme against it, called penicillinase, emerged. The outcome is that a person infected by penicillin-resistant bacteria cannot be helped by penicillin. In spite of the penicillin, the bacteria grow unchecked and may give rise to grave pathological conditions.

Penicillin-resistant bacteria strains, often *Staphylococcus aureus* (the most common bacterium in pus), are greatly feared at large hospitals. The picture to the *right* (4) shows the extent of isolation in which a sufferer must be kept: everyone around him wears a mask; he remains in isolation in his room, receiving his food there; his

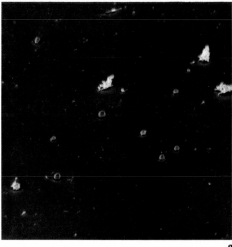

4

relatives are not allowed beyond a closed glass door.

Before a case of penicillin resistance can be treated, a culture of the patient's bacteria must be grown and tested with various antibiotics, which are placed on the dish containing the bacterial culture. The antibiotic surrounded by the broadest zone of destruction is the most effective.

The series of photographs *above* (1–3) depict the normal situation: bacteria that are sensitive to penicillin. In the middle picture, the drug has killed most of the bacteria, and in the third picture there are only a few left.

The picture series *below* (5–7) shows what happens when penicillin-resistant bacteria are treated with penicillin. There is virtually no effect, and in the picture to the *right* (8) we see the colonies of resistant staphylococci expanding in spite of the penicillin treatment.

5

6

7

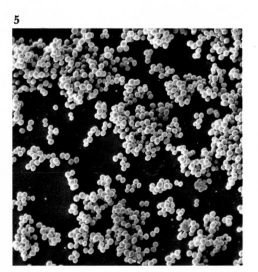

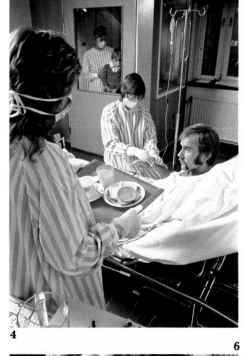

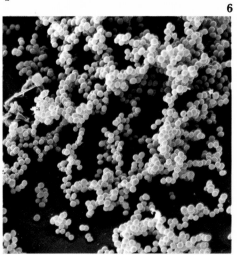

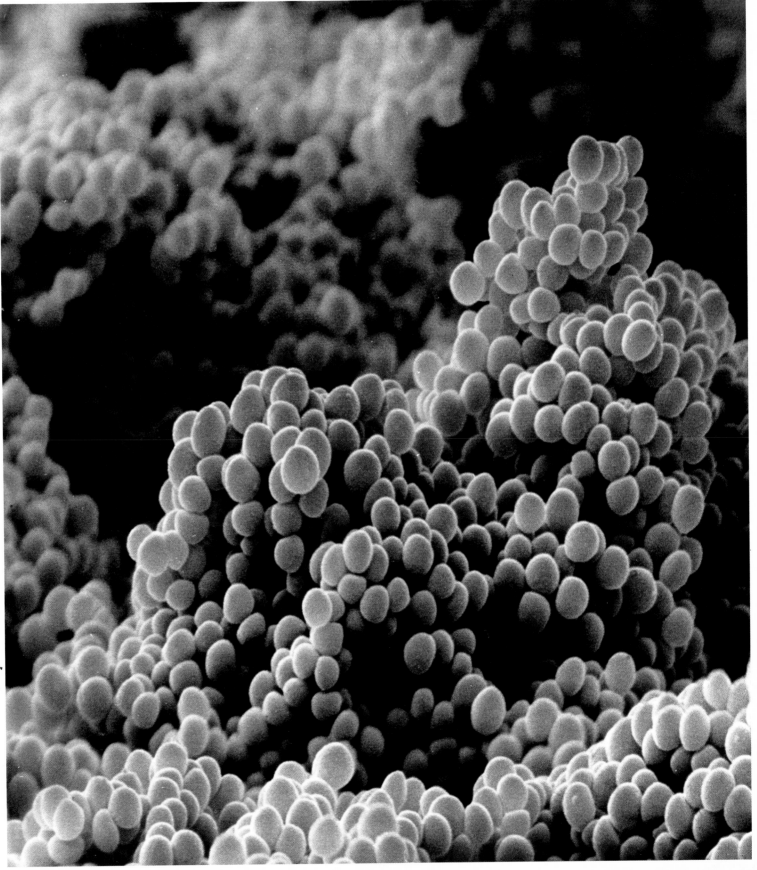

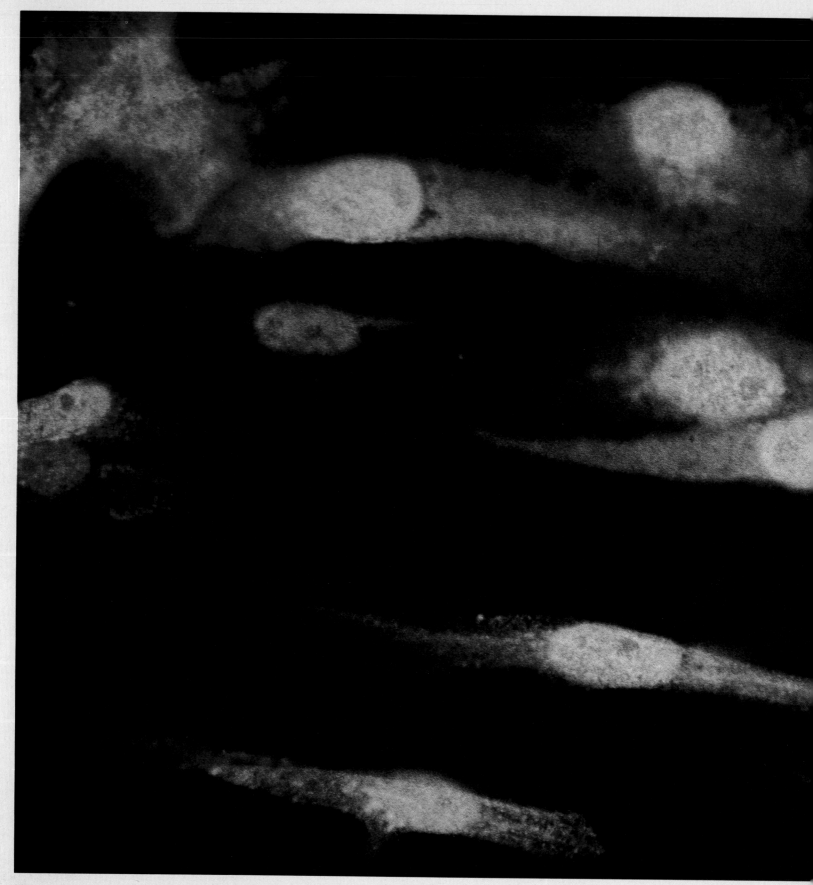

Epithelial cells of the throat, infected with influenza virus. (The bright areas are cell nuclei.)

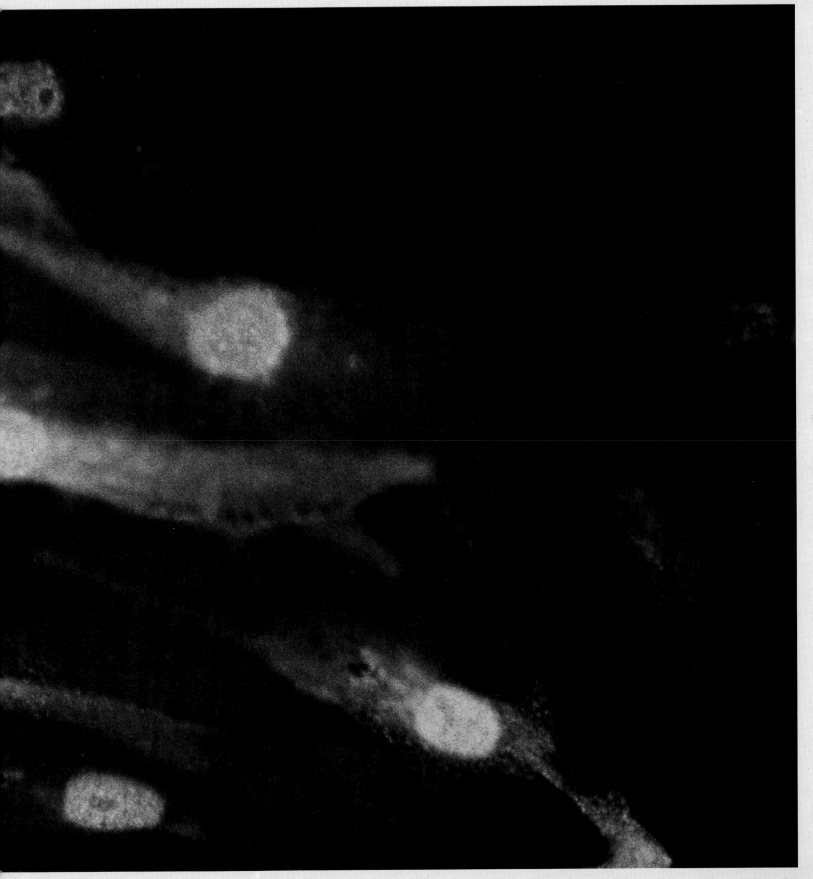

Viruses

A virus is something unique, composed partly of nonliving and partly of living matter. In their inactive form, the particles of a virus can be dried or deep-frozen for years and then—in appropriate environmental conditions—suddenly and in full strength assume their active form and infect living organisms, from bacteria and plants to animals and man.

A virus is thus something of a biological enigma. Its name is the Latin for "poison," and although its peculiarities were not discovered until the 1930s, its effects were known even to the Romans. They imagined that the bite of a rabid dog transferred the same sort of poison as that of a snake. This is not so, but not even the great late-nineteenth-century bacteriologists Pasteur and Koch succeeded in finding the causes of smallpox, rabies, measles, or any of the other infectious diseases we now know to be viral in origin.

It is hardly surprising that they did not succeed, despite their cell culture techniques and light microscopes. Viruses are so unimaginably small that they pass through the finest filters, and so close in size to the wavelengths of visible light that they virtually float past them.

No virus exceeds a few millionths of a millimetre in diameter. To a virus, even a bacterium is as large as a house is to us, and the human cell is like a whole city block. A single red blood cell is about 150 times as large as an ordinary virus. In the world of viruses, all living things are larger—and everything smaller is nonliving matter.

As elsewhere, however, there is considerable variation in size. The largest virus—300 millionths of a millimetre in diameter—is about twenty times larger than the smallest, the polio virus, which measures only 16 millionths of a millimetre across. Virus shapes also vary: most are spherical, but some are shaped like elongated rods or airships and others like tadpoles. A remarkable design is that of an insect virus with twenty triangular facets on a sphere.

What does a virus consist of? The answer is not surprising: protein and nucleic acid. The nucleic acid contains virus genes, DNA or RNA, enclosed in a protein coat that protects the hereditary material. This simple construction is not sufficient for independent life. In order for the transition from the inactive to the active form to take place, and for the virus to be able to live and reproduce, it must enter a living cell. It depends for its development on the cell's metabolism. The virus is a parasite—a sponger.

There are viruses in water, air, soil, dust, and foodstuffs. It is thus easy for us to inhale or ingest them, or absorb them through our skin. Once inside the body, virus particles land on cell surfaces. Previous exposure to virus attacks may render us immune, and then nothing happens: the virus is neutralised by circulating antibodies. If we are not immune, the virus is activated, and it sets to work by inserting its genetic material through the cell wall. It is able to dissolve the latter and fuse with the cell contents. Others permit themselves to be swallowed by the defence system's feeding cells, inside which they proliferate. One virus type, which specialises in assailing intestinal bacteria, functions along the lines of a hypodermic syringe, injecting its hereditary material into the bacterium through a narrow tube—an enemy take-over at its most perfect.

The viral genes destroy those of the cell or bacterium, totally incapacitating them. In due course, the whole apparatus of the cell is working to support the virus. Take, for example, the T4 virus: after about twenty minutes, the cell bursts and a couple of hundred new virus particles pour out. Each one of them can infect an additional cell. Every twenty minutes, infected body cells thus shed thousands, and soon millions, of these particles. In twelve hours a single virus can give rise to a progeny of astronomical proportions: 10^{73} (ten followed by seventy-three zeros)! And in twelve hours an unprepared immune system cannot possibly mobilise countervailing weaponry: we fall ill.

Although a virus is the simplest of all existing life forms—a cluster of genes in a protective protein sheath—it is at the same time an example of great refinement. By reducing its equipment to the absolute minimum and dispensing with the apparatus of metabolism that characterises a living cell, a virus can tolerate and survive conditions that otherwise rule out normal life. In return, the virus is dependent on the enzymes of the living cell for its continued existence.

There are probably several thousand viruses, of which a few hundred are pathogenic in man. A small number are harmful to both animals and man (e.g., the influenza virus), but the majority parasitise particular species. Human viruses often specialise in attacking certain cell types.

The common cold and influenza viruses most often parasitise membrane cells, whereas the mumps virus travels to glandular cells—in the salivary and sexual glands—and the polio virus to nerve tissue. The smallpox virus, like

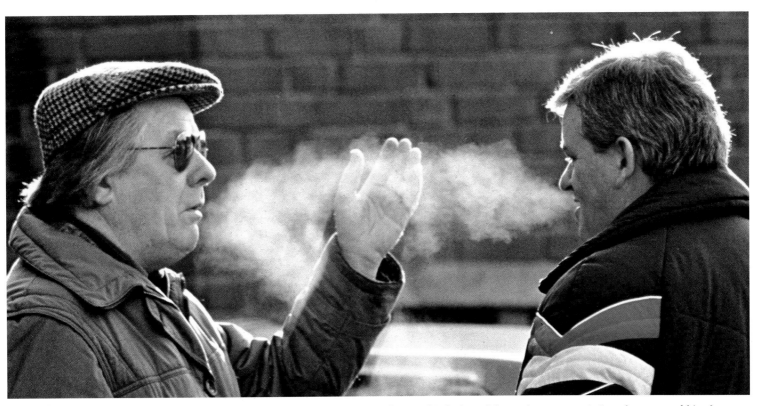

In cold weather, the droplets of moisture in our breath are visible. A person with a viral infection of the respiratory tract infects those around him because viruses by the million are borne by the droplets.

rubella (German measles) and measles, is initially active in the membranes of the respiratory tract but then migrates to the skin. The rabies virus attacks peripheral nerve cells and then "eats its way" up to the brain.

The onslaught of a virus causes the cell's normal functioning to cease. If, for example, the virus assumes command of the insulin-producing beta cells in the pancreas, the result is diabetes. In some cases the cell's protein-dissolving enzymes, normally enclosed in "sacs" called lysosomes, are released, whereupon they attack and damage nearby cells. If red blood cells are assailed by a virus, their walls may admit fluid, causing them to burst. The blood's ability to transport oxygen is thus impaired, and the body cells' metabolism suffers: the organism is enfeebled. In extreme cases, the result may be internal asphyxiation.

If a pregnant woman becomes infected by certain viruses, such as rubella and cytomegalovirus, the fetus may be damaged. The frequency of deformities resulting from rubella—normally a somewhat innocuous childhood illness—is as high as one in ten. The damage suffered varies but in severe cases may manifest itself in blindness, deafness, and heart defects. The fetus is infected via the mother and lacks the ability to defend itself against the virus. For this reason, girls are now vaccinated against rubella at about the age of thirteen. Expectant mothers, on the other hand, must not be vaccinated against either rubella or smallpox, since the virus in the vaccine can be transferred to the fetus. Rubella in a pregnant woman is generally regarded as grounds for abortion.

Certain viruses, including influenza, spread rapidly and on occasion give rise to pandemics, as they are called. A worldwide epidemic of this kind, called "Spanish flu" because the Spanish court was smitten, occurred at the end of World War I. The epidemic killed about 20 million people—more than those who fell in battle. Influenza returns periodically, in different guises—"Hong Kong," "Asian," and so on—and causes epidemics in whole continents. The reason for this cyclical pattern is thought to be that certain characteristics of the influenza virus change, so that immunity built up in the body against one type is ineffective against another.

"Stable" viruses such as measles, mumps, and yellow fever, however, impart lifelong immunity. The body's only general defence against viruses (unless it is immune from a previous infection) is interferon, which the cells produce when attacked by viruses. It prevents the virus from reproducing and the cell from dividing.

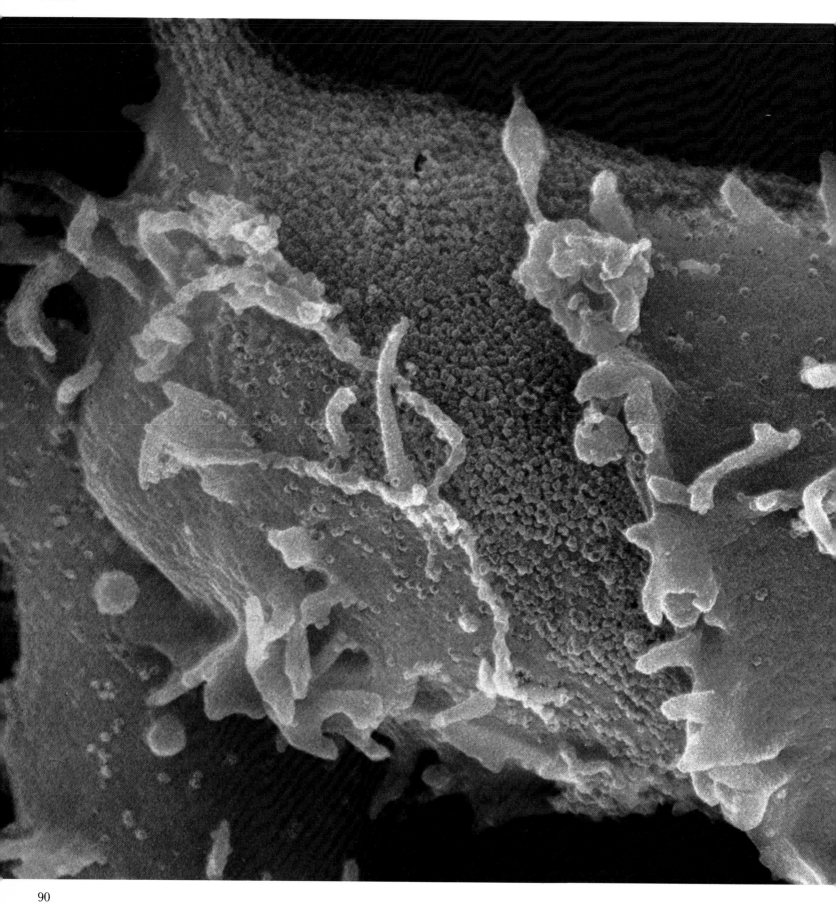

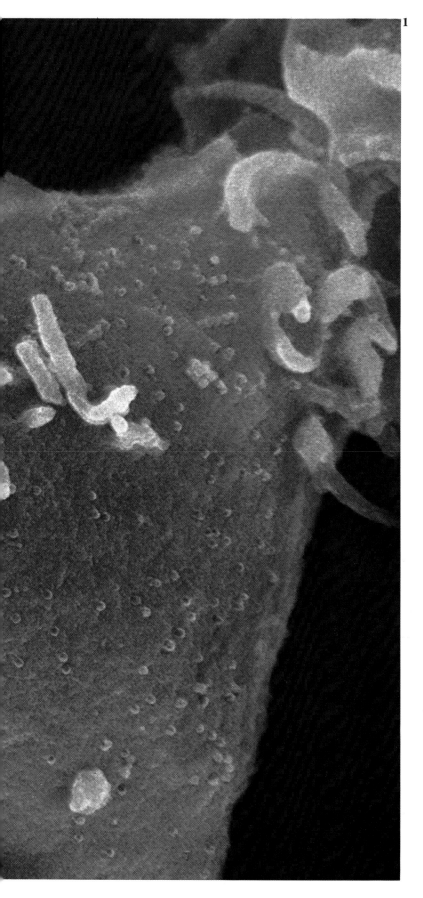

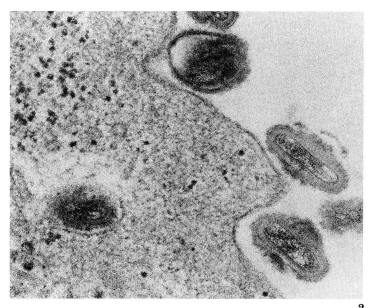

Thousands of new virus particles are born

Above **(2),** a virus penetrates the cell membrane. One particle is already inside, others await their turn. The first to arrive in the cell nucleus takes command, reorganising the cell's production for a sole purpose: to make new viruses. A mere nine hours later, thousands of new virus particles flood out through the cell wall, which may sometimes be perforated **(1).** The small blue points on the cell surface are the particles on the way out. The cell is so full of virus that it has split down the middle. The emerging particles immediately attack other cells—unless the immune system succeeds in forestalling them. *Below,* four different types of virus: **(3)** *herpes,* **(4)** *influenza,* **(5)** *polio,* and **(6)** *adenitis.*

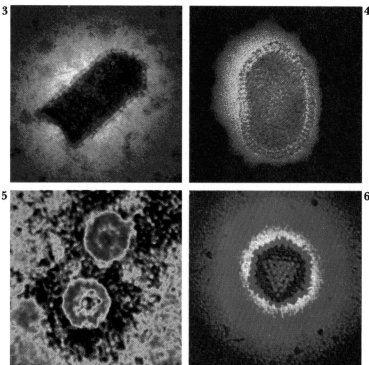

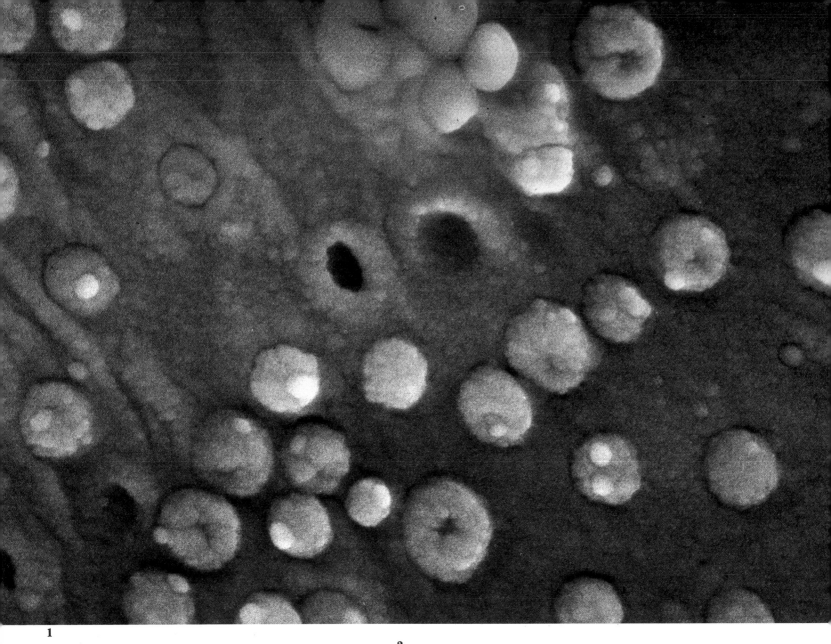

1

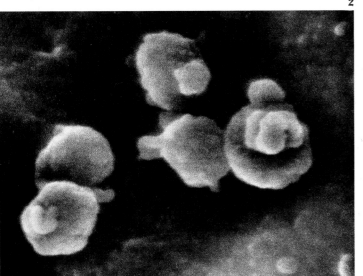

2

1. *Cell surface with herpes simplex virus. Some virus particles are in the process of emerging through the cell membrane.*
2. *Detail of herpes simplex virus. Inside the virus particle's membrane is the genetic material DNA, surrounded by a protein sheath.*
3. *Herpes lip sores. Sores like this heal in a week or two.*
4. *Herpes-infected cell. The tiny, light points on the central portion of the cell are virus particles.*
5. *A herpes virus.*

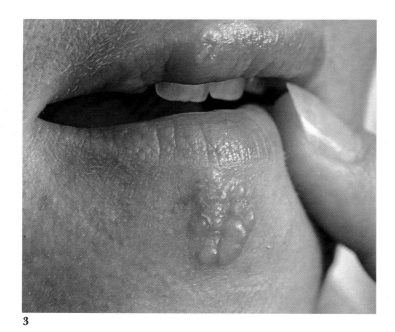

3

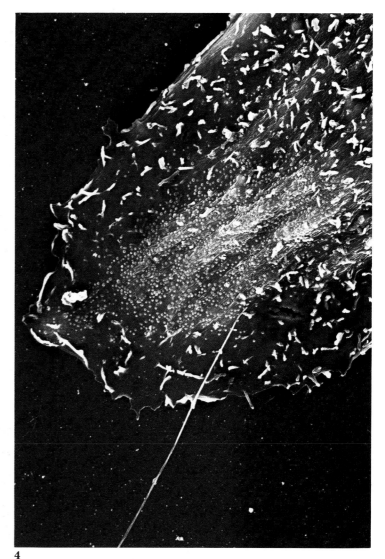

4

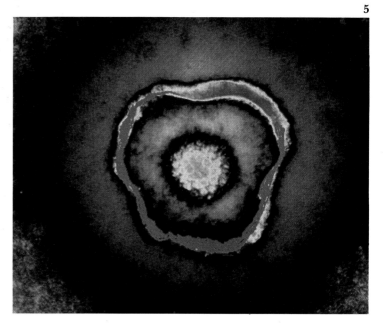

5

A dormant virus awakes and launches an attack

Virtually everyone is infected with herpes simplex virus early in childhood, and carries it in a dormant form throughout life. At times of illness, stress, and other strains—even too much sun in the spring—the powers of the immune system are reduced, and the herpes virus has its chance. The symptoms are relatively innocuous, the main one being watery blisters or sores around the mouth and nose. In a minority, however, herpes causes injuries to the cornea that, in unfavourable circumstances, can damage a person's sight. The picture *above* shows typical herpes lip sores. The *upper right* picture shows a herpes-infected cell, with virus particles emerging, eight hours after the onset of infection. The *lower* picture shows a herpes virus with genetic material in the middle.

The name "herpes" denotes a group of fairly large viruses. Their diameter measures about 180 millimicrons (millionths of a millimetre). Not all are as mild in their effects as herpes simplex: one common variant gives chicken pox, another shingles (a relatively rare ailment), and a third, cytomegalovirus, results in fetal injuries. One particularly feared form is herpes simiae, which spreads to man from monkeys and can be fatal. In animals, the herpes virus can cause tumour formation.

Six hours after the herpes simplex virus has infected the cell in the large picture, *opposite,* and has reached the nucleus and incapacitated the cell's own organs of control, new virus particles start emerging from the surface. Certain types of virus cause the cell to burst when they have no further use for it, but the herpes virus pushes its way out by a budding process on the cell surface. In the *upper left,* we see a virus in the process of emerging through the membrane; in the middle, there are crater-like holes presumably made by departing virus particles and, beneath the holes, herpes virus particles at different budding stages.

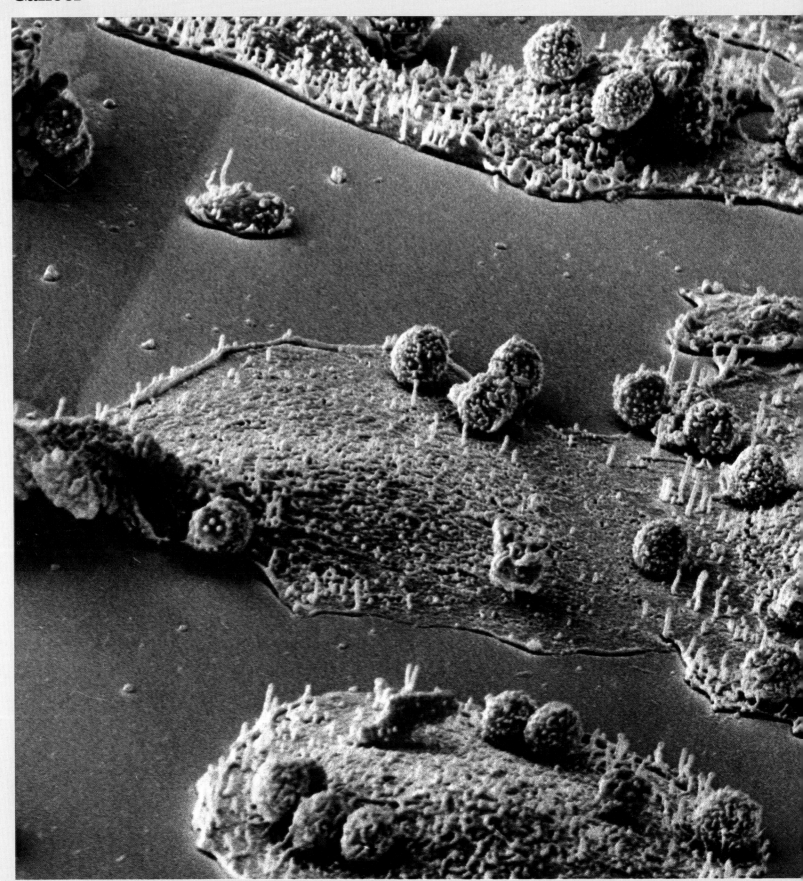

Cancer cells resembling islands in the making, with spherical killer cells adhering to them.

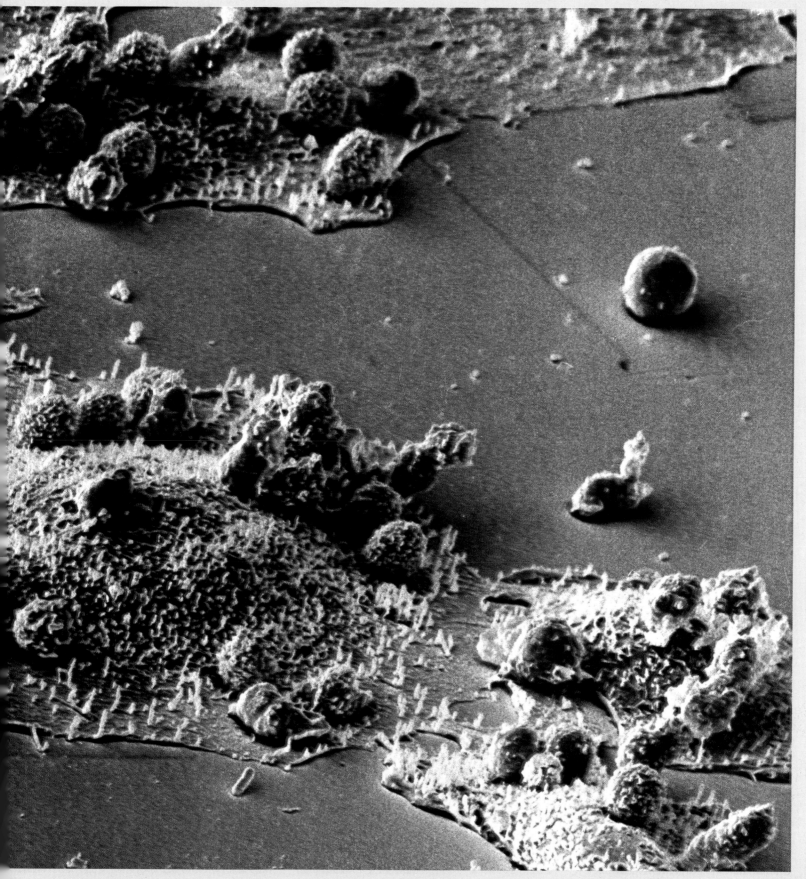

Cancer

Cancer, or malignant tumour disease, is one of the most feared diagnoses of our time—although between 45 and 50 percent of all cancer cases are restored to full health with modern medical care. This fact is easily forgotten. Cancer is often taken as a death sentence.

In spite of extensive research over the last few decades, man has not been able to establish with certainty why an ordinary cell in the body is transformed into a tumour cell. Suddenly, it shakes off the dictatorial control of the cell apparatus, starts an uncontrolled division, becomes a lump, and can send forth tumour cells via the blood and lymph. These in turn form secondary tumours *(metastases)* in various parts of the body.

The above course of events is well known, but what triggers it is still open to discussion. Certain facts are well established—for example, that a genetic disposition toward tumour mutation is inbuilt in the cells, in the form of oncogenes ("tumour genes"). It is also known that radiation, viruses, and certain carcinogenic chemicals are involved when a cell deviates from the normal cell pattern, becoming a tumour cell. Chemicals of this kind occur in our food (e.g., nitrosamines in meat, certain mould toxins), in tobacco smoke (benzopyrenes and cyclic hydrocarbons), and in certain workplaces (bituminous substances, asbestos, plastic raw materials).

What all these factors have in common is a capacity to alter the genetic material of the cell nucleus. The control apparatus of the cell changes course, and if the process is not thwarted, it may destroy the whole organism.

One thing, however, is certain: that the frequency of cancer would be considerably higher if the body itself had not developed methods of suppressing unruly cells. Many pieces of the jigsaw are still missing, but we know that the immune system can employ interferon, antibodies, and—above all—killer cells in the fight against tumour cells. It is in this immunological field that researchers are concentrating on the search for methods to supplement modern cancer treatments (surgery, chemotherapy, hormonal treatment, and ionising radiation therapy).

One enigma is the immune system's failure to attack *all* tumour cells, although their behaviour is so sharply distinct from that of normal cells. During their constant patrolling of the tissues, the soldiers of the immune system pass by and disregard these deviants. The life-threatening process continues unrestrained, either because these tumour cells lack the antigen properties that normally provoke the immune system to attack or because suppressor cells curb its assaults.

This nonchalant, uninterested attitude on the part of the immune system is in strong contrast to its actions in cases when the tumour cell is identified as hostile. The killer cells of the body's defences, the T-lymphocytes, then hurl themselves on the tumour cells, kill them, and comb the tissues, like bloodhounds on a scent, to find cells that have loosened from the original tumour and dispersed in the organism. The killer cells are the immune system's special combat units in the war against cancer. Ordinary feeding cells follow them to clear away the debris, swallowing and digesting the tumour cells.

However, the body's defences against cancer do not consist solely of killer cells. Certain tumour types have characteristics that prompt the body to form antibodies against them in the traditional way. The antibodies then adhere to the tumour cell's surface and the various factors of the complement system shoot holes in it, making it an easily identifiable target for the feeding cell.

Cancer is not *one* disease but a whole range, with varying characteristics. In some cases, the altered properties appear so clearly on the tumour cell's surface that the immune system immediately finds and attacks it. In other cases, the change is less apparent; the tumour can then obtain an advantage timewise, growing until it constitutes such a large conglomeration of cells that the immune system—once it gets started—finds it difficult to keep up. In this situation an operation to reduce the tumour mass can sometimes enable the immune forces to gain the upper hand and restore the patient to health.

Experience shows that, in addition, it is possible to stimulate the immune system and raise its efficiency by injecting certain irritants into the body. Live but weakened BCG *(Mycobacterium bovis)* bacteria improve results in the treatment of melanoma, a serious type of skin tumour. Dead bacteria, too, can promote the activity of the immune system, with the advantage that they do not proliferate in the body. If, for example, *Corynebacterium parvum* is injected directly into a tumour which, at the same time, is being treated with cytotoxins, the result is better than that achieved by cytotoxins alone.

Another method of stimulating the immune system involves chilling the tumour, with a view to making tumour proteins flow out into the circulatory system, thereupon possibly prompting the formation of antibodies.

T-lymphocytes are the body's principal weapon of defence against tumours. These killer cells are among the most aggressive fighters in the immune system; it is they which cause problems in the transplantation of kidneys and other organs. They are mobilised en masse at the site where the body's own tissues meet the foreign tissues of the transplanted organ. To decrease the risk of rejection of the new organ, surgeons are therefore obliged to suppress the immune system by various means.

The disadvantage of immunosuppressive treatment, as this is called, in which cortisone preparations play an important part, is that it increases the risk not only of infections but also of tumours developing. Statistics show that malignant tumours occur about one hundred times more often in people who have received transplants than in people of the same age who have not. It is partly owing to these complications that other, more selective measures to deal with undesirable immune reactions, directed specifically against the T-lymphocytes, are being tested. Experiments are also in progress with the special lymphocyte hormones called lymphokines, which participate in regulating the immune system. If they meet expectations, it is hoped that they will enable certain immune reactions to be "switched off" without others being affected.

Advances in immunology in the 1980s may also bring success in the form of new, improved methods of treating tumour diseases. Expectations are focused primarily on monoclonal antibodies, which can on the one hand make a cancer diagnosis more reliable and, on the other, function as homing missiles, loaded with cell toxins which they discharge, with great accuracy, in the core of the tumour.

A successful breast cancer operation need not impede a normal existence. Shortly afterward, a woman can resume her everyday life.

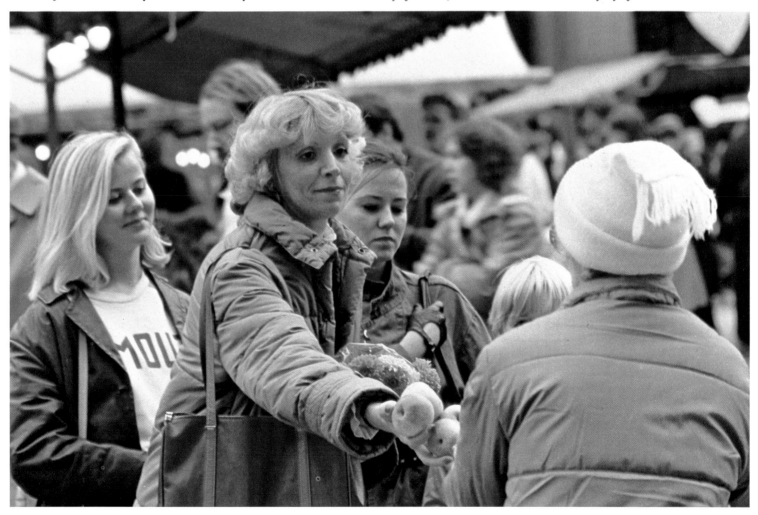

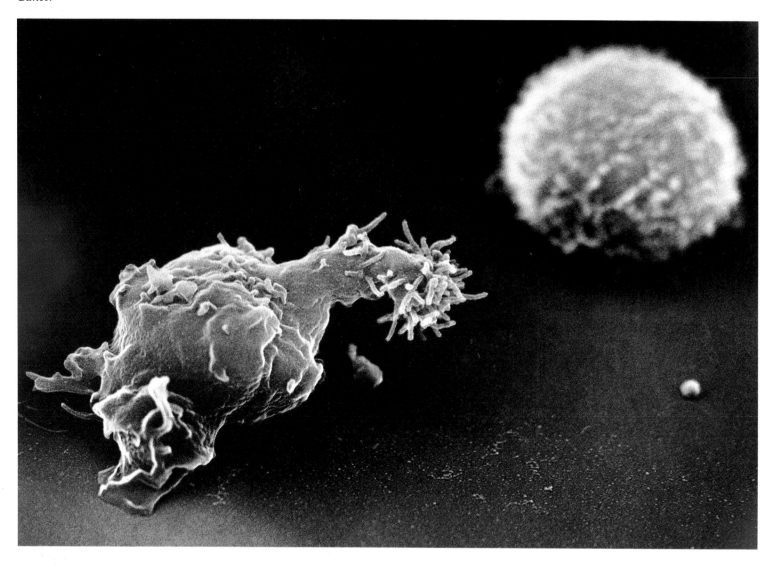

The killer cell on the warpath

Although the main task of the immune system is to protect us against the multitude of external microorganisms and other foreign perils, some of its weapons are reserved for combating abnormal cells. The task is strongly reminiscent of the secret police in a dictatorship. Killer cells move incessantly through the body's tissues, combing the tissues for deviant cells. *Above,* we see two of them in different guises, one spherical and the other resembling a creature from a science-fiction film. Killer cells, which are a variant of T-lymphocyte, are capable of altering their appearance.

The killer cells receive their training in the thymus gland, behind the breastbone. T-lymphocytes originate in the bone marrow, enter the bloodstream, and settle in the thymus for a while. Here, they become immune-competent, that is, ready to play their part in the immune system. Some of them are classed as helper T-cells, others, as suppressors, and a third, exceedingly aggressive category, as killer cells. The last mentioned are equipped with a potent toxin with which (in some unknown way) they assail the deviant cell. It then dies.

But how do killer cells locate their victims? For the rest of the immune system, it is the foreign antigens on, for example, the bacterium's surface which reveal the enemy. The killer cell, however, requires something else. It is programmed to track down not only a foreign antigen but, at the same time, the body's own antigens. For this reason, it attacks only diseased body cells. Very often, for example, a virus conceals itself inside body cells, safe from antibodies, complement factors, and feeding cells. It is protected by the antigens of the vanquished cell, to which the body's defences do not respond. However, on its arrival the killer cell detects the virus in its hiding place for this very reason: the cell bears on its surface both the body's own antigens and foreign, virus antigens. Instantaneously, the killer cell strikes. The same response is triggered off by certain tumour cells: only an insignificant change in antigen characteristics is required to provoke the killer cells' assault.

Right, we see a killer cell before it attacks the large tumour cell.

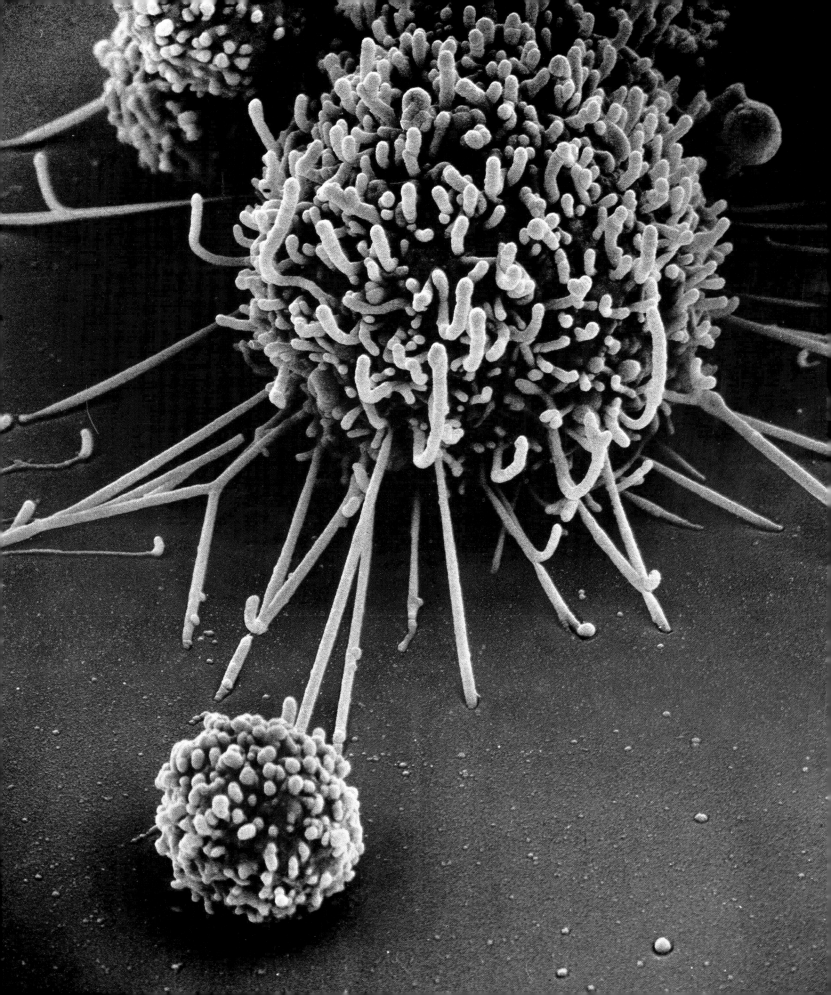

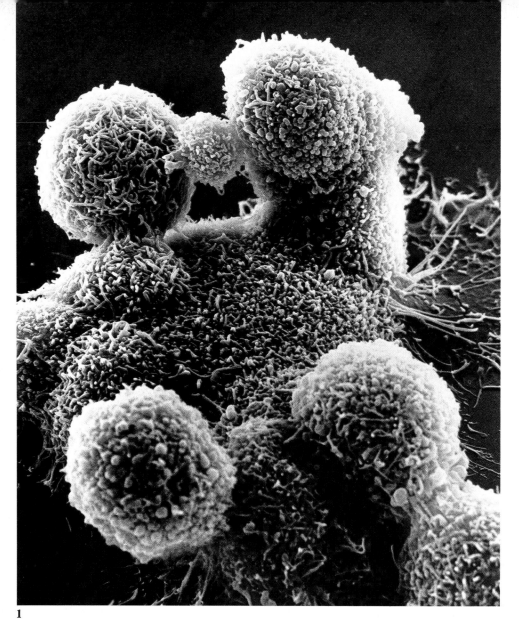

Deviant antigens seal the tumour cell's fate

The tumour cell *above left* is fated—at least five killer cells are attacking it simultaneously. After being transported to the tumour by the blood, they have entered it, reacting against its combination of the body's own antigens and those of foreign origin. The killer cells' special task is to annihilate those body cells which in some respect deviate from the norm. In addition to the body cells' normal antigens, these also have antigens which are unique to them—and which seal their fate. The killer cells latch on to the cell surfaces; toxin penetrates the cells and they die.

Below left, a benign tumour in the stomach originating in nerve tissue, photographed as it appears to the naked eye. It consists of millions of tumour cells which, however, unlike those of malignant type, stay put, neither infiltrating other organs nor forming secondary tumours.

Right, a killer cell—here in monstrous guise—grips a protoplasm thread of the large tumour cell and starts to penetrate the enemy. Goliath meets David: the giant seldom survives the encounter with the little killer cell.

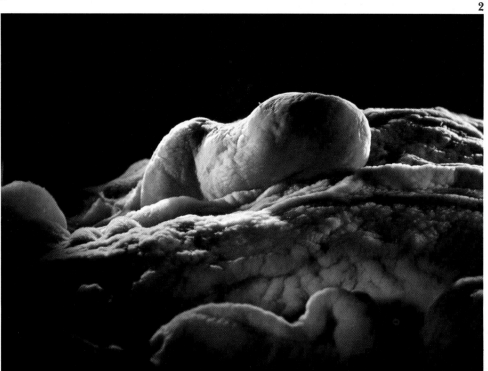

1. *A small killer cell tucked in between two cancer cells is seen in the upper part of the picture. Beneath, several more cancer cells.*
2. *Benign tumour in stomach.*
3. *A cone-shaped killer cell,* bottom left, *assails a far larger cancer cell.*

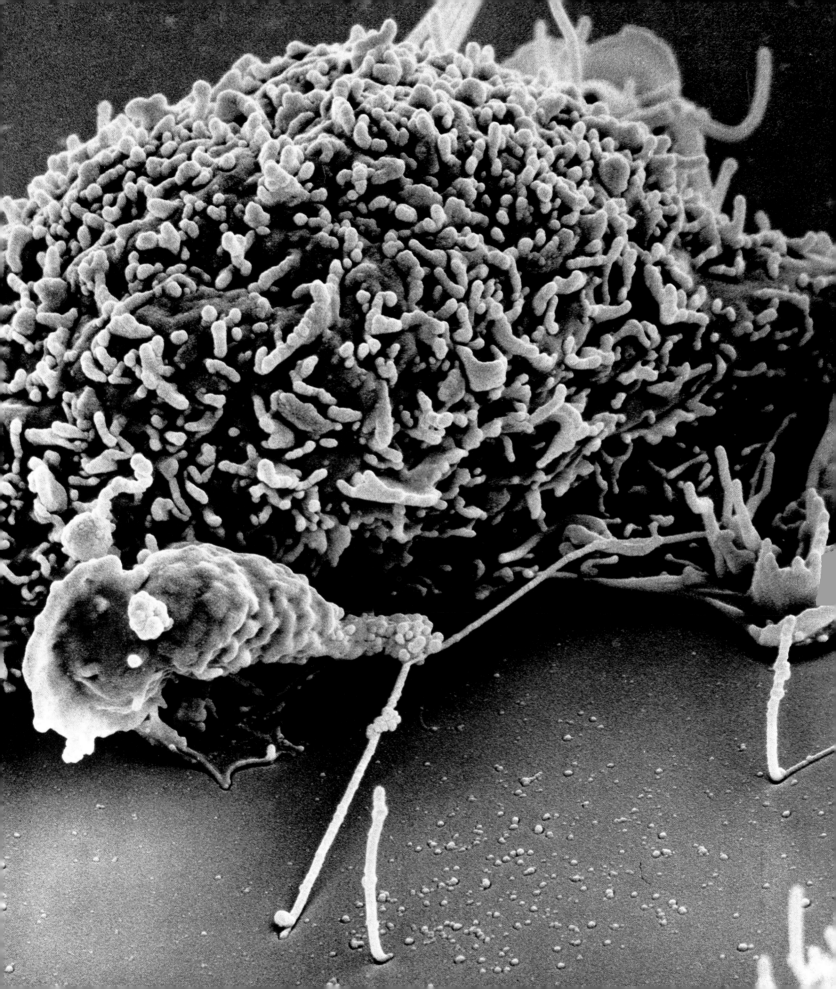

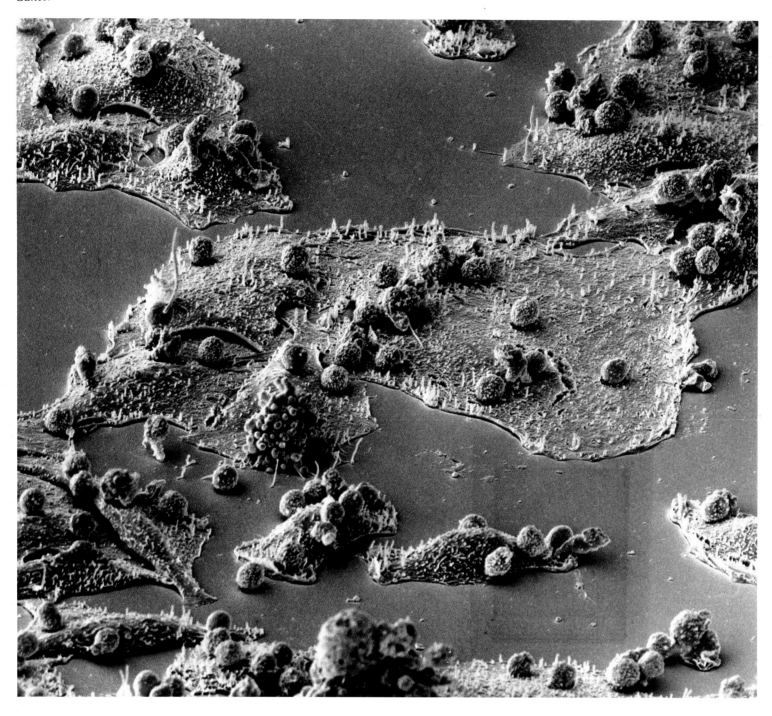

Landscape of tumours

Here, tumour cells repose on a slide, resembling islands. But this is no peaceful scene: the islands have been invaded by killer cells. *Above,* the spherical killer cells dominate the picture. *Right,* they resemble prehistoric animals, extending their necks to reach the tumour cell and give it the coup de grace. The objects resembling bare tree trunks on the islands' edges are protoplasm outgrowths from the tumour cell. The elongated killer cells are active and in the process of releasing their poison. The cancer cell dies very soon afterward.

One might assume that such a mortal enemy to tumours as the killer cell should itself be immune to cancer, but it is not. In certain regions of Japan, a virus has been isolated—possibly originating from monkeys—which attacks killer cells and produces a tumour, the T-lymphoma.

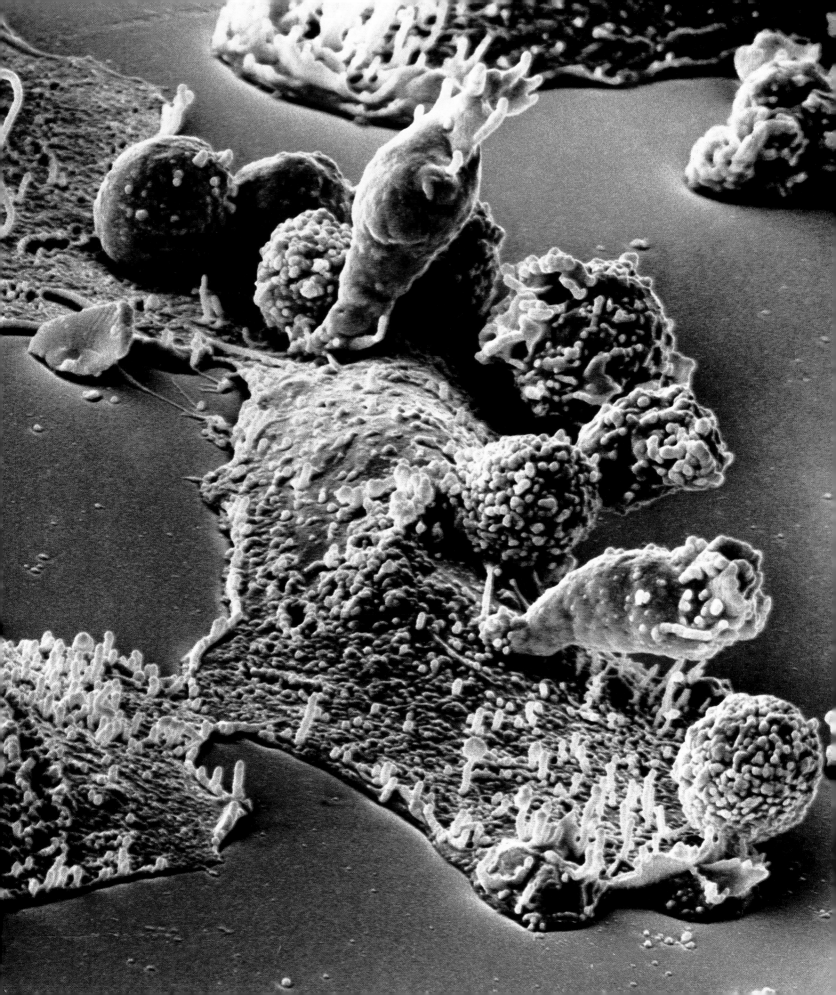

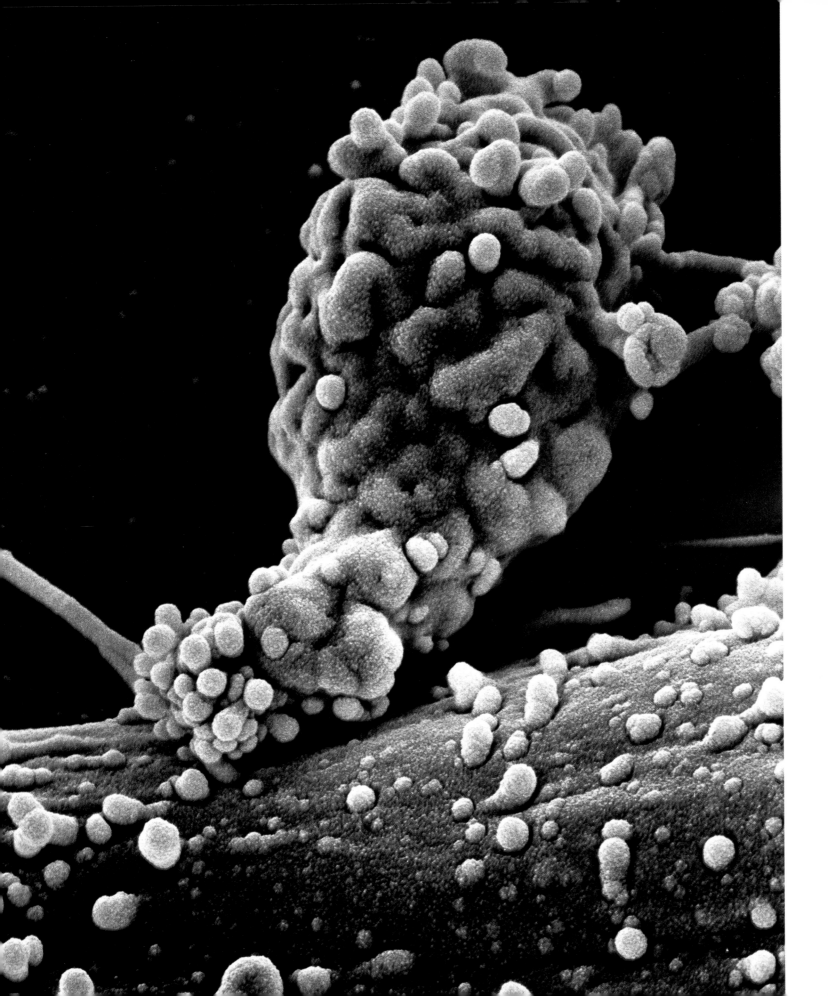

A kiss of death—the killer cell in action

Left, we see how a killer cell gives the tumour cell the poisonous "kiss" that dispatches it. We do not know exactly how the toxin is transferred, only that the encounter between the two cells leads to the tumour cell's death.

Below, a dying cancer cell, its entrails—the smooth, bladder-like formations—extruding. Above, to the left and right of the large bladder, we see a few killer cells. We thus know for certain that the immune system has at its disposal armed forces directed against body cells that get out of hand, start an uncontrolled growth, and develop into tumours. But if this is the case, why do so many people get cancer? How powerful are the immune defences against tumours? Dare we hope for a vaccine against cancer?

To begin with, we may pose the question of why *everyone* does not get cancer. The probability of changes in the genetic blue-print arising in one or more cells, in a body containing many billions of cells, is large. These diseased cells, which are capable of developing into tumours, are nonetheless eliminated in some way in most of us, probably by killer cells of T-cell type, or by their relatives the NK cells (natural killers).

However, cancer becomes more frequent with advancing age. Certain researchers believe the explanation—at least a partial one—to be a weakened immune system.

Surveys show that approximately half of patients with various types of cancer, for example, lung cancer, have in their blood killer cells which are attacking the cancer cells. The concentration of these T-lymphocytes is not high but it is measurable. Perhaps the truth is that unaided they are incapable of defeating the cells of a tumour, which are often proliferating at great speed, but that they can do so with help from outside. Perhaps, after surgery, radiation therapy, or chemotherapy have reduced the number of tumour cells, the immune system can deal with the rest. This is the background to research efforts to devise methods of reinforcing the killer cells' effect on the tumour cells.

There is little chance of our developing any generally effective vaccine against cancer, because of the great variation in antigen properties that tumour cells display. To be effective, the cancer vaccine would need to contain antibodies against them all—something beyond the bounds of reason.

Monoclonal antibodies—for the discovery of which a Nobel prize was awarded in 1984—offer another path of development. Experimental attempts have been made to load these "homing missiles" with radioactive isotopes and cell toxins, in the hope that they will track down the tumour cells and then "explode" in them. The method may possibly become important in the future.

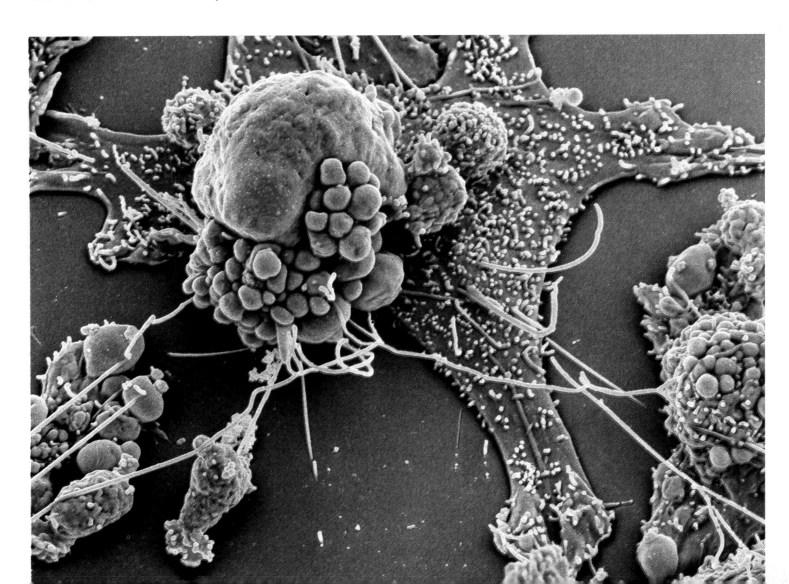

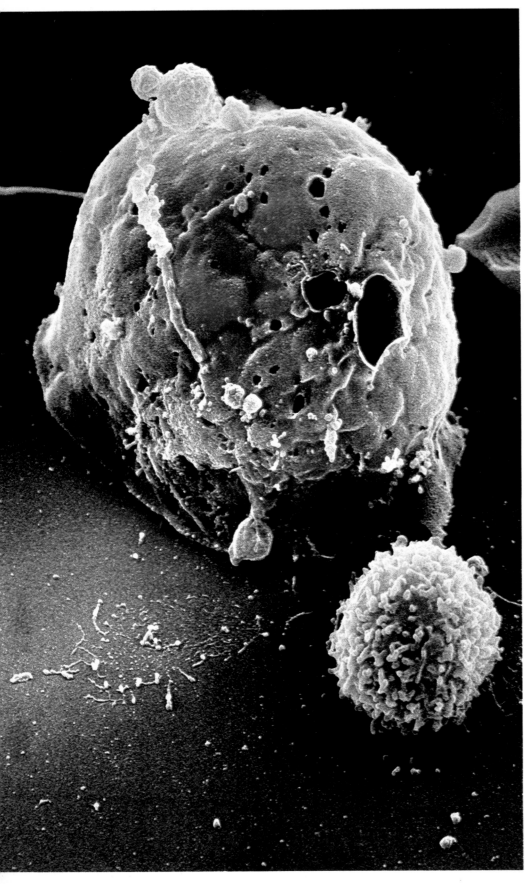

Victory—death of the tumour cell

Two stages in the tumour cell's destruction after it confronts the killer cells. *Left,* the empty shell of a cancer cell. The perforation made by the "kiss of death," when the defender emptied its toxin into the adversary, remains. With a leak in its membrane, no cell can survive: the high salt content of its interior means that fluid is absorbed from the surroundings and, in the end, the cell usually bursts.

One of the many types of weapons of the immune system—the complement factors—are specialists in puncturing their enemies in this way.

In front of the empty tumour cell lies a spherical killer cell. Its duties completed, it has resumed its resting shape.

Right, only the cell skeleton remains. Each cell contains fine, thread-like structures whose task is to stabilise the construction. Despite its tiny size, the cell nucleus contains the genetic blueprint, mitochondria, ribosomes, and many other cell elements with essential functions. The cell is the smallest unit of the body, and yet a whole factory. In the *bottom right* are two of the victors—the killer cells. Sometimes, however, it is the killer cells that are defeated in battle.

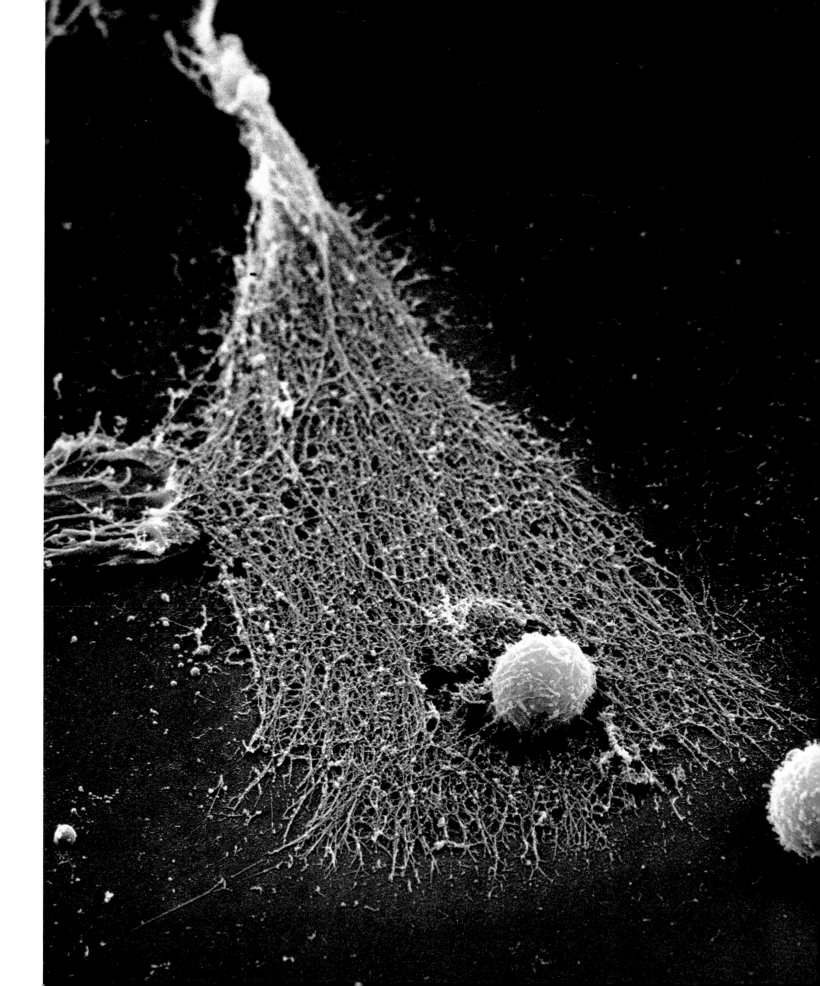

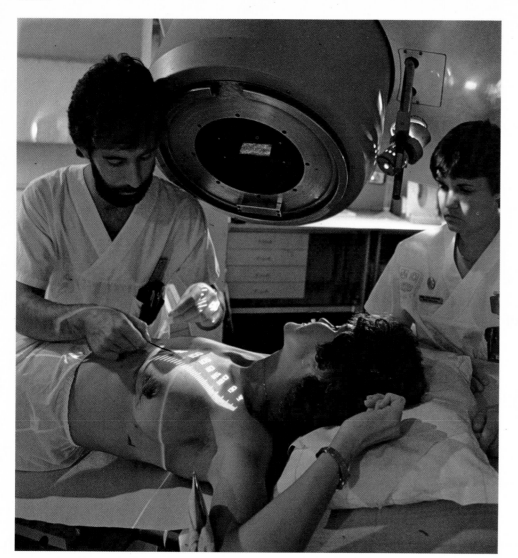

After the radical mastectomy, i.e., removal of one breast and the underarm lymph nodes, the patient is treated with telecobalt radiation therapy (left).

Below, *the radiation dose is checked against calculations already performed. It is important to get the dose exactly right: too little radiation would permit tumour cells to survive, while too much could damage the healthy tissue.*

Below left, *the woman who has undergone mastectomy wears a brassiere with an inbuilt external silicon prosthesis. The artificial breast is modeled on the other breast and given the same weight.*

Time to return to everyday life! The removal of a breast is a psychological ordeal for many women, but most surmount their problems and find that a completely normal life is possible after mastectomy.

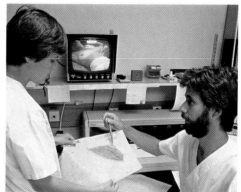

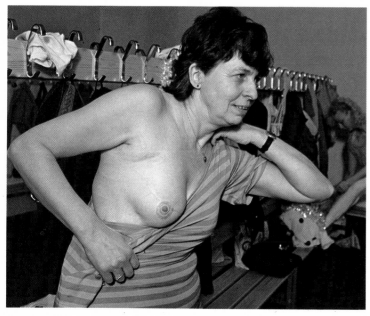

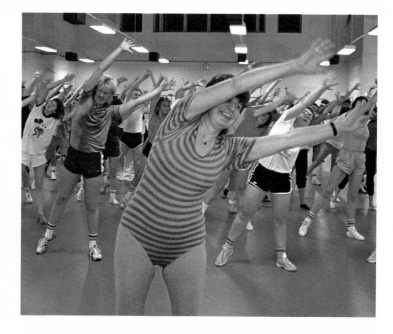

Normal life is possible after the removal of a breast

Tumours in the female mammary glands are relatively common, but the majority are benign. Of women in industrialised countries, however, 7 or 8 percent develop malignant tumours. Causes are thought to include both high levels of the female hormone estrogen (oestrogen) and elevated intake of cholesterol, the latter being a consequence of our immense consumption of fats in the West. Hereditary factors also play a part: if the mother has had breast cancer, the daughter runs three times as great a risk of succumbing to the disease as women whose mothers have not had breast cancer.

All lumps, and changes in the breasts in general, should be checked by a doctor. More and more women have learned to examine (*palpate*) their breasts systematically, and tumours are therefore discovered sooner than they used to be. In general, the tumour displays no symptoms during the first stage. When the woman, or her doctor, first detects a patch of hardened tissue, it is about the size of a pea (half to one centimetre in diameter). X-ray investigations of the breasts (mammography) can reveal tumours even smaller than this.

Early detection of tumours is of immense importance to the result of treatment. Breast cancer is no exception, particularly if the tumour is of a type which produces *metastases*, secondary tumours, at an early stage. When a change in the mammary gland tissue is discovered, its position is ascertained by X ray, whereupon the doctor, using a fine hollow needle called a cannula, punctures the suspected tumour and extracts a sample of its contents. Under the microscope, he can then see which type of cells the tumour contains, that is, whether it is benign or malignant. If the latter, an operation is performed as soon as possible. Another method is the surgical removal, and microscopic examination, of a small portion of the suspected tumour tissue. This is called a *biopsy*.

If the malignant tumour is small and there are no metastases, the surgeon may decide on a limited operation (*lumpectomy* or *partial mastectomy*), in which case only the tumour and a sufficient margin of surrounding tissue are removed. When this is done, the appearance of the breast may be restored with the use of silicon inserts (breast reconstruction, or "internal prosthesis"). Otherwise, the surgeon may choose to perform a *radical mastectomy,* which means removing the whole mammary gland plus the lymph nodes in the underarm region—the latter in view of the risk of metastases. Radiation therapy is usually given after the operation to destroy any metastases in remaining lymph nodes of the chest region.

Many women experience the loss of a breast as a disabling amputation. In recent years, the importance of psychological counseling both before and after the operation has been realised. Women who have undergone the same operation, among others, are therefore enlisted to help fellow sufferers. The potential for constructing a cosmetically acceptable replacement for the amputated breast is nowadays good, thanks to internal and external silicon inserts, modeled on the other breast and given the same weight. With such inserts, it is entirely possible to live a normal life—people are unaware of any difference, unless they are told.

One forceful argument in favour of the surgical treatment of breast cancer is, of course, the enhanced survival rate. Statistics show the survival rate after ten years, in a group of women with breast cancer who did not receive treatment, to be only 5 percent. Of women who are treated for breast cancer with modern methods, on the other hand, approximately 75 percent are alive ten years later, provided that the tumour has been discovered and treated at an early stage.

Mastectomy patients should undergo medical check-ups for the rest of their lives—initially every three months, then twice a year and finally once a year. The operation site, the remaining breast, lymph nodes, and certain internal organs are then investigated with a view to detecting recurrent tumours.

"Nature's method" of treating cancer is based above all on killer cells, either of T-lymphocyte type or NK cells (*natural killers*). They are programmed to detect body cells that bear foreign antigens in addition to the body's own antigens. These may originate from viruses hiding inside cells, but also from cancer cells with deviant antigen patterns. When the killer cells find such a pattern, they adhere to the cell and kill it with toxin. One explanation of why tumour cells nonetheless succeed in evading these death patrols in the bloodstream is that their surface antigens are not sufficiently deviant to attract the killer cells' attention.

As is described elsewhere in this chapter on defences against cancer, the efficiency of the immune apparatus may in some cases be raised by the injection of bacteria. Another possible future method is that of targeting monoclonal antibodies on cancer cells, wherever in the body they occur. In addition, the method of activating the immune system with leukotrienes—a variety of immune hormones—appears to promise well for the future. Otherwise it must be admitted that, to date, experimental work on immunological methods of curing cancer has not yielded convincing results—with one exception, namely the type of tumour arising in B-lymphocytes, the cells that produce antibodies. Here, a method of dealing with the tumour cells by means of monoclonal antibodies has been found. These new methods are discussed in more detail in the last chapter.

Medical treatment of breast cancer includes, in addition to surgery, radiation therapy with telecobalt equipment, hormonal treatment, and cystostatics, that is, substances which inhibit the growth of fast-growing cells (including cancer cells), and which are also called cell toxins.

Radiation therapy is effective because it causes the genetic material in the cell nucleus to disintegrate. Since tumour cells divide faster than most normal body cells (except those in bone marrow and intestinal membrane, for example), they are damaged more quickly by the radiation than is the surrounding, healthy tissue.

Hormonal treatment is aimed at "starving" tumour cells, which need the female sex hormone estrogen (oestrogen) for their growth. The treatment is adopted when a tumour has metastasised. Generally speaking, both ovaries—which are the chief producers of estrogen (oestrogen)—are surgically removed. Experiments are also in progress with medicines which block the cells' estrogen (oestrogen) receptors.

Cytostatics are substances which suppress cell growth. Tumour cells are particularly sensitive to cystostatics, just as they are to radiation therapy. Varying and combining different types of cystostatics has enabled excellent results to be achieved in many cases. Development in this field is rapid and promising.

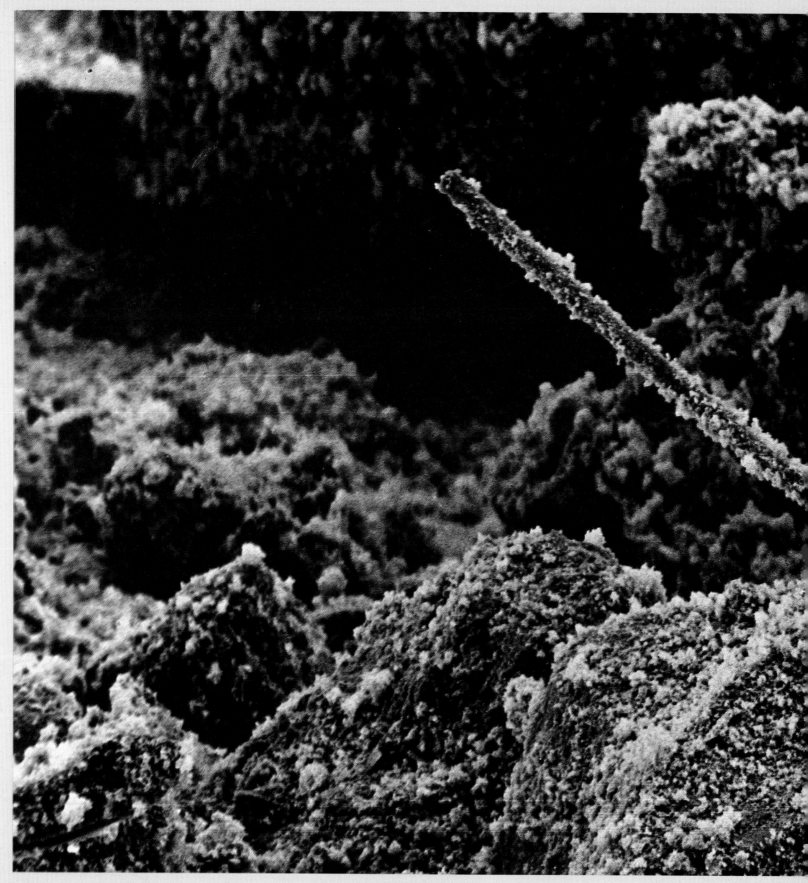

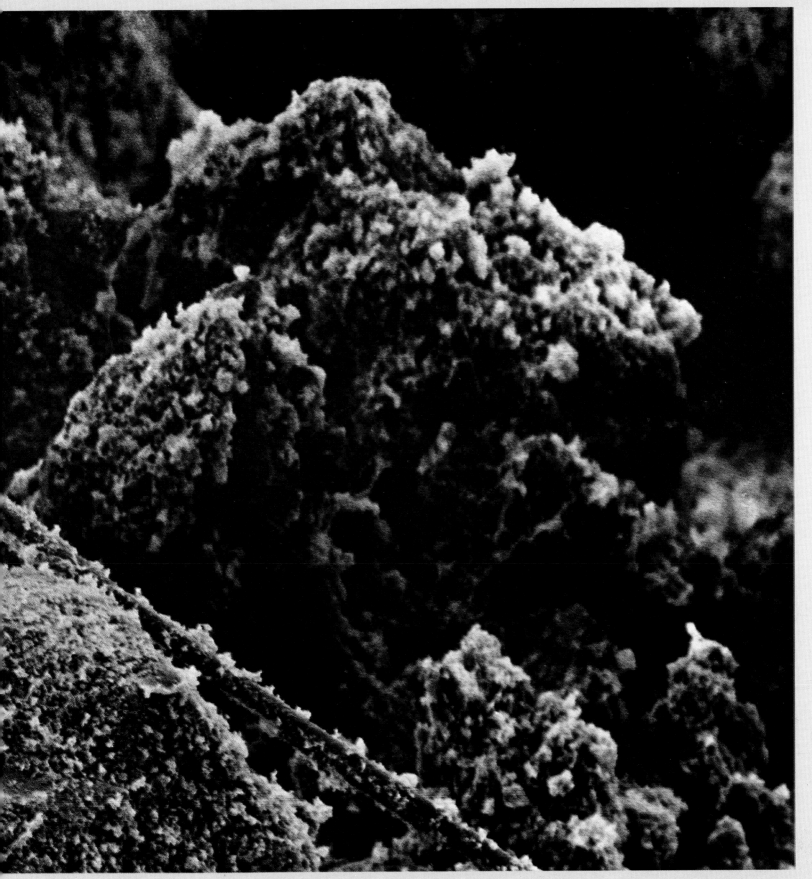

The respiratory tract

Clean air is rare nowadays, occurring almost exclusively in the polar regions. Most of us are therefore obliged to subsist in an atmosphere polluted by impurities from traffic, domestic heating, and industrial combustion. In urban areas, the air we breathe is for the most part a hazy mishmash of soot, dust, airplane emissions, metal dust from vehicle wear and refuse incineration, silicate, fertilisers, sulfur compounds, nitric oxide and carbon monoxide, halogens, bacteria, viruses, microscopic fungi, and radioactive dust. In addition, there are those impurities which arise from various natural processes: pollen from plants, sand from desert storms, ash from volcanoes, or cosmic dust from meteorites. Fortunately, however, the respiratory tract is equipped with various protective devices, from the nostrils to the air sacs (alveoli) inside our lungs, and thanks to these most people manage to survive, even in the city.

Protection in the respiratory tract is based on mechanical, chemical, and immune devices. When air enters through the nose, large particles are impeded by hairs in the nostrils. The nasal passages are anatomically designed in such a way that air becomes turbulent and particles are cast centrifugally outward, to the walls, where they stick in the mucus continuously produced by tiny glands. The mucus contains antibodies and chemical substances effective against both bacteria and viruses.

The epiglottis, positioned at the top of the larynx (voice box), and thus of the trachea (windpipe), closes at lightning speed in emergencies—if, for example, some morsel of food has "gone down the wrong way," or if we inhale a corrosive gas like chlorine or ammonia. The pharynx (throat) also contains two of the immune system's biggest lymph nodes, the tonsils, as well as an abundance of lymphoid tissue, in which there are myriad white blood cells. In this heavily armed region most airborne particles come to rest, whereupon they can be tackled by the immune system.

The trachea and the two large bronchi are clad with a fitted carpet of cells bearing cilia, tiny hair-like protuberances that constantly sweep a thin layer of mucus up toward the throat. The cilia—which are barely one-hundredth of a millimetre long—stroke the trachea and bronchus walls between 1,000 and 1,500 times a minute, shifting the particles and bacteria about sixteen millimetres upward in that time. When the mucus reaches the throat, it is swallowed or coughed up; in the stomach, the bacteria are killed by gastric juice, which has a high hydrochloric acid content.

The size of inhaled particles determines how far they penetrate the respiratory tract. Analyses show that those which exceed ten-thousandths of a millimetre in size remain in the nasal passages, while those between two- and ten-thousandths of a millimetre in diameter are borne down into the trachea and large bronchi, where they become attached to the walls. Beyond the large bronchi, turbulence declines, and the air travels more slowly in the smaller bronchi and bronchioles. Only extremely small particles (less than two-thousandths of a millimetre across) are able to remain airborne all the way into the network of alveoli, where gaseous exchange with the blood takes place.

The alveoli are surrounded by blood capillaries, through whose thin walls carbon dioxide is released into the air we exhale and fresh oxygen absorbed from air inhaled. For this process to be efficient, the surfaces must be kept clean, and the alveolar cleaning staff are feeding cells of various kinds. They track down foreign particles, including microorganisms, and swallow them. The material they cannot—or fail to—break down into a form enabling it to be transported out of the body remains in the lung tissue. This is why the lungs of city dwellers, and particularly smokers, are dark or even black with soot.

Two more protective mechanisms should be mentioned: coughing and sneezing. Both are controlled by nerve reflexes and are designed to thrust out irritants.

The coughing reflex is triggered by extremely small particles, which provoke constriction of the air passages. This leads to nerve impulses that, on the one hand, cause the vocal cords to shut and, on the other, force the breathing muscles to contract. Since the vocal cords seal the trachea, a high air-pressure level is built up in the lungs. Suddenly, the vocal cords open and a violent rush of air expels the irritant particles. The air velocity at the moment of coughing can reach an increcible 900 kilometres per hour—the speed of a jet airplane. It is like a hurricane in the lungs, propelling viruses, bacteria, pus, lumps of phlegm, and foreign particles out of the respiratory tract.

The sneeze reflex resembles that of the cough, but with one difference: The vocal cords do not close. No pressure builds up in the lungs, and the rush of air is unimpeded. Irritation arises in the sensory nerves of the nasal membrane, and impulses pass from them, in a roundabout way, to the muscles involved in breathing. Unavoidably, as the saying goes, "coughs and sneezes spread diseases": infected material is effectively transferred, in the air, from one person to the next.

Certain illnesses assail the defence system of the respiratory tract, making the sufferer particularly sensitive to particles in the air inhaled. Chronic inflammations of the respiratory tract—bronchitis and sinusitis—are the result, often with further complications. Since the attack also affects the cilia, and it is also cilia which propel sperm cells, this may reduce fertility or cause sterility in men.

A much more common consequence of inadequate defences in the respiratory tract, however, is hypersensitivity, that is, allergies. Allergies are caused by airborne particles that set off a kind of "false alarm" in the immune system. Such particles include pollen from birch trees and grasses, which provoke hypersensitive responses in many people. An allergic person need only breathe in a minute amount of pollen to be affected, within a few minutes, by sneezing, an itching nose, and swollen, watering eyes. Asthma is the most troublesome of all allergic ailments: the narrow air passages swell, making it difficult for the sufferer to breathe. Not only pollen from plants, but also dander from fur-bearing animals, dust, and certain foodstuffs precipitate asthma symptoms.

The mechanism underlying the allergic response functions, in brief, is as follows: The irritant substance (the allergen) enters the body, prompting the immune system to produce antibodies of a particular kind, which we have seen before, called immunoglobulin E (IgE for short). These antibodies bind to specific cells in connective tissue and around blood vessels called mast cells, which contain the biologically active, hormone-like substance histamine.

The immune system is thereby mobilised against new attacks by the irritant—but, unfortunately, in a way that can have disastrous results. The antibodies have an extraordinarily good memory, and react swiftly next time the allergen enters the body. They trap the allergen, simultaneously transmitting a signal to the mast cell, which literally explodes, shedding histamine, serotonin, leukotrienes, and other tissue-irritating substances into the blood. The histamine, for example, causes the air passages of the lungs to contract, thus giving rise to an asthma attack.

The allergic diseases are a growing problem, and researchers are working hard to find a way of curing or alleviating them. One approach is to ascertain, by allergy tests, which substances cause the symptoms, so that the sufferer can avoid them or gradually habituate himself by what is called desensitisation.

Since vehicle exhaust fumes are heavy and sink downward, toward the ground, it is children who are most exposed to their ill effects (the same, of course, applies to pet dogs). Exhaust fumes contain substances such as lead, carbon monoxide, and hydrocarbon compounds—all extremely toxic in high concentrations. Sampling of air in urban traffic is carried out in many countries, and test filters from streets exposed to heavy traffic turn black. Fortunately for us, the human respiratory apparatus is superior to the testing apparatus, which cannot rid itself of "inhaled" material. Our air passages contain mucus, in which larger particles become stuck, to be conveyed upward on the carpet of cilia and finally expelled by coughing or clearing of the throat. Particles that are borne into the recesses of the lungs are dealt with by feeding cells. However, the load on the lungs in, for example, industrial towns is so great that the dirt-consuming macrophages cannot fully cope with it. Black patches then develop in the lungs from the accumulated pollutants.

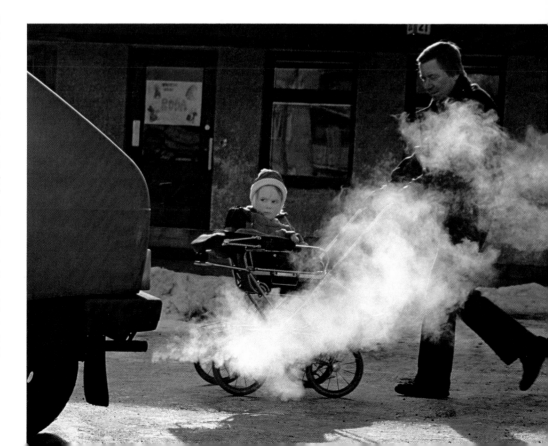

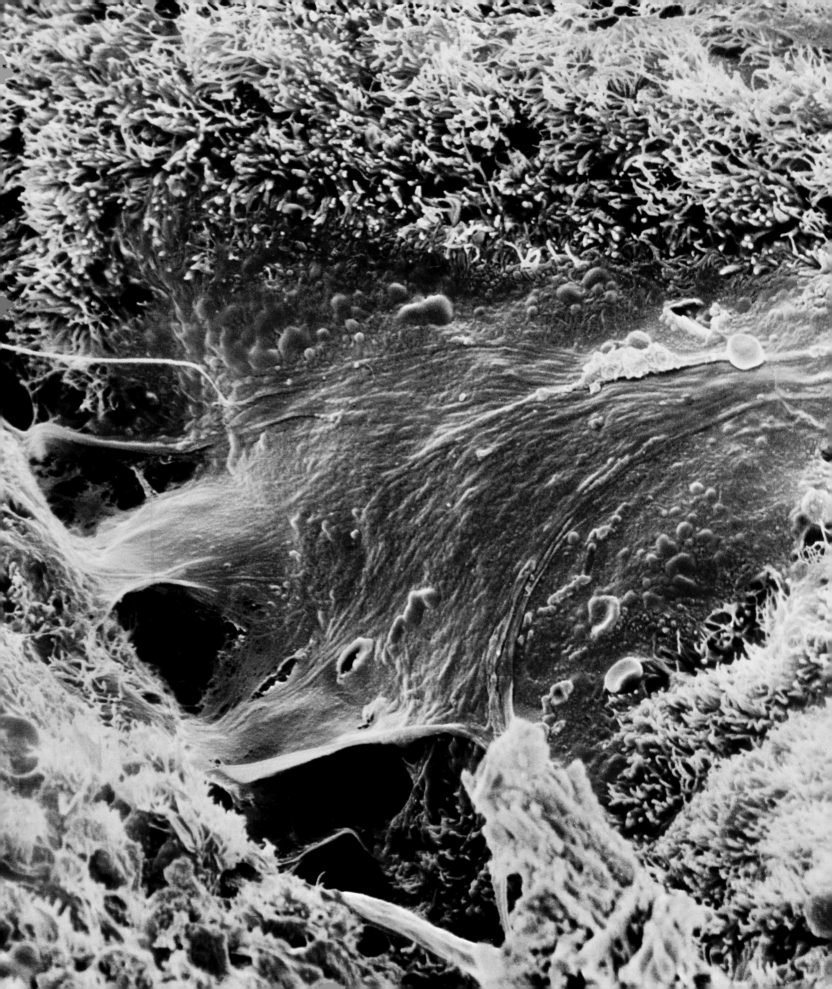

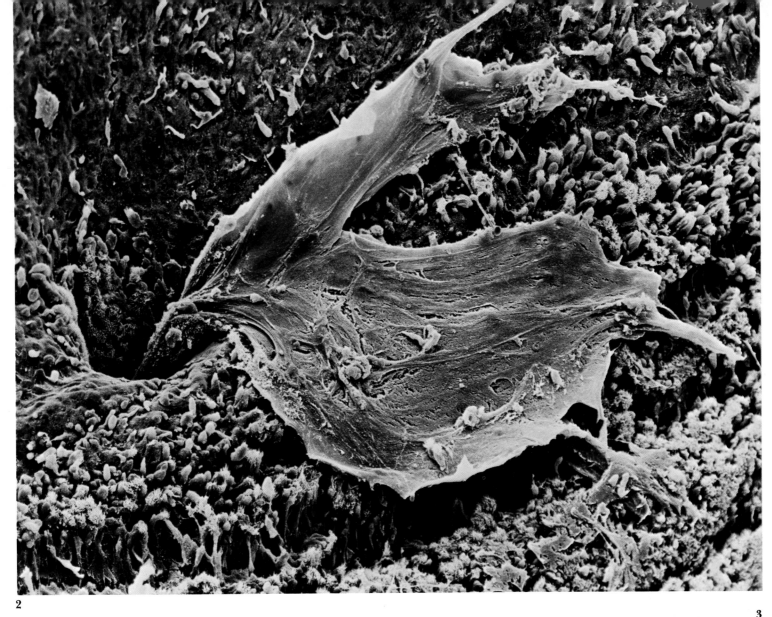

2

3

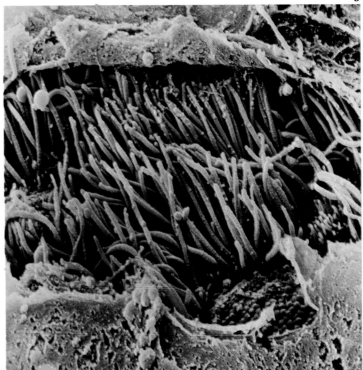

A fitted carpet of cilia

The respiratory tract is lined with a carpet of cells equipped with millions of tiny, hair-like cilia which penetrate the mucus. In perpetual motion, they push the layer of mucus upward. Inhaled dust particles are trapped in the mucus and thereby expelled from the lungs. During its passage through the nasal cavity, trachea, and large bronchi, the air becomes turbulent owing to the organs' anatomical construction; heavier particles are flung against the sides, where they are trapped in the mucus. Some lighter particles are carried out again when we exhale, but others remain in the lungs, where they are eaten by macrophages. *Left,* we see the carpet of cilia in healthy bronchi, covered with a mucous layer. Mucus is secreted by a gland *(2)* and spreads out to form a sticky layer covering the carpet of cilia. When our respiratory tract becomes infected, the mucus glands increase their production to aid the removal of bacteria and dead cells. The mucus, normally clear and transparent, thickens and turns yellowish green with the casualties from the battle between microorganisms and defenders. *Right (3),* we see the cilia through an opening in the layer of mucus.

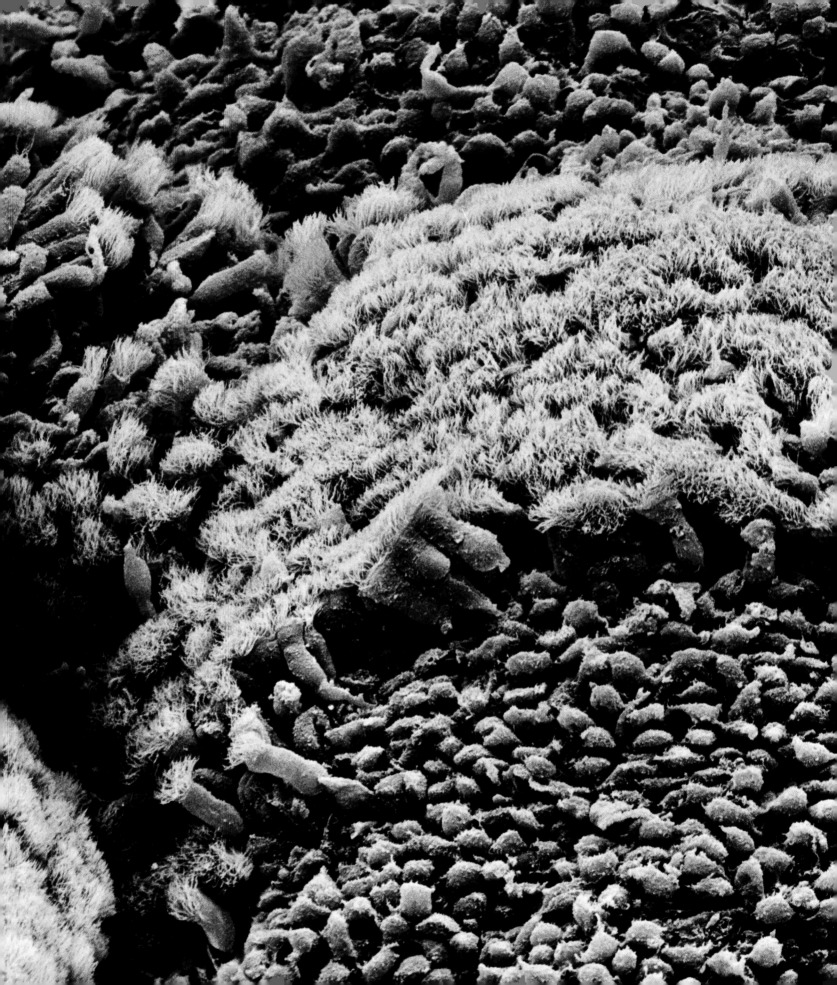

The carpet of cilia becomes "threadbare"

Infections, inhaled toxins (for example, solvents), and—above all—long-term tobacco smoking damage the ciliated cells which line the passages of the respiratory tract. In the middle section of the picture, *left,* they remain, surrounded by damaged areas from which the cilia cells have entirely disappeared.

Right, the pictures show ciliated cells progressively magnified. *Above,* the remains of damaged cells resemble a forest clearing, in contrast to the upper area with still healthy ciliated cells. The *middle* picture shows healthy ciliated cells, with their brush-like protuberances, and two damaged ones, naked and drooping. *Below,* we see a group of damaged cells, without cilia, incapacitated by protracted tobacco smoking and unable to play any useful part in the work of cleaning the respiratory tract.

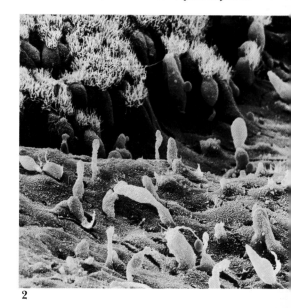

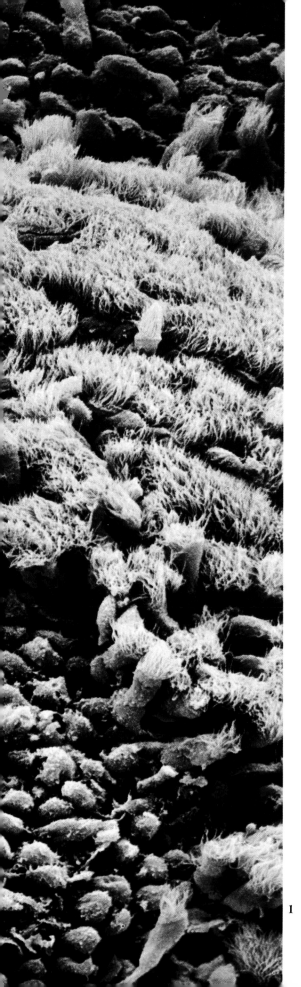

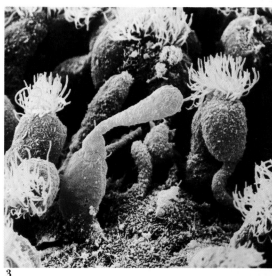

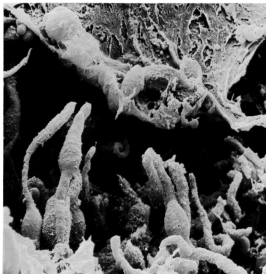

1. *The ciliated cells of the respiratory tract are partially destroyed by smoking: in the middle, cells with intact cilia; above and below, portions which have lost their ciliary cells.*

2. *Severely damaged ciliated cells, in the lower half of the picture.*

3. *Close-up of some healthy ciliated cells and, in the middle, two damaged ones that have lost their cilia.*

4. *Dead ciliated cells, detached from the layer of mucus which lies in the upper part of the picture.*

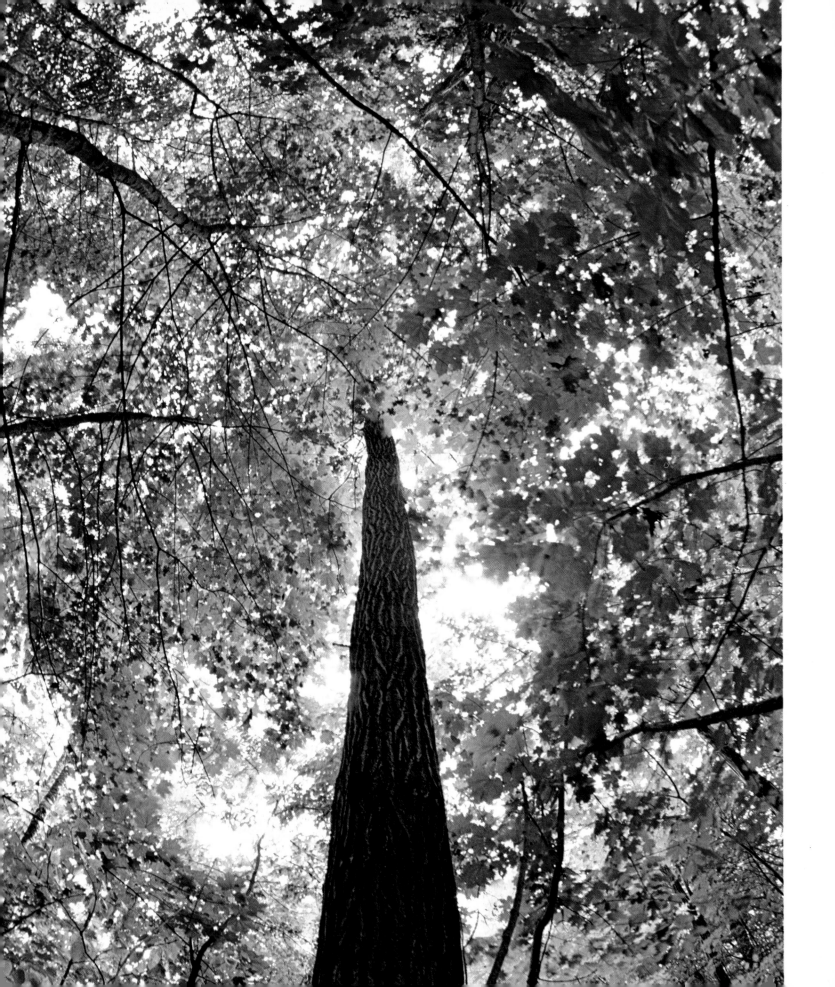

Country air can cause problems too

From the contaminated air of a large city, with its dust and fumes, we like to escape to the countryside. But not even the health-giving country air is entirely innocuous—particularly not for a person who is hypersensitive to plant pollen and other organic substances.

Pollen is to plants what sperm is to animals. It is pollen which fertilises flowering plants. In the spring, tree pollen floods the atmosphere; in early summer, grass pollen takes over. The pollen grains, often microscopic in size, are proteins. They function as allergens, that is, substances that stimulate the immune system in hypersensitive people to produce reagins (antibodies). Allergens thus have the same effect as antigens on the surface of a bacterium, and reagins are IgE antibodies. The allergic response is described in more detail in the following pages.

Certain allergens are so strong that they stimulate the production of antibodies in almost all individuals, provided they have been exposed to the allergen's effects previously. Usually, however, only particularly susceptible individuals react with allergic symptoms to the substances to which they have developed sensitivity. Hereditary traits play a prominent part in this disposition.

Hay fever is an allergic response to pollen. The symptoms include a runny nose and watering eyes, facial swelling and redness. Pollen from broad-leaved trees, above all, birch, is more allergenic than pollen from conifers. In the United States, hypersensitivity to ragweed—plants belonging to the *Ambrosia* genus— is strongly predominant. Some individuals are sensitive to only one pollen type, others to several. Allergic responses can also be triggered by certain thread-like elements in fungi, mould spores, and the epithelial cells from animals—dogs, cats, horses, and cattle. Allergies to animals are often highly specific: for example, one can be allergic to Alsatians but not to other breeds.

Right, an array of substances that can provoke allergic responses in hypersensitive individuals. *Above*, microscopic plant fragments and pollen mixed with dirt and wastes from factories and towns, transported over long distances. The *middle* picture shows pine pollen; *bottom*, we see flakes of metal on the surface of a grain of pollen. Metals occurring as fine particles in the atmosphere include cadmium.

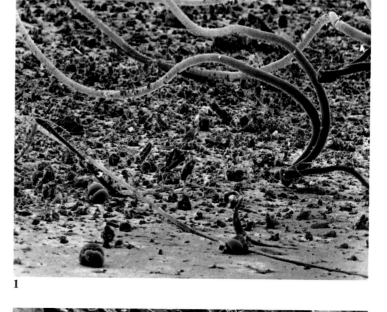

2

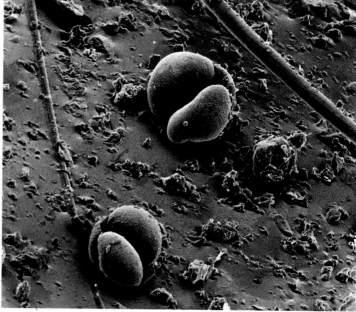

1

3

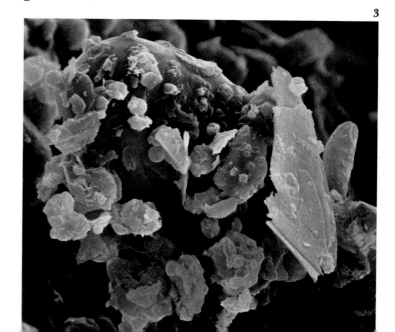

1. *Tiny fragments of plants and dirt.*
2. *Pine pollen.*
3. *Flakes of metal (the angular, light shapes), attached to the surface of pollen grains.*

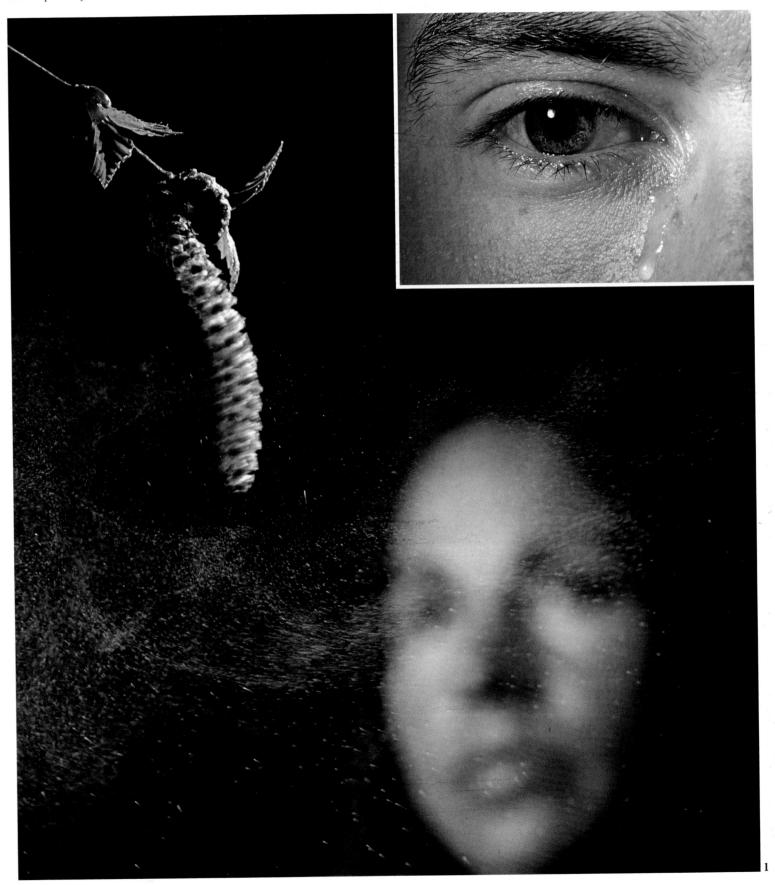

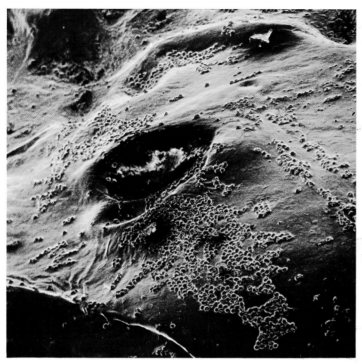

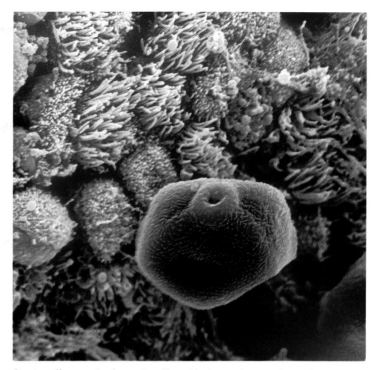

2. *The mucus on the nasal membrane is liberally sprinkled with birch pollen carried by the inhaled air.*

1. *A silver birch* (Betula pendula) *catkin, aided by the wind, releases its pollen in the spring.*

4. *Cross-section of the nasal membrane.*

3. *A pollen grain from the silver birch on the nasal membrane cells, greatly magnified by the electron microscope. In these tissues, as in many others, there are mast cells, which in an allergic person discharge histamine and other substances when they come into contact with pollen. It is the histamine that gives rise to the symptoms; pollen is their indirect cause.*

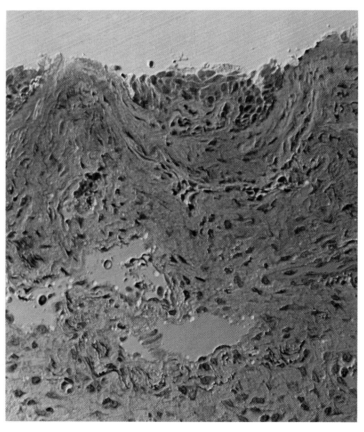

Plant pollen provokes an immune response

The allergic response is a remarkable biological phenomenon. Pollen grains shed by the birch catkin, *left,* which enter the respiratory passages, are not the direct cause of symptoms characterising pollen allergy. It is when they adhere to the antibody-laden surface of mast cells, as they are called, that a reaction arises. Theoretically, it may be described as a "false alarm," causing the immune system to react against itself. Irritated by the pollen grains, the mast cell discharges its contents, including histamine, into the tissue. Inflammation and swelling rapidly ensue. However, not all of us are affected: for most people, walking through a birch forest is an unadulterated joy. Immunologists suspect that the faulty response of the immune system which produces these symptoms is a manifestation of activity originally directed against parasites. The type of antibody which reacts with pollen is, in fact, one found in abundance in persons suffering from parasitic diseases. In modern society, parasites are unusual and the body, with misdirected zeal, assigns its surplus defence capacity to dealing with essentially harmless invaders.

The mast cell—the body's histamine bomb

One of the specialists of the immune system is the mast cell (*right*)—one of the granulocytes, the small feeding cells which are the first to tackle a hostile invader.

Mast cells are stationary and distributed throughout the body's tissues, but are most abundant in the skin, the respiratory tract, and the digestive tract. They contain biologically highly active substances in the form of small granules. One such substance is histamine, a tissue hormone that can (for example, in those who are allergic) have dramatic effects. It causes the blood vessels to expand and their walls to become more pervious, so that blood is pumped out into the tissues. Inflammation is one result of this, when tissues redden and swell.

Histamine has a contracting effect on smooth muscle, such as that of the respiratory passages and bronchi. An asthmatic attack, when the bronchi contract and make breathing more difficult, is caused by the histamine outflow from mast cells in the membrane of the respiratory tract. This reaction, in turn, is caused by the detonation of the body's histamine bomb in response to an allergenic substance.

Right (*1*), two mast cells are shown: one (on the left) is intact and "loaded"; the other (on the right) has released its tissue-irritating granules.

On its surface, the mast cell has receptors which attract antibodies of a particular type, IgE, targeted on the allergenic substance, that is, birch pollen. When, in a hypersensitive person, such pollen becomes attached to the IgE antibodies, the mast cell receives a signal to empty itself—and the histamine flows out.

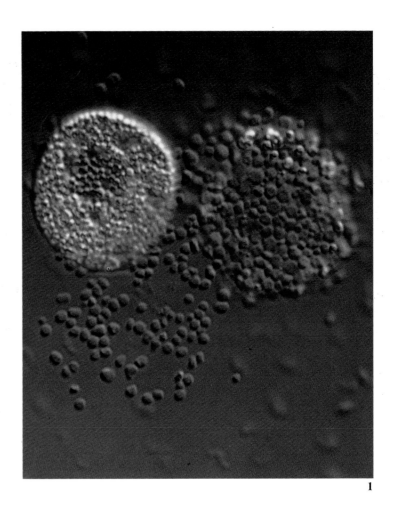

1

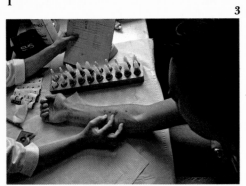

1

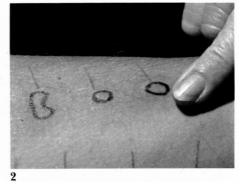

2

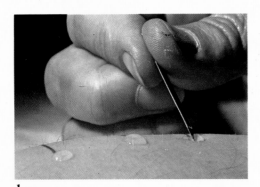

3

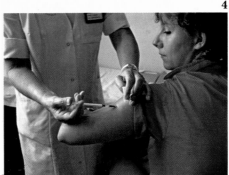

4

Skin tests and treatment

Which environmental substances are we sensitive to? The answer is obtained by a skin test, in which drops of various allergenic substances are placed on the skin. A light scratch with a needle (**1**) is enough for the substances to penetrate the skin. (**2**) The answer is provided: the irritant substance is the one producing redness and swelling.

Hypersensitivity to pollen is nowadays treated by successive habituation. A purified extract of the relevant pollen, in ampoules in the bottom left-hand picture (**3**), is injected over a long period, in increasing dosages (**4**). The immune system can thereby produce antibodies against the irritant. When the allergic person then encounters it in the natural environment, he possesses powers of resistance and does not fall ill.

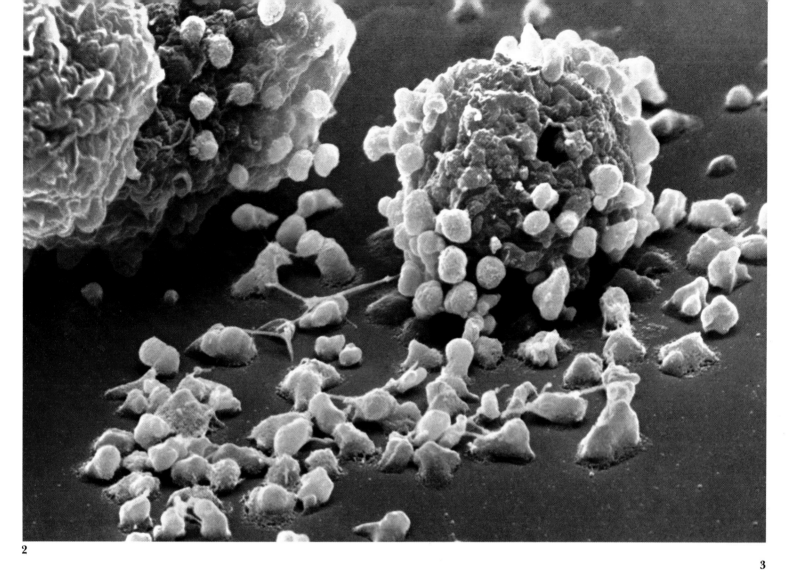

2

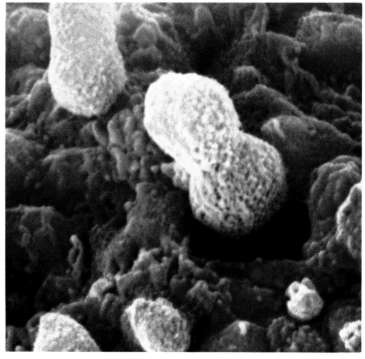

3

Above (2) is shown, greatly magnified, a mast cell which has emptied its powerful granules of histamine and other substances. Pollen grains enter the body with the inhaled air. Most of us are not hypersensitive to it, and do not notice anything in particular, but to the allergic person, pollen is a torment which provokes symptoms of various kinds: swelling membranes, watering eyes and runny nose, breathing difficulties, and so on. Other substances, such as almonds, fish, or animals' hair, can also give rise to allergic symptoms.

The immune system produces antibodies against foreign antigens in all of us; it is only in the person who is hypersensitive to these antigens that the antibody-antigen combination triggers a different response. The mast cell *(above)* has on its surface thousands of antibodies directed against the pollen grains invading the body. When the pollen binds to the antibodies, the mast cell of the allergic person releases its contents, notably histamine, and the characteristic allergic symptoms arise.

The picture on the *right (3)* shows the magnified surface of a mast cell as a few of its particles are being expelled.

Pharmaceuticals called antihistamines, which block the tissue cells' receptors where the histamine molecules otherwise settle, are now available. However, their effectiveness is limited—and against asthma, nonexistent.

What the urban population inhales

Domestic heating, traffic, and refuse incineration in large cities are the major sources of air pollution. In addition, certain parts of Europe continually receive large quantities of industrial emissions from industrialised areas on the Continent and in the British Isles. The widespread destruction of European forests is one indication of this fact. The combustion of fossil fuels releases, above all, sulfur and heavy metals, which are borne by winds over large areas and fall to the ground with precipitation. The large picture *below* shows, greatly magnified, the results of air sampling, using filters, at different traffic-density levels—low, normal, and high. Particles deposited on the filter in a period of low-density traffic are shown to the left, and particles collected during a period of high-density traffic, to the right.

Right, the pictures show air pollutants in close-up: soot and carbon particles, fine grains of sand, glass, asbestos fibres, and a metal particle. Many metals, such as cadmium, vanadium, tungsten, mercury, and iron oxides, are released during refuse incineration. Unchecked by purification plants, they are dispersed in the atmosphere. Living organisms have not encountered them in this way in their previous development; this is why most animals and plants lack specific systems for breaking them down and rendering them harmless. Some substances, like mercury, cannot be excreted at all, or only at an extremely slow rate. They accumulate in the tissues and can cause poisoning.

Filters exposed to urban air pollution from early morning (left) *until the evening rush hour* (right). *(Magnification × 30).*

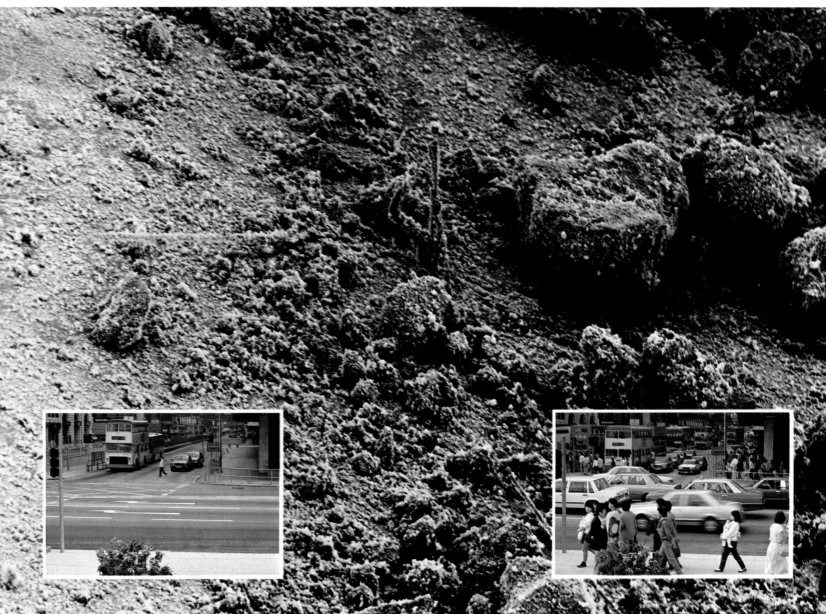

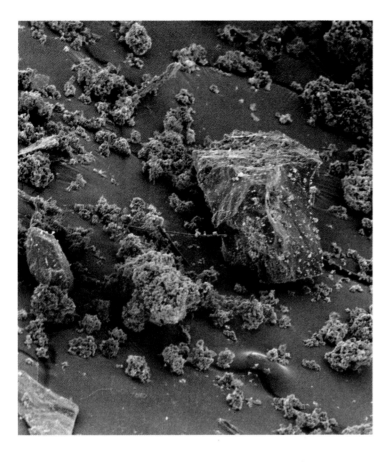
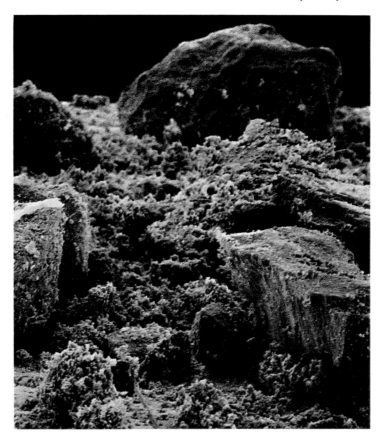
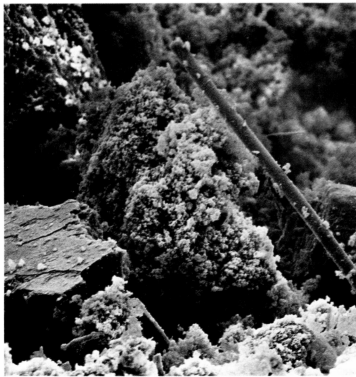
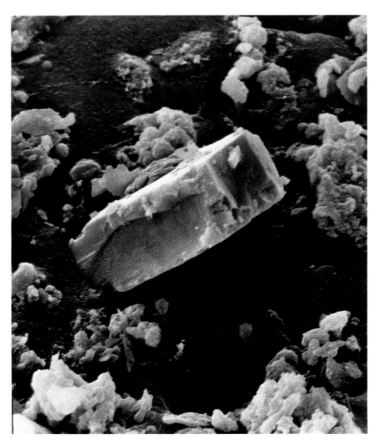

Urban air pollutants: soot and carbon particles, sand, glass, and asbestos fibres. Bottom right, a metal particle. Magnification: top left × *50,* top right × *100,* bottom left × *1,000 and* bottom right *4,000.*

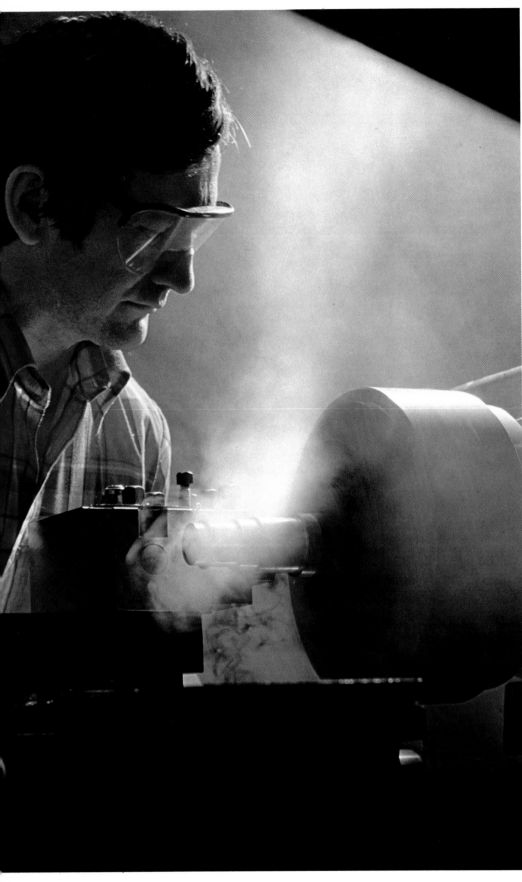

The high probability of injury in certain occupations

When the lathe operator *(left)* uses oil-impregnated metal in his work, the high temperature converts the oil into a vapour, which he breathes in. Fine droplets of oil are borne into his lungs in the inhaled air, eventually coming to rest in the air sacs, the alveoli. Since mineral oil contains substances deleterious to health, the immune system immediately tries to neutralise it. In the picture *(opposite)*, a macrophage—a large feeding cell—gathers oil droplets and consumes them.

It is hardly surprising that a person exposed at his place of work to high concentrations of dust and chemical substances, over a long period, runs a greater risk of ill health than other people. Combinations of different substances can also augment the risk of ill health. It is well known that heavy smoking and an excessive alcohol intake greatly increase the general risk level. For example, the probability of lung damage resulting from the inhalation of asbestos fibres is several times greater for smokers than for non-smokers.

The rapid proliferation of chemicals in our environment—thousands of new compounds every year—has placed modern man in a situation analogous to playing Russian roulette. We do not know if the pistol is loaded, or whether a new combination of substances in our environment is harmful. Moreover, it will be a long time before we have any answers: latency periods for exposure to weak toxins may be a matter of decades, and the person affected may have changed his environment so many times that it is impossible to trace the origin of his injury. Nor is an effect always specific to a particular substance. All we can do is to try and follow the old maxim "Better safe than sorry"—reducing the discharge of chemicals into our environment in every conceivable way. At the same time, we can attempt to cut down poison risks under our control, namely tobacco and alcohol. An epidemiologist at the University of California has pointed out that a person would need to spend a full year in the smog of Los Angeles to absorb the same quantity of carcinogens as a heavy smoker receives in a single day!

Right: *The feeding cell, a white blood cell, in the process of ingesting oil droplets that have entered the lungs with inhaled air.*

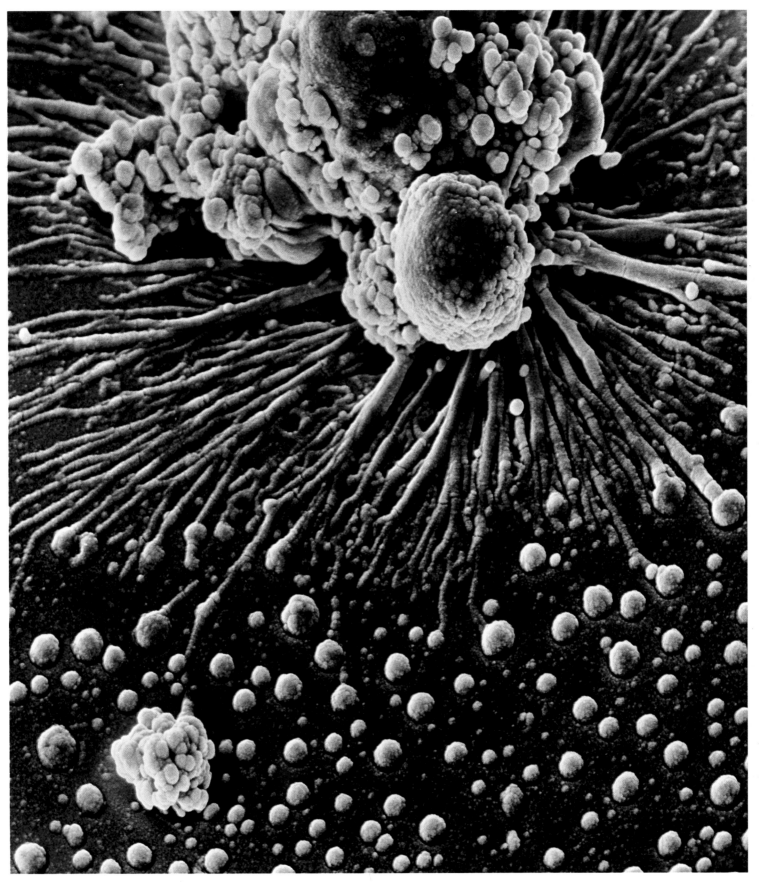

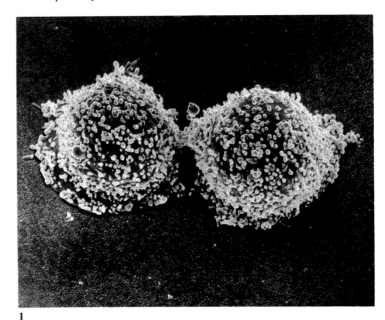

1

Macrophage activity

The immune system has at its disposal several kinds of cells that break down and ingest foreign substances in the body. Their generic name is phagocytes, which means feeding cells. There are three types of "small feeding cells" (microphages), all being varieties of granulocyte (granula = grain), which kill by spreading their grains over an enemy. Or they can simply—with speed and efficiency—swallow bacteria, for example, which have entered a skin wound.

There are two kinds of "large feeding cells," macrophages and the related monocytes. *Left,* a macrophage in the final phase of division stands at the ready. Macrophages are prepared to strike as soon as they apprehend the "scent" of an enemy. The scent consists of substances excreted by bacteria and damaged cells.

When the macrophages are in pursuit of foreign particles and organisms, nothing stands in their way—they can pass straight through tissues, squeeze through the intercellular spaces, and penetrate one layer of the body after another. Their fighting spirit is enhanced by the appetising antibodies that have bound to, and marked out, the enemy.

2

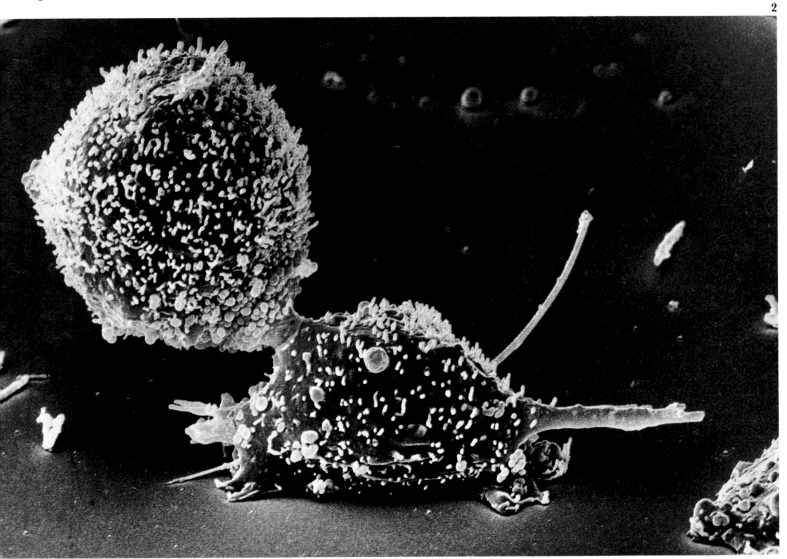

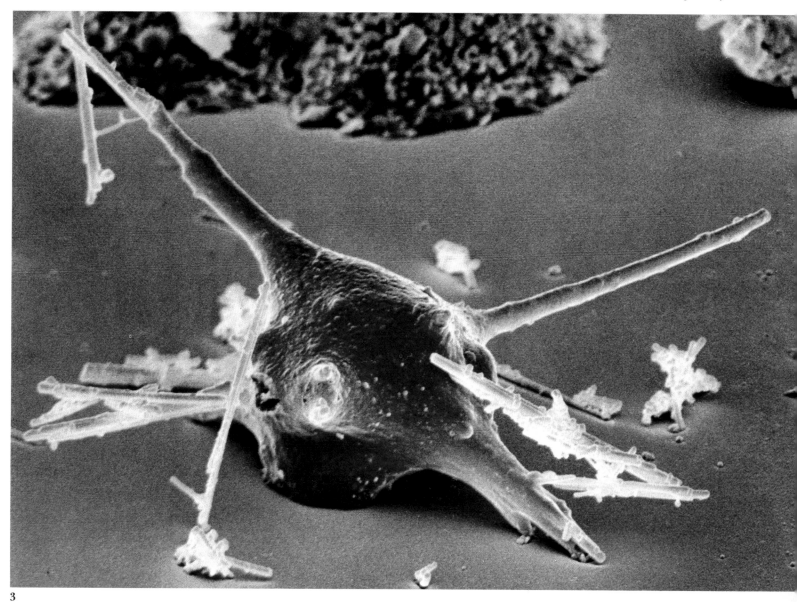

3

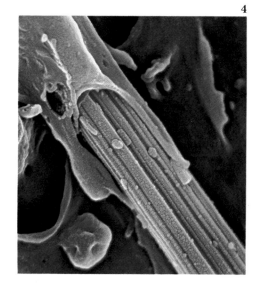

4

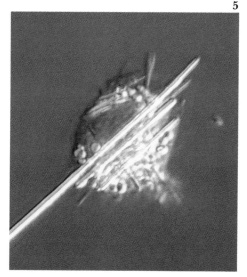

5

1. *A macrophage in the final phase of division.*
2. *Although the macrophage in the picture has ingested asbestos fibres, it can still divide. Here, we see the final stage of division: one daughter cell contains all the fibres.*
3. *However, it is no use: the asbestos does not break down, and the macrophage is defeated. Finally, the fibres are enclosed in the tissue, forming a lump.*
4. *Detail, showing how the macrophage's cell membrane (top left) surrounds the fibre. Asbestos fibres come from building materials and vehicle brake linings.*
5. *A macrophage riddled with holes from asbestos fibres, under a microscope.*

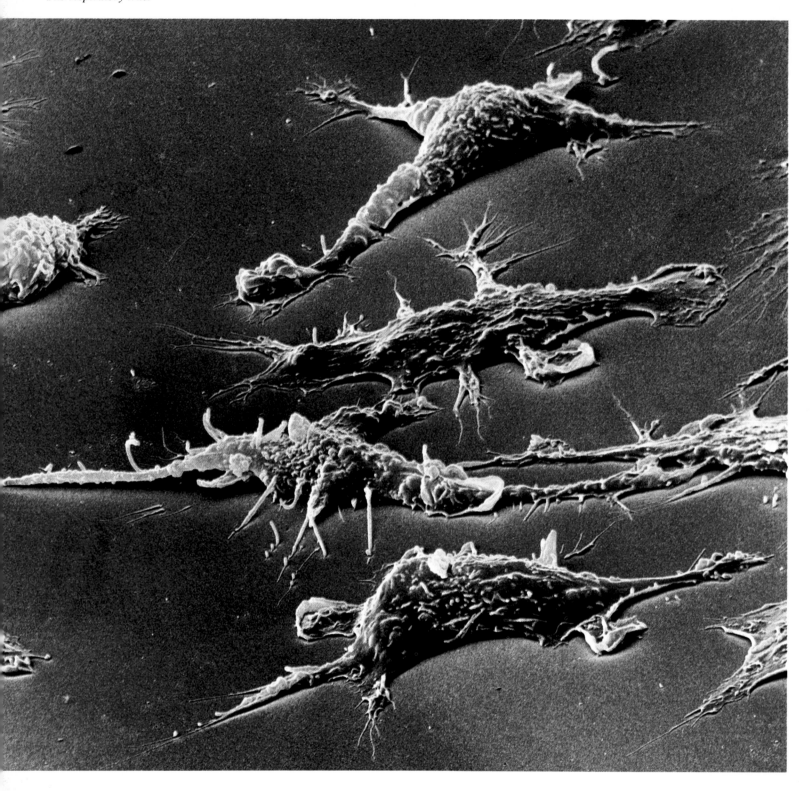

Like prehistoric animals lying in wait for the enemy

Here, like a group of dinosaurs from millions of years past, lie the strongest defenders of the immune system—macrophages. They can take numerous shapes, and here they may be seen under the electron microscope, floating on the base of a glass dish. When a macrophage encounters an enemy, it tries to float around it and in this way swallow it.

Right, *a macrophage with problems: it is trying to ingest a stone flake considerably larger than itself.*

130

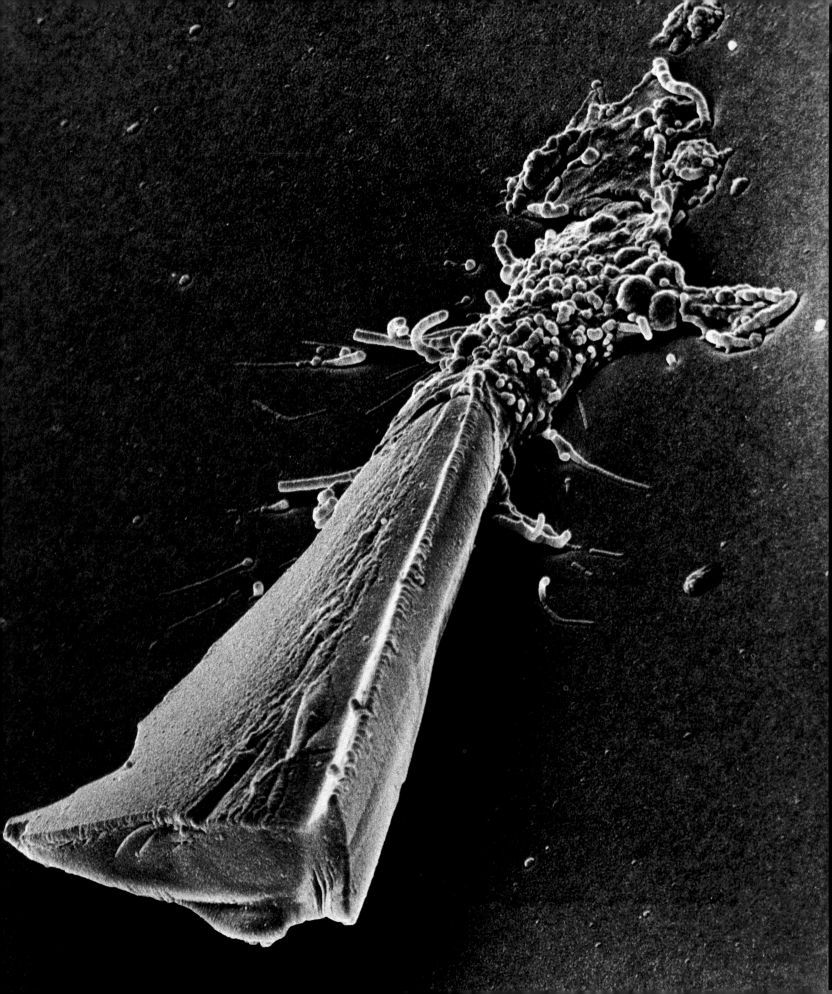

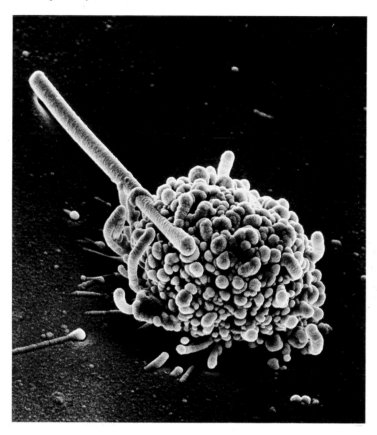

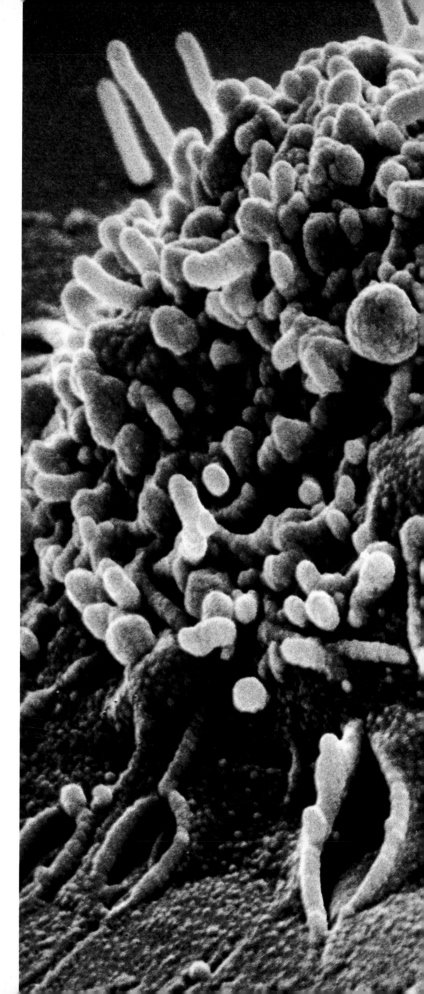

Armoured tanks of the immune system

Macrophages move more slowly than granulocytes but, on the other hand, are tougher and can handle larger prey. They are the armoured tanks of the immune system. Here, in both pictures, they are in the process of enclosing microscopic glass fibres, which are also indigestible and can only be captured and transported away. The macrophages move by means of their "false feet," pseudopodia, which are shown clearly in the picture *above*.

Feeding cells are—in terms of the history of its development—among the oldest parts of the immune system. Much farther down the chain of development, they may be found even in worms, in the tissues surrounding the intestine. Born in the bone marrow, macrophages are sent to serve in tissues of all kinds. The majority circulate with the blood, but some are stationary, for example, beneath the skin where, linked by their thread-like outgrowths, they form a fine net barrier against invading micro-organisms.

When the macrophage attacks a bacterium, a concave hollow forms in its wall. Surrounding the bacterium, it closes the "door"—and starts showering it with strong enzymes and hydrogen peroxide. The bacterium dies and disintegrates into its simple components. The macrophage takes up what it can use in its own metabolism; the remainder is cast out of the body.

However, the macrophage's task is not limited to dealing with foreign organisms and material: it is the body's refuse disposal worker. The macrophage cleaning patrols see to the disposal of damaged and dead cells in an infected wound, veteran red blood cells, and other such debris.

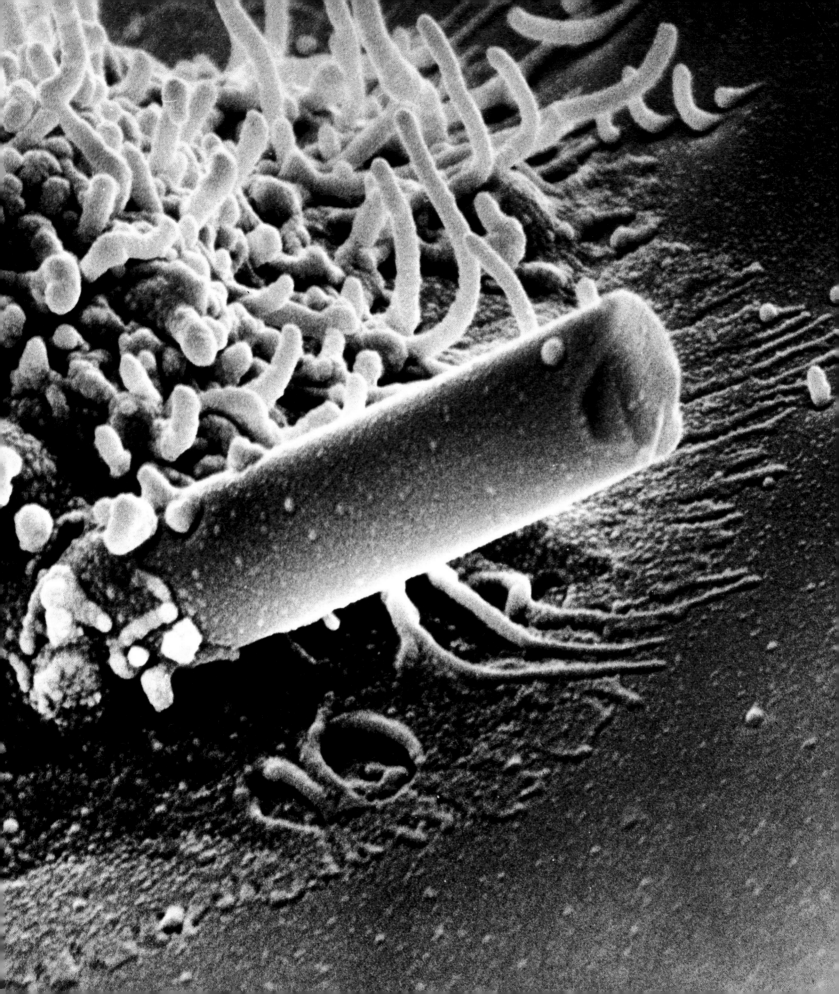

Cigarettes—a modern pestilence

For most of his long history, man was a nonsmoker. One may lament the fact that he did not remain so. In the sixteenth century, the Spanish *conquistadores* returned from the New World, bringing with them among other things the Indian invention of burning the leaves of the tobacco plant in a pipe and inhaling the smoke. However, it was not until the habit of rolling shredded tobacco in paper came into general use, at the end of the nineteenth century, that smoking became a widespread addiction. It became very popular in the era of World War I, and a few decades later, in the 1950s, ill-health statistics reflected the consequences of cigarette smoking in the form of a rapid rise in lung cancer frequency.

Ongoing research shows that cigarette smoking has deleterious effects on a number of different bodily organs—in addition to the lungs and respiratory tract, it also damages the heart and blood vessels, (digestive tract), liver, and pancreas. Moreover, it is evident that not only the smoker himself but also those in his surroundings run the risk of injury from "passive smoking." The children in the picture *below,* traveling in a car with both parents smoking, are thus in the danger zone.

It takes a long time for the harmful effects of smoking to be revealed—apart from the acute nausea an unaccustomed smoker suffers when he smokes too much. Nor do all smokers suffer symptoms. This may be explained by, for example, the size of the "dose," hereditary factors, enzymes such as AHH, the method of smoking, and so on. Combinations of smoking with other toxins, such as air pollutants and alcohol, may play a part.

Now that we are aware of the risks of smoking, one may ask why anyone ever starts—and, above all, continues—to smoke. The initial experience with tobacco is generally unpleasant, but peer group pressure, curiosity, and the desire to appear grown-up push youngsters the other way. As the body gradually learns to tolerate the toxins entering it, ill-effects decrease, and after a while the cells become accustomed to functioning with nicotine and other substances present. A physical need arises in addition to the psychological one. One gets stuck in a rut—and it is extremely difficult to get out. There are people who refuse to give up cigarettes although they have had to have a leg, or even both legs, amputated as a result of vascular damage and consequent gangrene caused, or exacerbated, by cigarette smoking.

Over 2,000 different substances in tobacco

What, then, makes cigarette smoke so hazardous?

There are more than two thousand chemically distinct substances in tobacco, many of which become harmful to living cells when they are burnt—and some of which become carcinogenic. In addition to particles, smoke also contains dangerous gases in concentrations hundreds of times higher than those permitted at workplaces. Depending on his method of consumption, the smoker's intake includes a greater or smaller proportion of the substances released in the cigarette embers, where the temperature is between 600 and 700°C (over 1000° Fahrenheit). It is, of course, smokers who inhale who receive the largest proportion.

The biological effects of most of the constituents of smoke are unknown, but certain substances have been studied in detail.

• *Nicotine* is a nerve poison that in a high dose (fifty-thousandths of a gram or more) can kill an adult. A cigarette contains between one half to two-thousandths of a gram of nicotine, of which up to 90 percent enters the smoker's lungs if he inhales. From there, the blood disperses it in the body. Nicotine has a constricting

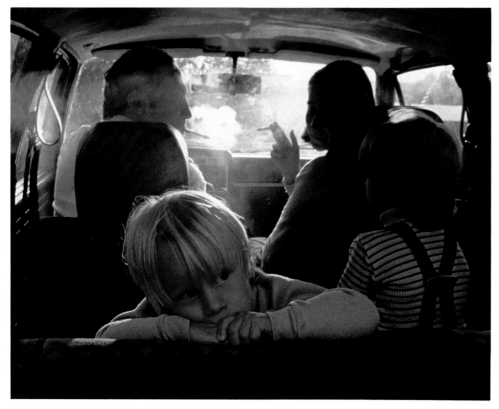

Here, the parents are smoking in their car. The air they exhale contains billions of particles. The children in the backseat cannot help becoming passive smokers, inhaling nicotine and carcinogenic substances, as well as small doses of carbon monoxide, which reduces the blood's ability to absorb oxygen.

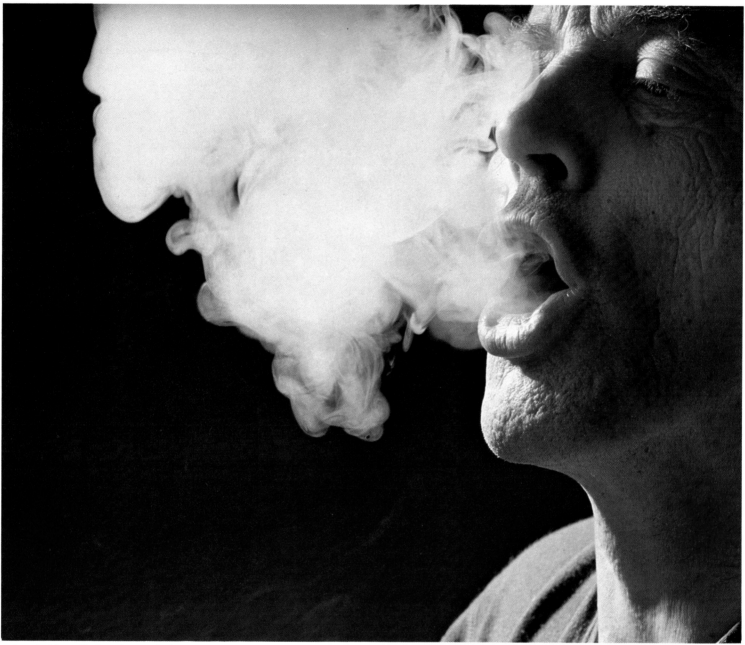

Though this puff of smoke may look innocuous, it contains around two thousand different substances, many hazardous to health.

effect on the blood vessels, increases adrenaline secretion from the adrenal (suprarenal) glands, accelerates the heartbeat, and stimulates the brain and nervous system. If a person's blood vessels are calcified and narrow already, the extra constriction produced by nicotine may well be serious; sometimes it is fatal. Blood flow deteriorates, and if the coronary vessels of the heart are affected, a heart attack may result.

It is above all the nicotine that is habit-forming: nicotine provides the "kick," while tar constitutes the taste.

• *Carbon monoxide* outrivals oxygen in the red blood cells, since it binds to their hemoglobin about one hundred times more easily, thereby depriving the body cells of large quantities of oxygen.

• *Acreolin* and *nitric oxide* attack the cilia of the respiratory tract,

in time creating large bare patches and as a result inpairing the mucus-transport capacity. Eventually, chronic bronchitis is a further complication.

• *Benzopyrene,* a hydrocarbon, is one of the many carcinogenic substances in tobacco smoke. Like soot particles and other substances, benzopyrene is one of the ingredients of tar, which collects on the air passage walls and can start processes culminating in lung cancer.

Intensive information campaigns about the harmful effects of smoking have led to decreased consumption in large parts of the world. The smoker who kicks the habit, even after fifteen or twenty years, can fairly quickly return to the same risk level as the nonsmoker.

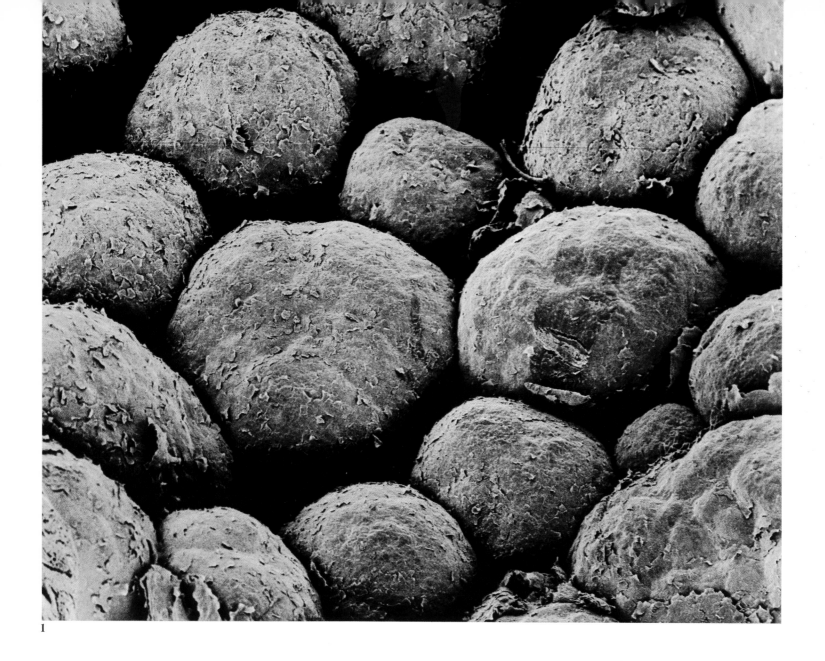

1

Smoking impairs the sense of taste

Every puff on a cigarette fills the mouth with smoke which is then, in most cases, drawn down into the lungs. The concentration of toxic substances is, of course, highest in the mouth, where the membranes are affected. The rounded formations *above* are healthy papillae on a nonsmoker's tongue. Saliva containing flavourings penetrates between the papillae, affecting the taste buds on their sides. *Above right*, we see the corresponding tongue area of a person who has smoked long and heavily. Between the papillae lies tissue which has been deformed by smoke. Heavy smokers frequently lack the senses of both smell and taste, and the scene depicted here suggests the reason why. On the opposite

page *(bottom left)* we see how smoke passes over the surface of the tongue, and *(bottom right)* how a portion of the tip of the tongue has been damaged by long-term smoking. Pipe smoking, tobacco chewing, and snuff taking cause cell changes in the mouth membrane, leading to cancer in some individuals.

1. *Healthy tongue papillae.*
2. *Taste papillae severely damaged by tobacco smoke.*
3. *Inhaled smoke passes over the tongue.*
4. *Tip of the tongue, damaged by long-term smoking.*

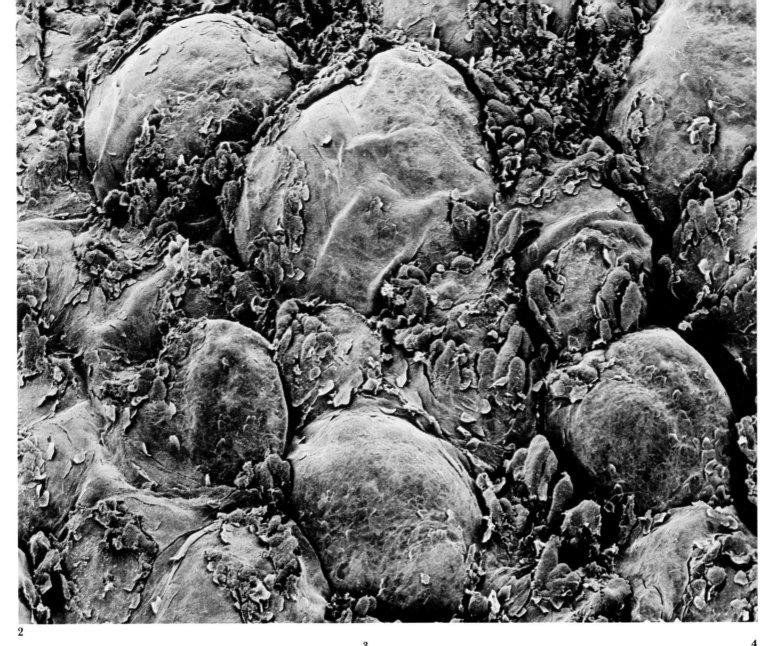

2

3

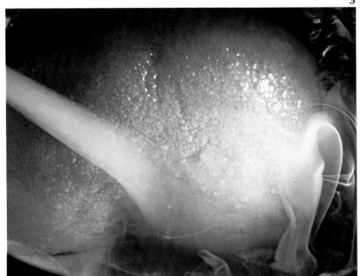

4

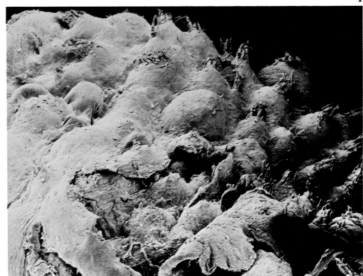

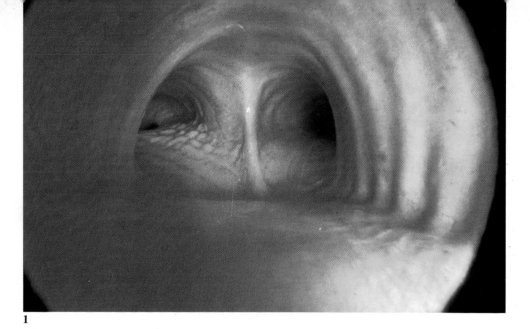

1

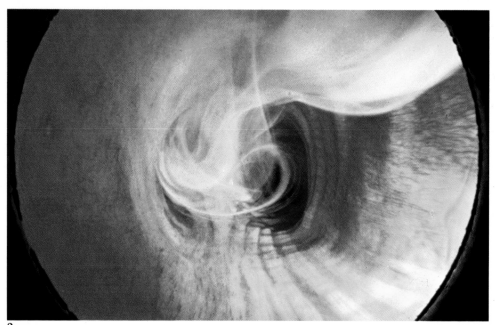

2

3

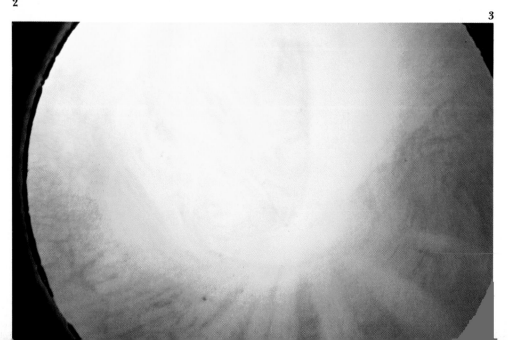

4

Smoke whirls into the lungs

The respiratory tract is shaped so that inhaled air becomes turbulent as it is drawn down into the lungs. This is clearly shown in the series of illustrations, *left*, depicting the smoke's whirling downward motion. The turbulence has two purposes—to warm up the cold inhaled air against the air passage walls, and to throw inhaled particles centrifugally against the sticky membrane. The smoker's respiratory tract walls shown here are covered with a thin layer of tar.

Opposite, the amount of nicotine and tar in the smoke from a single cigarette is shown. The mound of nicotine and tar was produced in what is called a smoke machine. The hot smoke is channeled toward a cold glass slide, on which it condenses. When we smoke, the tar particles are dispersed throughout the lung surface, where feeding cells do their best to remove them. In the lungs of a heavy smoker, the macrophages cannot possibly keep up: the tar is stored in the outermost layer of the lung tissue.

The fact that soot and tar contain carcinogens was discovered as early as the end of the eighteenth century, when the British surgeon Percival Pott described the cancer afflicting chimney sweeps. Localised on the sex organs, it was ascribed to deficient personal hygiene. When chimney sweeps began to wash more thoroughly, their occupational illness disappeared. Confirmation of the carcinogenic properties of tar products came when Japanese researchers, at the beginning of this century, painted mice's ears with tar and thereby experimentally produced cancer. Modern analyses of tobacco smoke show that it contains at least fifteen different carcinogens and, in addition, substances that do not themselves cause cancer but that hasten the cell changes carcinogens produce. Phenols and fatty acids are examples of such substances, which are termed cocarcinogens.

1. *Here, the windpipe divides into the left and right bronchi, leading to the lungs.*
2. *As the smoke is sucked down, it moves in a whirling spiral and particles are flung centrifugally against the air passage walls.*
3. *The smoke now fills the air passages completely.*
4. *With the aid of a smoke machine, as it is called, the nicotine and tar content of a cigarette has been collected on a filter.*

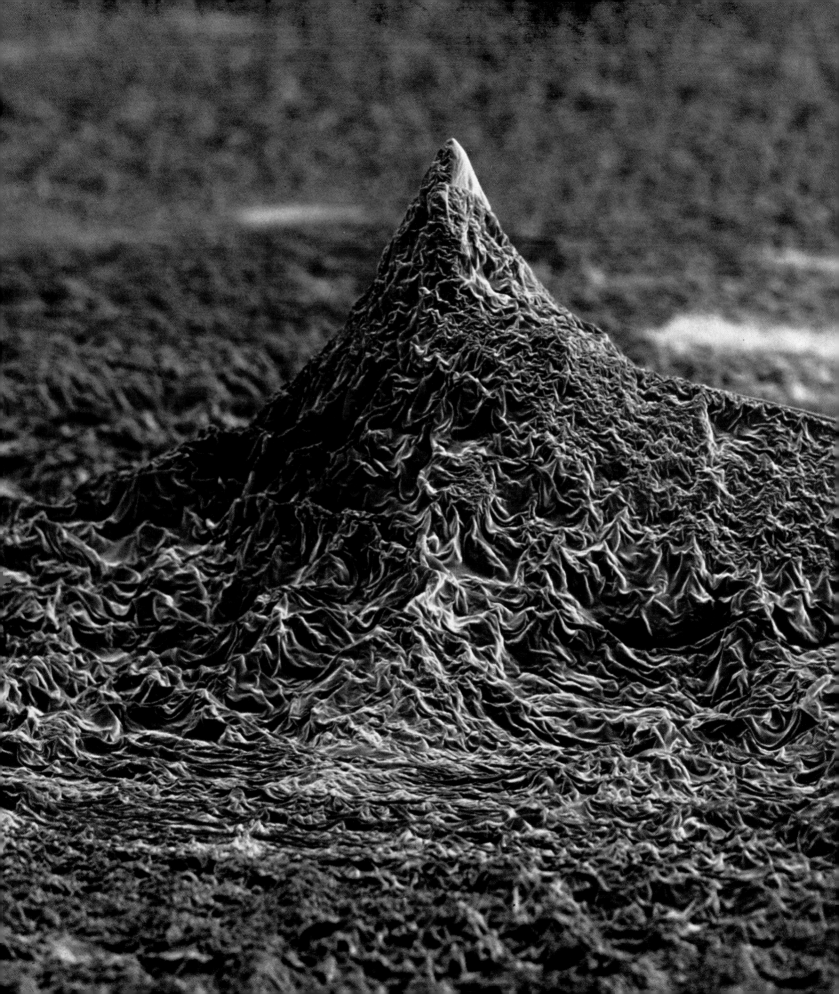

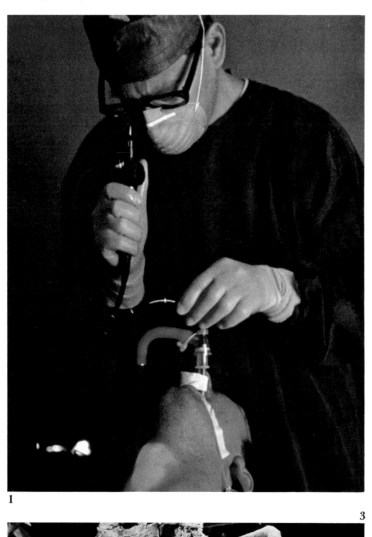

1

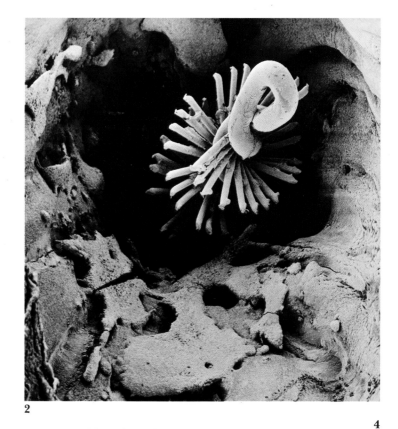

4

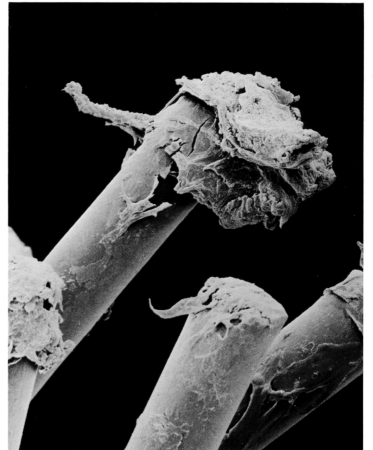

2

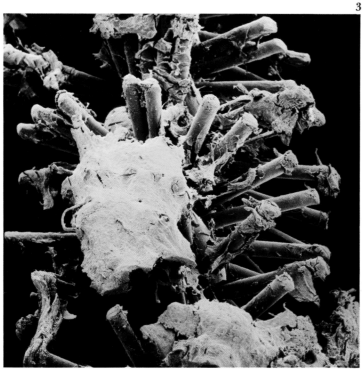

3

Taking lung samples with a brush

Lung cancer is an insidious disease with no warning symptoms. It is often discovered by chance on an X ray, when it may already be in a late stage of development. Unfortunately, lung cancer often metastasises (i.e., forms secondary tumours in other organs) early. Among the symptoms the sufferer may himself observe are changes in his coughing habits. A heavy smoker very often has a smoker's cough, and it is when the cough alters its character in some way that it may be significant: if it is more persistent, or becomes a hacking cough, or starts to wake him up at night, it should be investigated. The reason for the change may be the irritating presence of a bronchial tumour. Coughing is the body's way of expelling from the lung a source of irritation. Streaks of blood in the phlegm are another important sign; they need not imply cancer, but they may, and an investigation should therefore be made. Chronic wheezing and recurrent bronchitis or pneumonia may also be indications of a lung tumour.

The doctor has several methods to choose from in detecting cancerous changes in the lung. One is a microscopic inspection of phlegm coughed up—cytological sputum analysis, as it is termed.

The mucus contains epithelial cells; if any of them have turned into tumour cells, they can quickly be detected with the aid of the microscope. This method establishes the presence of malignant bronchial cancer in no less than 90 percent of cases.

Bronchoscopy—see photographs, *left*—is an important supplement to lung X rays. The instrument consists of a pliable glass fibre rod, with a light at the lower end. It is inserted through the trachea and bronchi, where it is manoeuvred in such a way as to enable the walls of the trachea to be scrutinised. This is made possible by the unique refractive ability of glass fibre. At the lower end of the rod, there is either an instrument with which the doctor can extract a tiny tissue sample for closer inspection or a minuscule brush which can collect samples from the membrane far down in the smaller bronchi.

The pictures to the *left* show how a brush of this kind is used. Under what is called an intubation anesthetic, the bronchoscope is inserted into the patient's trachea. The anesthetic is necessary to block the coughing reaction. Membrane samples are then extracted, by means of the brush, for analysis and cell culture.

1. *Under what is called an intubation anesthetic, the bronchoscope is inserted into the patient's trachea.*

2. *The brush, only a few millimetres wide, in a bronchus. To the left and beneath the brush, we see cancerous lumps in the bronchus wall. The tissue on the right is healthy.*

3. *Mucous membrane samples on the brush.*

4. *Cell samples at the ends of the brush strands.*

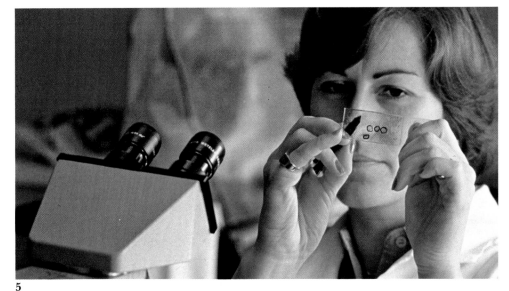

5

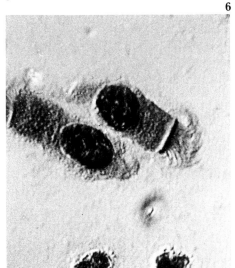

6

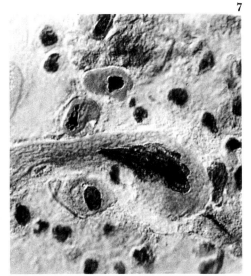

7

5. *Cell investigation by means of a microscope. Another kind of instrument is used to detect chromosome changes in the cell, if any.*

6. *Healthy cell under a microscope. The cell nuclei are the dark oval shapes.*

7. *Cells from advanced lung cancer. The diseased cells are deformed and swollen.*

In three decades, lung cancer has advanced from a fairly modest place in the cancer stakes to become the most common form of cancer among men in the United States and the British Isles. The increase is also steep in other Western countries. All surveys point to a clear connection between cigarette smoking and the sharp increase in lung cancer frequency. The incidence of lung cancer is rising among women, as their smoking habits increase.

Below left, the clean and unblemished lungs of a newborn child (*1*) and, below them, the lung of a person who has smoked a great deal over a long period (*2*). Patches of his lungs are entirely black from tar deposits. To the *right,* the picture shows lung emphysema (*3*), one of the lung diseases that smoking can provoke. It is characterised by extension of the air sacs (alveoli) as a result of inflammations and chronic bronchitis. The tissue changes, abundant mucus is secreted, and breathing is impaired in the diseased area.

Opposite, top, the photograph shows a malignant lung tumour

(*4*) taken under the electron microscope. The tumour cells (to the right of the picture) appear as a result of long-term (often lasting two or three decades) irritation of epithelial cells on the topmost layer. The tumour develops from cells that were originally normal but whose genes have been damaged by carcinogenic substances in tobacco smoke. The metamorphosis into tumor cells means that they are freed from all control, their growth is unchecked, and they infiltrate surrounding tissue. Cells from the tumour can, by various routes, move to the brain, bones, liver, and other organs, where they can develop into metastases. Abnormal cell changes resulting from smoking may spontaneously reverse themselves if the irritation, that is, the smoking, stops in time.

Below left, in the right-hand part of the picture, we see a spherical malignant lung tumour and, in the left of the picture, the normal, ciliated respiratory membrane (*5*). *Right,* tumour tissue as it appears through the bronchoscope (*6*).

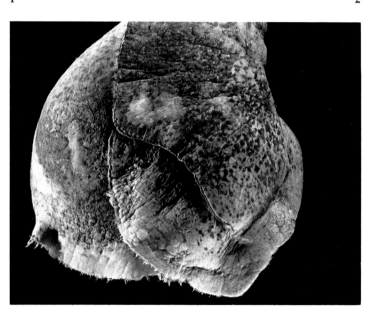

1

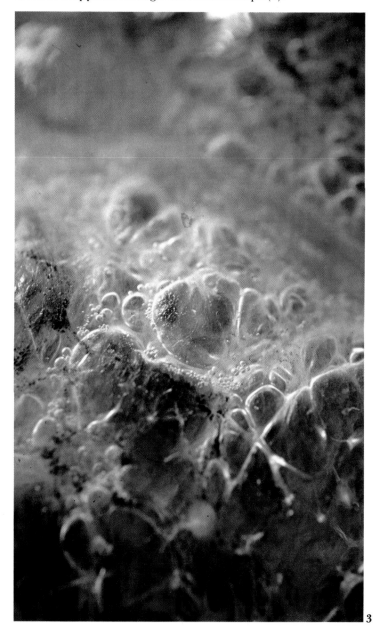

2

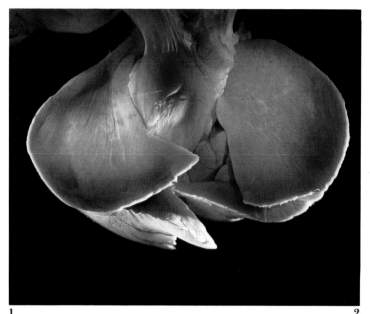

3

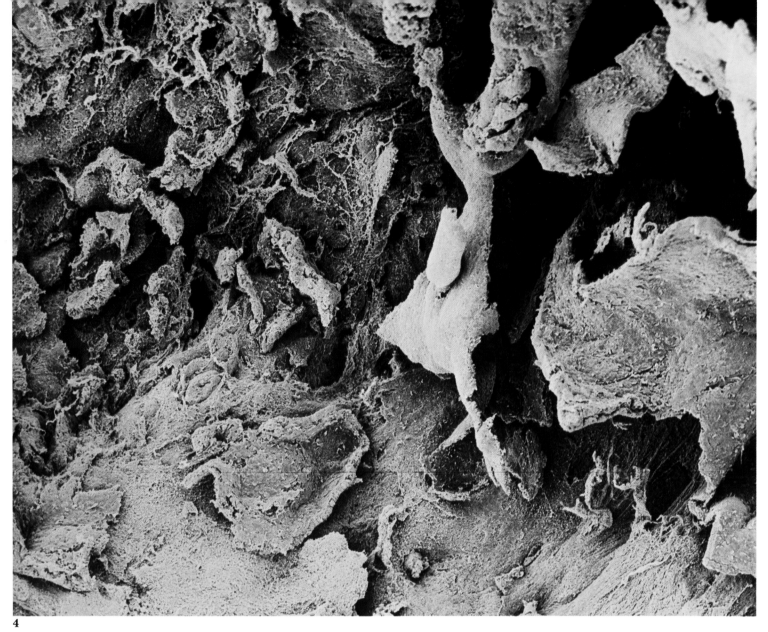

4

5

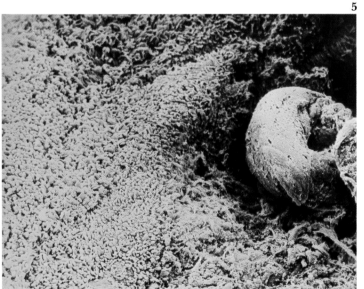

6

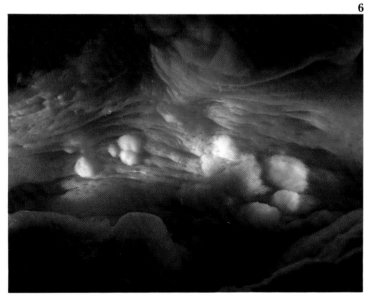

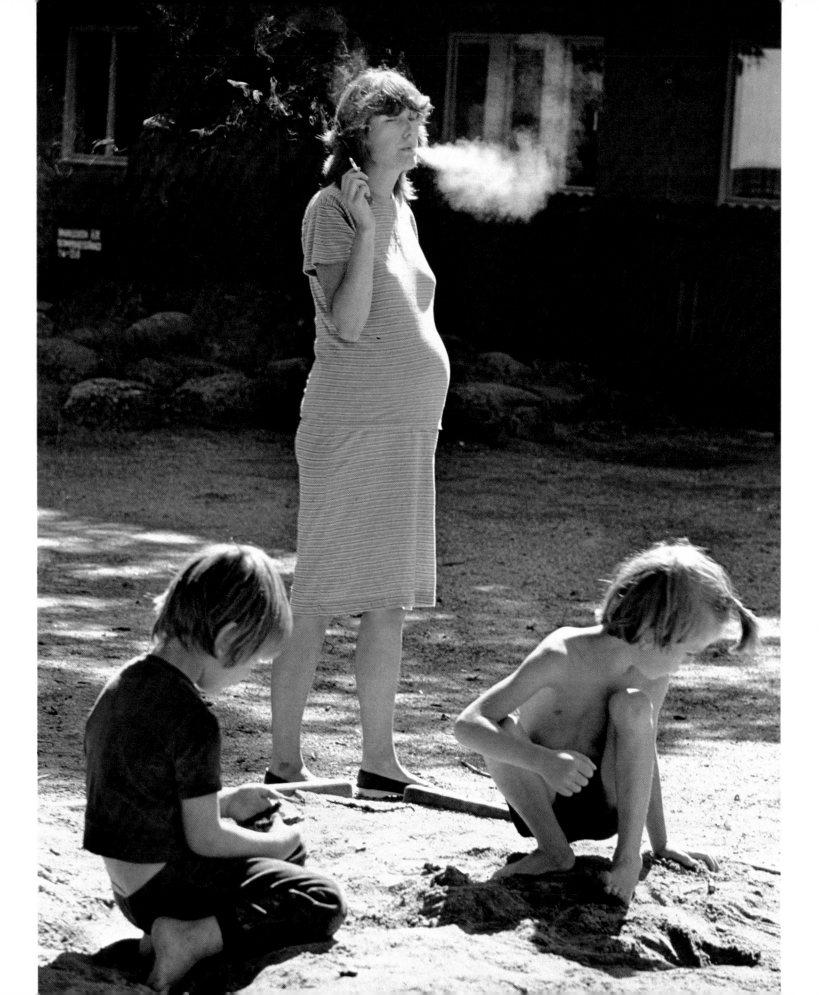

Fetal risk

The growing fetus is, in theory, well protected behind the placenta. Its filter constitutes a barrier which bacteria and the larger viruses and molecules are unable to penetrate. Unfortunately, the protection it affords against chemicals is less effective. If the mother drinks alcohol or smokes, the fetus becomes an involuntary consumer of alcohol and tobacco. Children of women who imbibe excessive quantities of alcohol during pregnancy show various signs of damage, from slight deformities to serious retardation.

The effects of smoking on the fetus are not known in detail, except for one: low birth weight. The children of women who smoke weigh less than the children of nonsmokers. A high proportion of babies with a birth weight of less than 2.5 kilograms (5.5 pounds) have mothers who smoked during pregnancy.

The fourth month of pregnancy constitutes a turning point: mothers-to-be who stop smoking before the fourth month usually give birth to babies whose weight is normal. It is smoking after this time that inhibits fetal growth. According to researchers, the probable cause is insufficient oxygen. As shown in the picture *below*, maternal smoking damages the blood vessels of the umbilical cord. (The umbilical cord in a nonsmoker is on the *left*, and in a smoker, *right*.) The blood vessels of the placenta are also damaged. Once the child is born and breast-feeding is under way, it may absorb nicotine in the mother's milk (if she smokes more than twenty cigarettes a day). The symptoms are vomiting, diarrhea, palpitations, and pallor. Children of mothers who smoke heavily are also affected three times as often as the children of nonsmokers by catarrh and pneumonia severe enough to require hospitalisation.

1. *Smoking in this late stage of pregnancy can damage the fetus.*
2. *Blood vessels of the umbilical cord are affected by smoking.*
3. *Healthy, intact surface cells of blood vessels in the umbilical cord.*
4. *Cells in the same vessels deformed by smoking.*

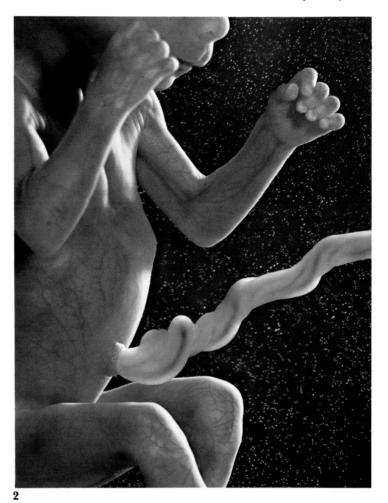

2

3

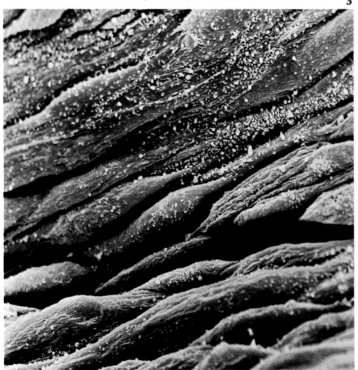

4

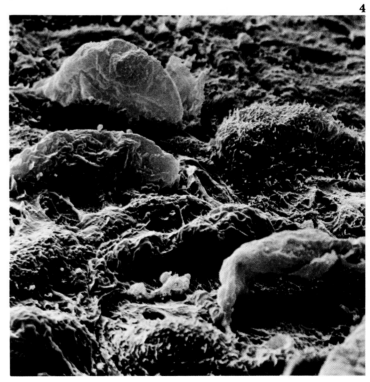

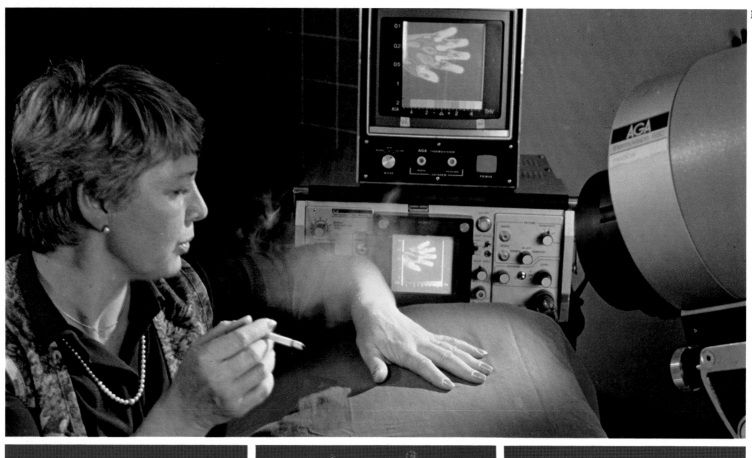

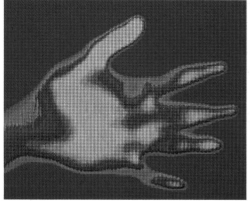

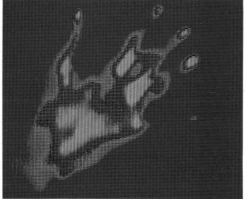

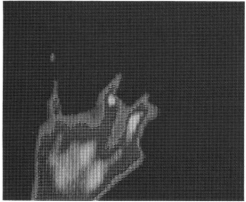

2   3   4

Nicotine strangles the blood vessels

It is above all nicotine that the smoker seeks, that gives him the "kick" he or she wants—the stimulus to the brain and nervous system, the increased alertness. But that is not all nicotine does. Via the autonomic nervous system, it affects the muscles of the blood vessel walls, so that they become constricted. In extreme cases this has dire results, as shown in the pictures *opposite*.

Above, a thermographic (heat) camera clearly registers the blood circulation in the hand during smoking **(1).** The camera renders temperature differences visible, by recording heat radiation. With the aid of electronics, it converts different temperature ranges into colours in a scale from white (warmest) to dark blue (coolest). Heat radiation thus provides the picture of the hand on the screen above. The camera (on the right in the picture) registers the radiation from the woman's hand at the moment she starts smoking. The circulation of blood is even, and the camera shows the warm hand as largely white.

The pictures *above* show what happens, particularly in the blood vessels of the fingers, during the smoking of a single cigarette. *Left (2),* the photograph shows the normal temperature distribution. In the *middle (3),* we see how the fingers almost vanish after three puffs on the cigarette: heat radiation falls by more than two degrees! *Right (4):* after several puffs, the hand's blood vessels are strangulated and the fingers are "gone."

The constricting effect of nicotine may be devastating when it coincides with factors leading to atherosclerosis. This disease begins with the depositing of fatty acids on the walls of blood vessels, which makes them narrower and impedes blood flow. At a later stage—true atherosclerosis—the fat deposits harden, the blood vessels become stiff, and the slow circulation of blood makes clots liable to form.

Atherosclerosis and blood clots are most serious when they affect the vessels of the heart and brain. Heart attack and stroke kill—or make a person an invalid. If the disease develops in the lower extremities, blood clots can lead to gangrene, necessitating amputations.

Smoking is what makes the blood vessels become constricted. Just as smoking has become more common among women in recent decades, so the frequency of atherosclerosis in the legs has increased among women.

One early sign of atherosclerosis in the legs is painful cramps in the calf muscles while walking. The sufferer stops frequently to alleviate the pain of this "window-shopping disease." Smokers do well to stop smoking when the disease has progressed this far. In severe cases, as for the woman to the *right (5),* it may reach a stage where amputation is necessary.

Bottom, three stages in blood vessel calcification are shown: *far left (6),* a cross-section of a healthy vein with its different muscular layers; *middle (7),* cholesterol deposits have reduced the space inside the blood vessel, the lumen, by three-quarters; *far right (8),* the vessel is blocked by a clot.

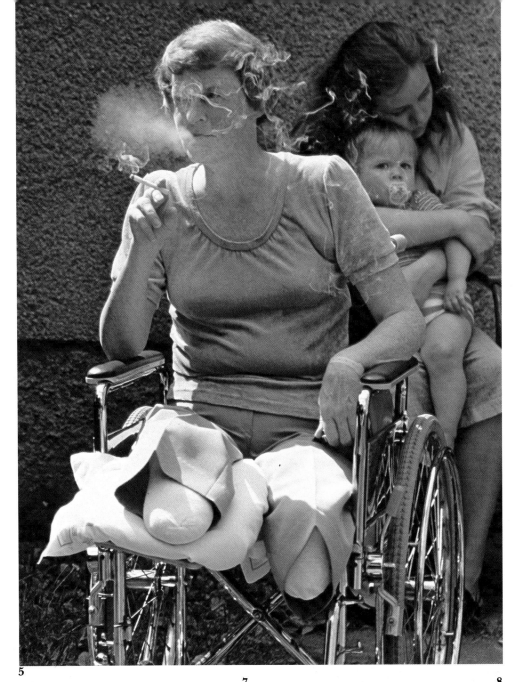

5

6

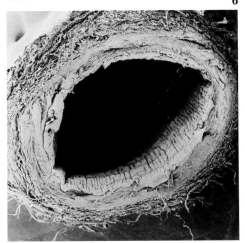

7

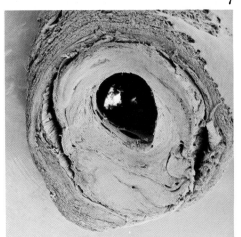

8

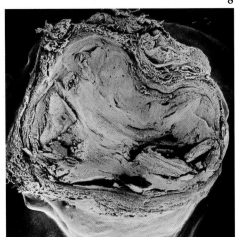

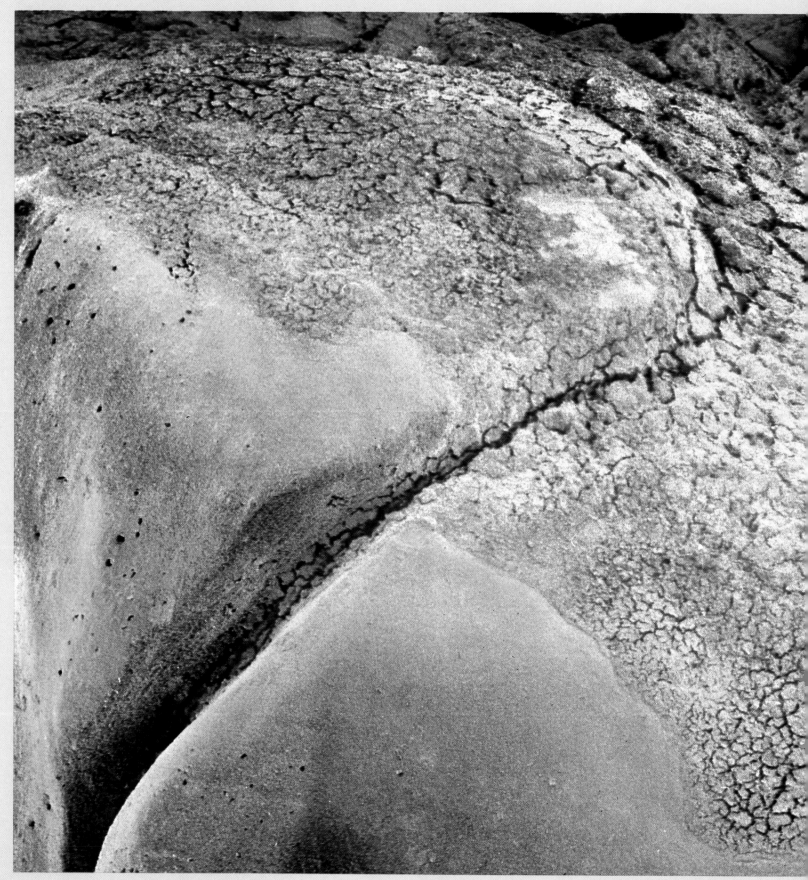

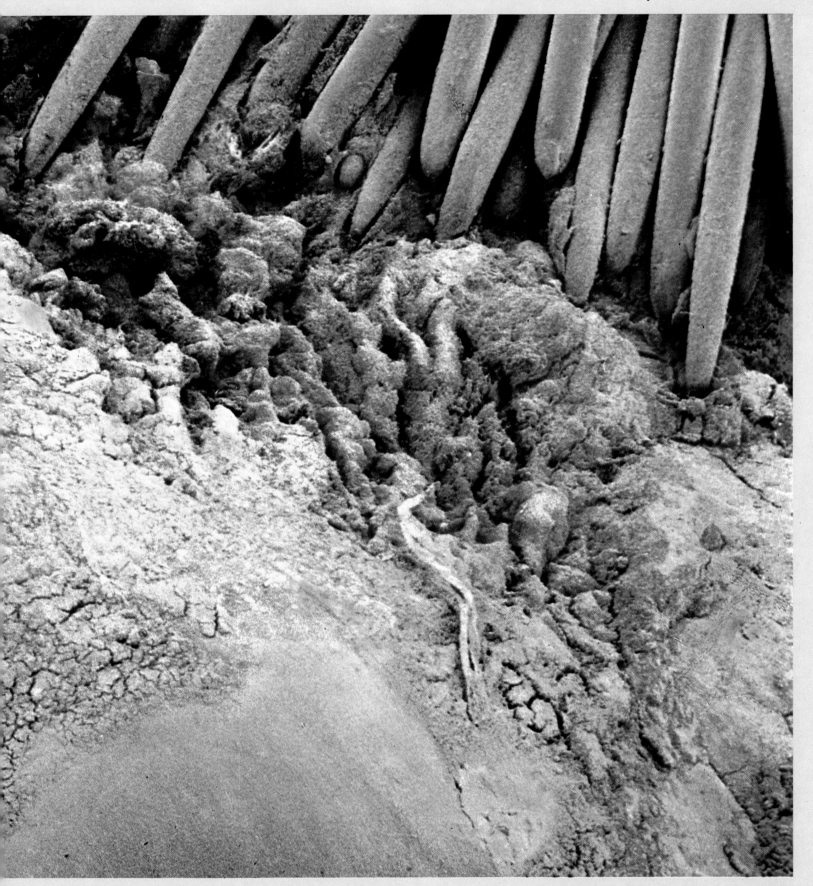

Teeth

The mouth and respiratory passages are the major openings in the body's defences. They are constantly subject to invasion attempts. Hordes of microbes, millions strong, enter them daily; some are dangerous and cause disease, but most are harmless and do not pose the slightest threat to health.

From a superficial viewpoint, the mouth is the ideal bridgehead for a bacterial attack. The supply of nutrients is abundant, it is warm and moist—in short, it is precisely the kind of environment bacteria like best.

Fortunately for us, this is only one side of the story. *Homo sapiens* could never have evolved if the body's defences had not developed methods of making life difficult for invaders. The salivary glands secrete a constant stream of saliva, which rinses microorganisms from membranes and tooth surfaces. But saliva is not only a mouthwash; it is also rich in antibodies of the IgA (immunoglobulin A) variety. These cause bacteria to clump together and make them more appetising for those white blood cells whose existence is one long hunt: the feeding cells. Incessantly, these inspect the gum tissues and ingest the bacteria they find, destroying them in the process. The feeding cells' work is accomplished faster and more easily if antibodies have latched on to the bacterium. The antibody functions both as tracer and as aperitif.

The flow of saliva, moreover, forces us to swallow even when we are not eating, and in the stomach most bacteria are killed by hydrochloric acid in the gastric juice. The mouth membrane has its own means of waging chemical warfare, *lysozyme,* a substance with the ability to break down bacterial cell walls. The teeth, in their turn, are protected by the hardest material in the body, tooth enamel, whose normally smooth surfaces provide an unsatisfactory foothold for bacteria.

The saliva, with its IgA antibodies and rinsing effect, the hard tooth enamel, and the lysozyme in the mouth membrane constitute the basic defences in one of the body's most exposed invasion areas. The investigation of skulls found in graves, many millennia old, show the effectiveness of these defences when man's diet was a suitable one: fine sets of teeth—worn, but free of decay. What is it, then, that has made tooth diseases the most common ailments of all in the civilised world?

The main culprit is *sugar,* industrially manufactured from sugarcane and sugar beet and easily accessible to all major population groups ever since the eighteenth century. Man's taste buds appreciate sweetness: if infants are allowed to choose between plain and sweetened water, most choose the latter. From an evolutionary point of view, this may be explained by the fact that carbohydrates (the group of nutrients to which sugar belongs) are rich in energy and that nature used taste signals to aid *Homo erectus* in selecting an efficient diet. At that time, carbohydrates meant certain fruits and, to some extent, honey.

The bacteria in our mouths also welcome sugar in our dietary intake. One such bacterium, *Streptococcus mutans,* forms an acid when it breaks down sugar molecules; this acid wears holes in the enamel, thereby paving the way for a whole range of bacteria to penetrate the nourishing dentine. This process is called *caries,* or tooth decay.

The process begins when sticky sugars and other carbohydrates adhere to the tooth enamel, forming what is called *plaque,* a yellowish layer containing bacteria in profusion—not only streptococcus, which dissolves enamel, but also other bacteria, spherical, rod-shaped, or spiral in form. If they are left in peace, they penetrate the enamel and dentine, reaching the nervous and vascular tissue (the pulp) and continuing down the root canal to the tip of the root, where an abscess develops. The process may, if unchecked, spread into the jawbone. Caries is never self-healing. The damaged tissue must be removed with a dentist's drill and replaced with fillings of some kind.

A reduction in saliva production makes caries worse. Certain medicines, including the majority of narcotics and other psychopharmacological agents, can after prolonged use lead to a diminution in the salivary glands' output, so that saliva no longer rinses the tooth surfaces.

Today, with our high sugar consumption, we cannot rely on our basic defences to keep the microbes at bay. We must reinforce them with oral hygiene and various measures. The toothbrush came into more general use at the end of the nineteenth century, but it does not counteract the formation of plaque in hard-to-reach places. Toothpicks, dental floss, and special brushes are necessary to remove the deposits from the interdental spaces. Bactericidal mouthwashes are available, and positive experiments have been made with vaccines against the enzyme that forms dental plaque and against *Streptococcus mutans.* Modern immunology is thus fighting caries too.

Seeing the dentist may not be fun, but it is necessary for good dental health. With annual checkups (preferably starting at the age of four or five), correct dietary habits, and good dental hygiene, we can prevent tooth decay (caries) and the gum inflammations that lead to loosening of the teeth (periodontal disease). Eating habits in modern society are hostile to our teeth. A high sugar content in the food, the sucking of lozenges and other sweets between meals, and inadequate brushing of teeth lead to the tooth's surface being covered with a gelatinous layer of carbohydrate-rich substances (glycoproteins) in which bacteria thrive; beneath it, acid develops which corrodes the tooth enamel. Through the patches of decay which eventually form, bacteria can then invade the tooth and attack the dentine. This kind of wound is not self-healing. The dentist's drill must remove diseased tissue, so that it can be filled with, for example, mercury amalgam.

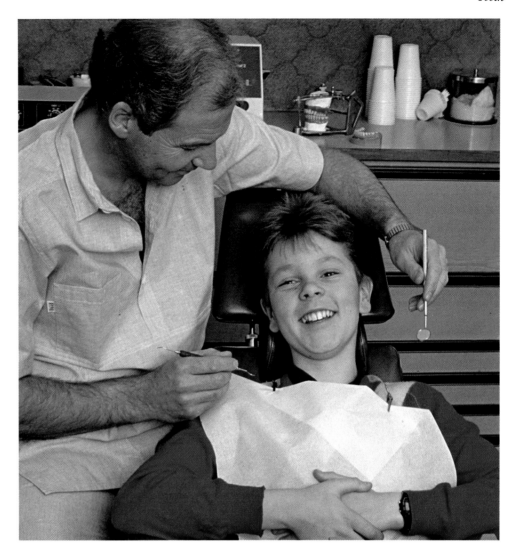

One measure which has stemmed the growing incidence of tooth decay—and even, in some countries, reversed it—is the strengthening of enamel with *fluoride*, a halogen element. "Painting" and rinsing the teeth with strong fluoride solutions, giving fluoride tablets to young children, and adding fluoride to toothpaste all help to harden the enamel layer and counteract caries.

The most serious threat to teeth nowadays is periodontal disease, or inflammation of the gums. Without treatment the teeth loosen and eventually fall out. This disease is, first and foremost, caused by inadequate oral hygiene: the teeth are not being brushed enough, or not in the right way. Plaque forms from food remains and bacteria, and hardens into tartar, or scale. Sheltered by the tartar, plaque bacteria assail the gum, penetrating between it and the neck of a tooth, hollowing out deep cavities in the gum and destroying the threads which connect the tooth with the jawbone. Swollen, bleeding gums and wobbly teeth are symptoms of advanced periodontal disease.

The disease can nonetheless be treated. A surgeon opens the gums and their inflamed cavities, and a dental hygienist scrapes away tartar from the necks of the teeth. The patient then sees to his own oral hygiene, with meticulous brushing, toothpicks, dental floss and small "bottle brushes" to clean the interdental spaces.

Prevention, however, is better than cure. Effective oral hygiene reduces the risk of both caries and periodontal disease. Fluoridisation strengthens the enamel, and vaccination increases the number of antibodies directed against enamel-destroying bacteria. Not least, better nutrition, with less sugar, does much to improve dental health.

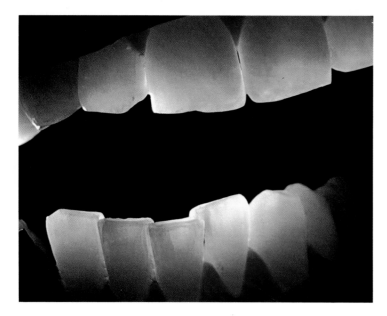

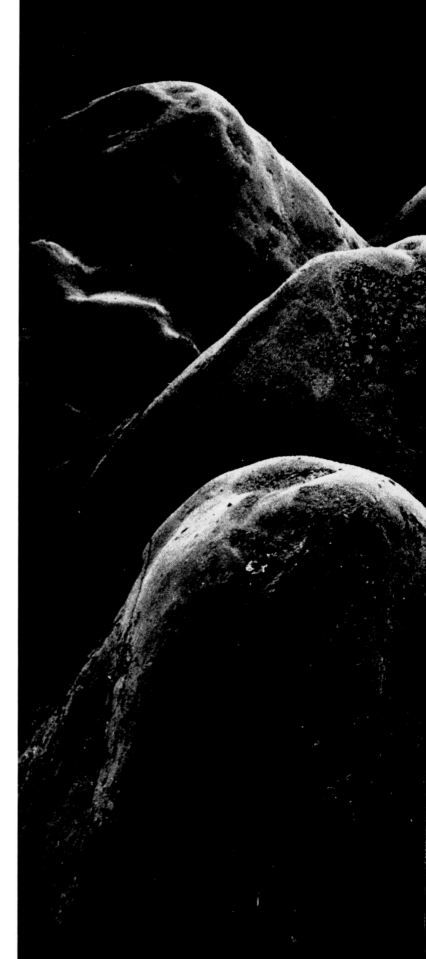

A dental landscape

Above, the chisel-shaped incisors, which cut the food into pieces. The task of the long, pointed canines is to secure a grip, while the premolars and molars *(opposite)* have an uneven surface suited to grinding the food. The purpose of chewing is both to break up the food so that it can pass the pharynx and to mix it with saliva—a preliminary stage in the process by which it is broken down into simple constituents.

The crown of a molar, *right*, magnified about 40 times, resembles a mountain landscape with ridges and valleys. We see how deposits collect in crannies which are hard to reach with a toothbrush. Under the deposits, the enamel is being damaged and in time caries will arise.

During chewing, the molars of the upper and lower jaws function as grindstones; the incisors, as scissors; and the canines, as forks. Breaking up the food mechanically in this way is a prerequisite for continued chemical decomposition in the gastro-intestinal tract, where the food is assailed by a large number of enzymes whose task is to make carbohydrates, proteins, and fats available to the body.

The process food undergoes in the mouth subjects the teeth to both mechanical and chemical stresses. Sand, tiny stones, and other hard material may, for example, accompany poorly rinsed vegetables into the mouth. Since the pressure between the teeth during chewing may be up to 200 kilograms (450 pounds) per square centimetre, a hard object may crack the teeth. Sand has an abrasive effect, scratching the tooth surfaces—something often observed, as we mentioned, in teeth from prehistoric man. When food is mixed with saliva (and the liquid we drink) the pH value of the mouth is altered by the release of certain substances. If the acidity level rises, the enamel is damaged.

However, the body has methods of counteracting these chemical assaults. During a meal, the salivary glands are active. Saliva contains calcium sulphate, which neutralises acids; in addition, it rinses the tooth surfaces. Nonetheless, saliva cannot easily penetrate plaque deposits, and particles of food—in which bacteria thrive—easily collect in the narrow interdental spaces and molar furrows.

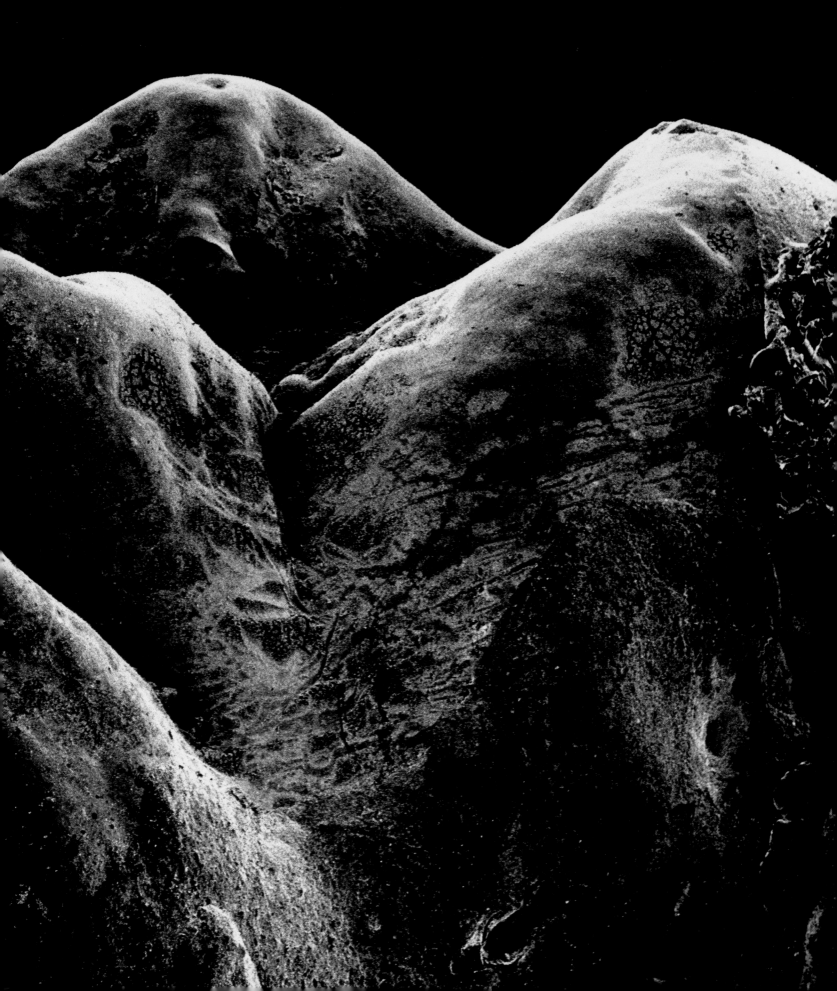

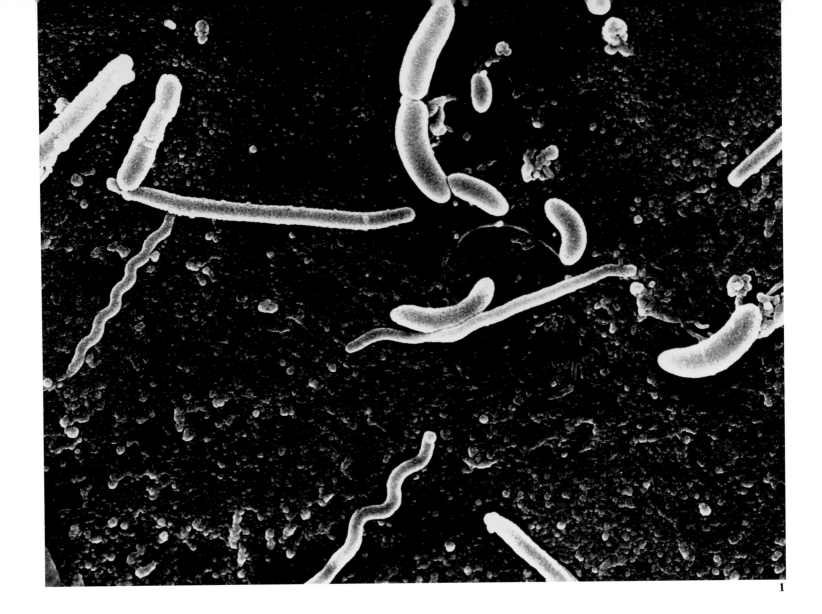

1

Bacterial port of entry

The mouth is a welcoming habitat for bacteria. It is moist, warm, and rich in nutrients. Particularly between the teeth and in the deep molar furrows, deposits of plaque easily accumulate. Plaque is to bacteria what a well-fertilised field is to crops. The points at which gums and teeth meet are another high-risk zone for bacterial invasions, especially when tartar has formed there.

Above, a microscopic snapshot of various bacteria—rod-shaped bacilli, spherical cocci, and spiral spirochetes—in the mouth. The saliva rinsing the tooth surfaces contains large quantities of IgA antibodies targeted on these bacteria, and the acid gastric juice is also lethal to them once they are swallowed.

The Dutchman Antonie van Leeuwenhoek drew the mouth bacteria he saw under his microscope in the mid-17th century: (A) a bacillus, (B) Selenomonas sputigena and the dotted line it makes on the glass slide, (E) cocci, (F) rod-shaped bacteria, and (G) a spirochete. This was the first time in history that bacteria were depicted.

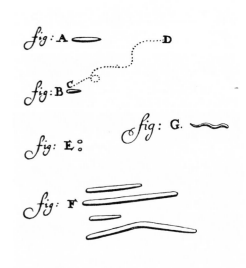

One of the biggest troublemakers in the mouth is the spherical *Streptococcus mutans* bacterium *(right)*. By eating sweets, many of us provide it with the cane sugar (saccharose) it loves, causing it to release substances that form dental plaque. Plaque contains an acid capable of dissolving the body's hardest material, tooth enamel. The attack takes place underneath the plaque, which prevents saliva from reaching the acid and rinsing it away.

The bacterial attack on the tooth enamel is exacerbated by disturbances in saliva production. Numerous medicines, notably the psychoactive drugs, reduce the salivary glands' activity.

Various attempts are being made nowadays to reinforce the body's defences against mouth bacteria. Several of them have proved successful—for example, "painting" the teeth with enamel-strengthening fluoride, adding fluoride to toothpaste, and vaccination against *S. mutans* and its plaque-forming enzyme.

Bottom right, a white blood cell tries to ingest a colony of streptococci in the gum.

1. *Various mouth bacteria. (× 6,000)*
2. *The first depiction of bacteria in history, van Leeuwenhoek's drawing of what he saw under his microscope in the 17th century.*
3. *Primary enemy of the teeth,* Streptococcus mutans. *(× 10,000)*
4. *Colonies of rod-shaped tooth bacteria.*
5. *Bacteria being attacked by a white blood cell.*

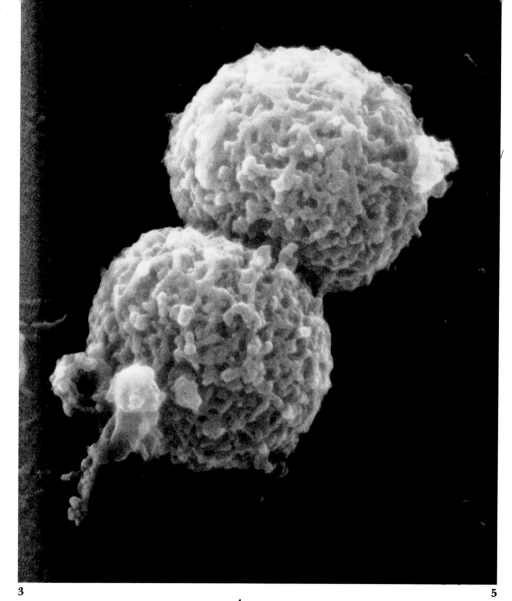

3

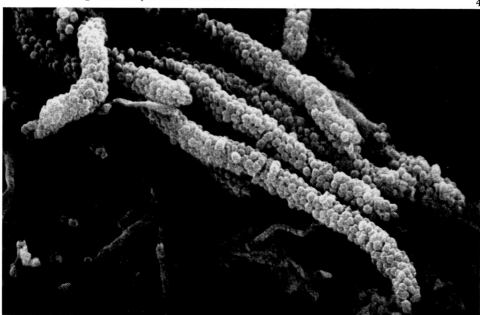

4

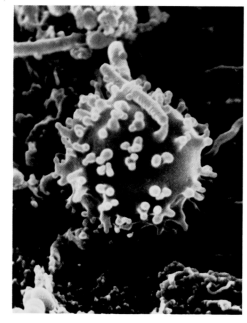

5

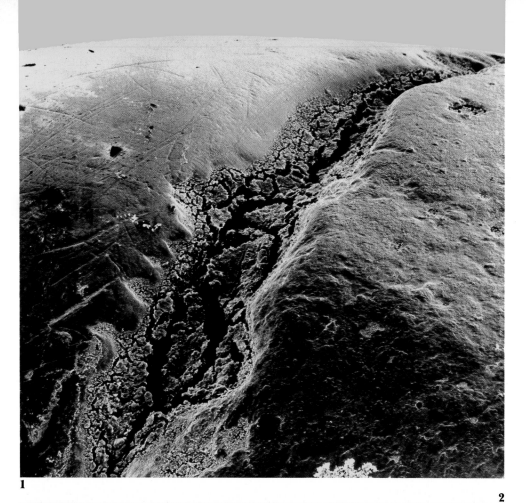

1

Caries

The pictures on these pages show different stages of tooth decay. *Left,* the scratches on the surface of a molar result from sand or other abrasive agents in our food. In the furrow there are traces of plaque, and the enamel around it shows signs of decay.

Below left, acid-forming bacteria have penetrated the enamel. At the bottom of the crater-like hollow, food particles and bacteria collect on top of the plaque, while the attack continues underneath. *Opposite,* the crater has become deeper: now the bacteria can invade the dentine and help themselves to its rich store of minerals. The hole becomes deeper still and the sensory nerves in the pulp—the nervous and vascular tissue in the tooth's central canal—sends disagreeable signals that all is not as it should be.

Caries is an extremely widespread ailment in the West, although its incidence has declined since fluoride treatment of enamel was introduced. Around 90 percent of the population is affected. However, as we stressed earlier, caries can be prevented—by proper eating habits (in particular, the reduction of sugar intake) and by correct care of the teeth, for example, brushing, the use of toothpicks, dental floss, or special brushes, and annual checkups.

When brushing the teeth, it is important to reach into every nook and cranny. The interdental spaces may be cleaned, for example, with floss or a toothpick.

Tartar develops from calcium deposited by the saliva. On its rough surfaces, bacteria and particles of food collect, particularly at the gum line. Bleeding gums and bad breath are often signs that tartar has contributed to the occurrence of periodontal disease, which is also very common, mainly among middle-aged and elderly people. Inflammation loosens the gums from the teeth, and even deeper cavities, in which bacteria thrive, are formed. These destroy the connective threads between teeth and jawbone, causing them to loosen and fall out.

2

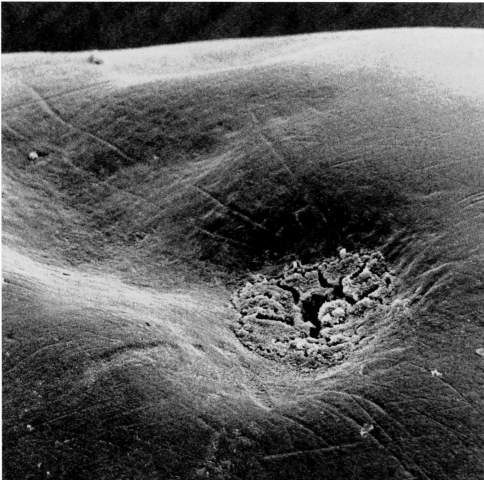

1. *Molar with fine scratches. (× 75)*
2. *Tooth enamel, penetrated by bacteria.*
3. *Once the hard enamel has been broken through, the bacterial invasion can proceed faster and more easily. (× 120)*

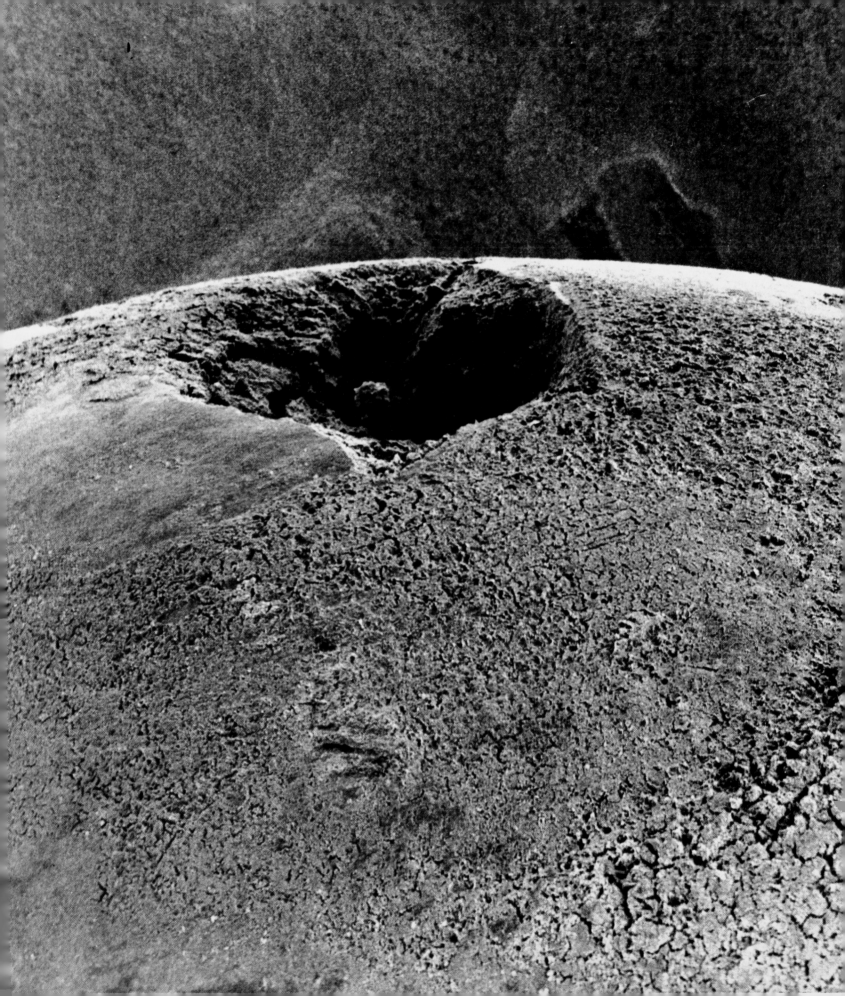

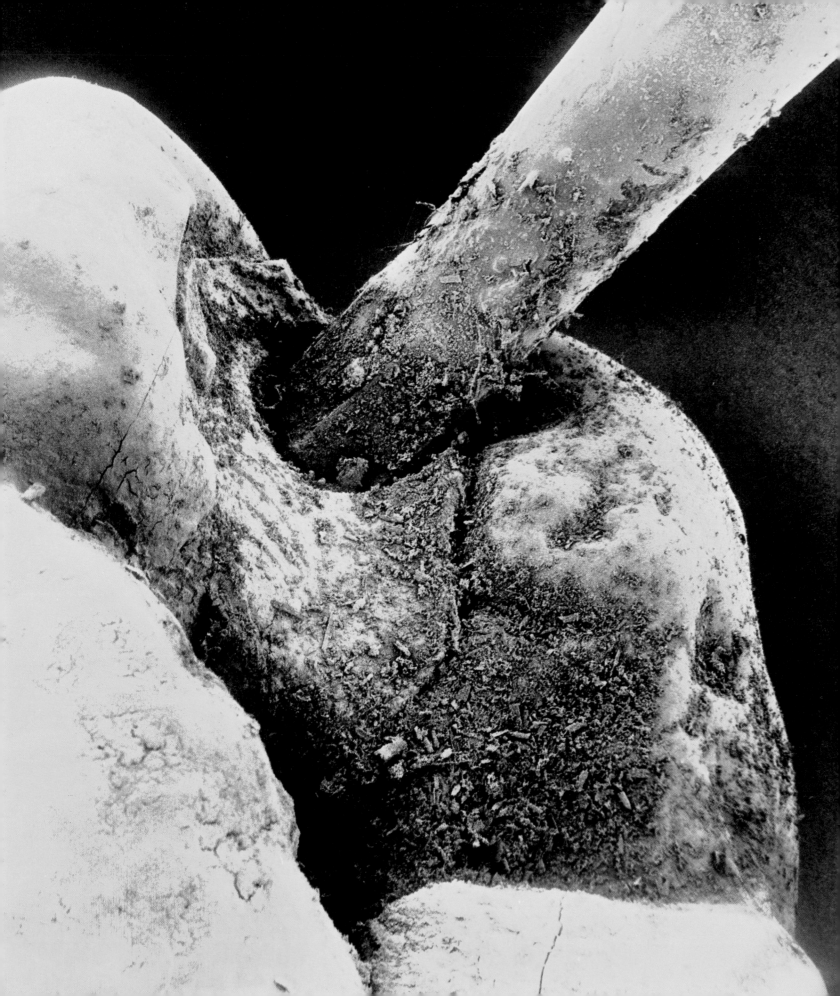

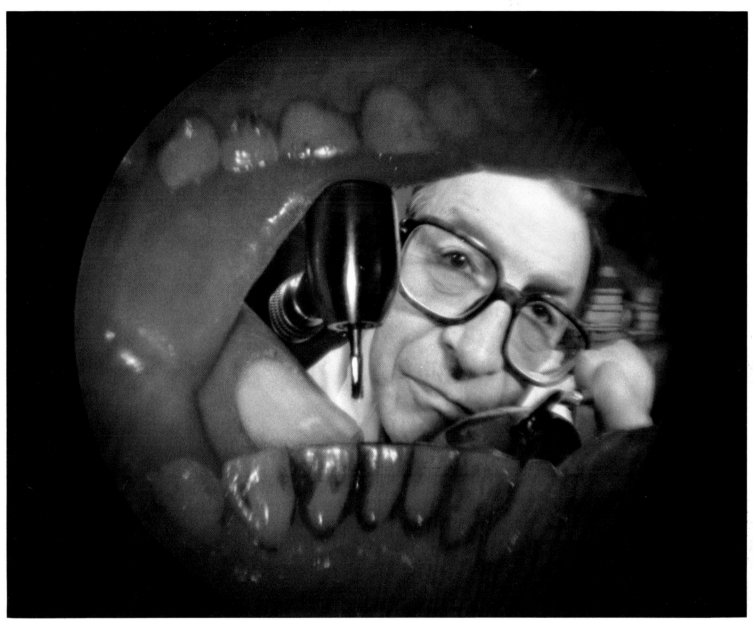

A dentist's drill seen from inside the mouth. Opposite, *magnified 50 times, the drill removes the decayed portions of a molar.*

Fighting caries—at 100,000 rpm

Tooth decay, unlike a skin wound, is not self-healing. It must be treated by a specialist, the dentist, who—with or without an anesthetic—drills away diseased tissue as far as the healthy dentine. The drill is usually water-cooled and turns at a rate of about 100,000 revolutions per minute. *Left,* the drill in a decaying molar; *above,* in an incisor.

If decay reaches the pulp, it becomes inflamed and an abscess forms at the tip of the root. To treat this, the dentist clears the pulp of soft tissue and fills the root canal with some sort of cement. The crown of the tooth is then rebuilt with amalgam or gold. An alternative is a pin tooth, where the crown is supported by a metal pin, or shaft, in the root canal.

If is is a simple case of decay, the cavity is filled with amalgam, which is a mixture of mercury and other metals. The filling hardens fast, and is then polished. Gaps in a row of teeth can be filled with bridging crowns of gold, often sheathed in porcelain.

The dentist or dental hygienist deals with loosening of the teeth by scraping away the tartar from right down in the gum cavities. In cases of advanced periodontal disease, the loose, inflamed gum line is cut away, which facilitates continued cleaning. If the teeth cannot be saved, removable false teeth are no longer the only alternative. One new method anchors false teeth by means of titanium screws in the jawbone.

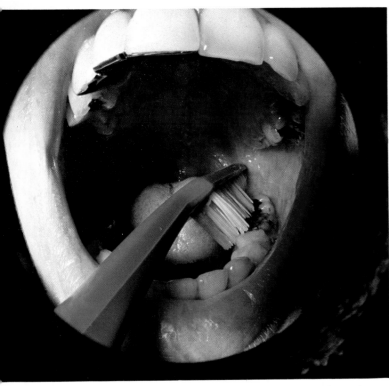

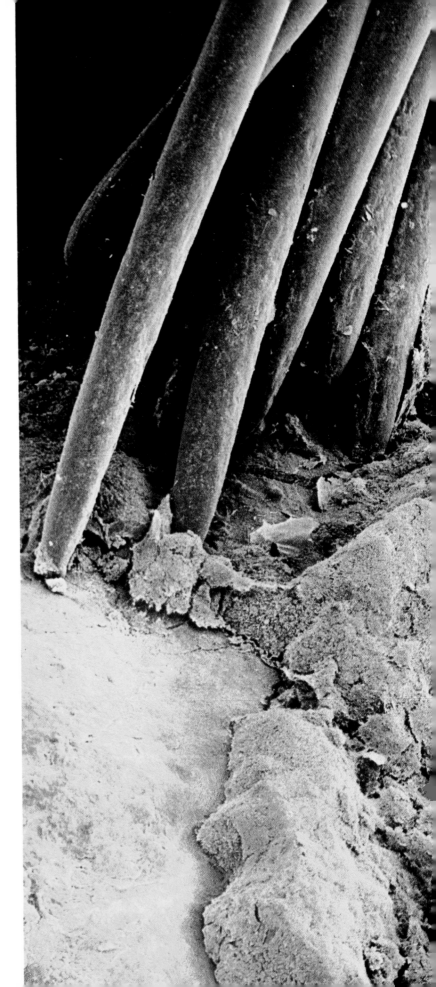

A soft brush with a small head is most suitable for brushing the teeth.

Some brands of toothpaste contain hard, abrasive particles, as shown, magnified c. 3,000 times, **below.** *They can damage the tooth enamel.* **Right,** *the toothbrush attempts to clear away a well-established plaque deposit with a superstructure of food particles and bacteria. (× 50)*

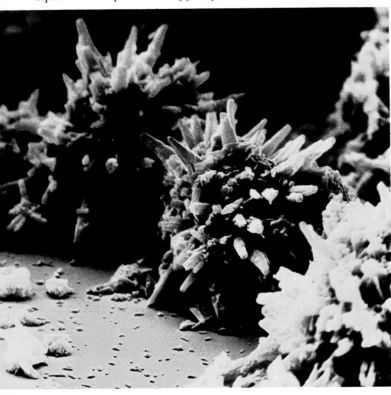

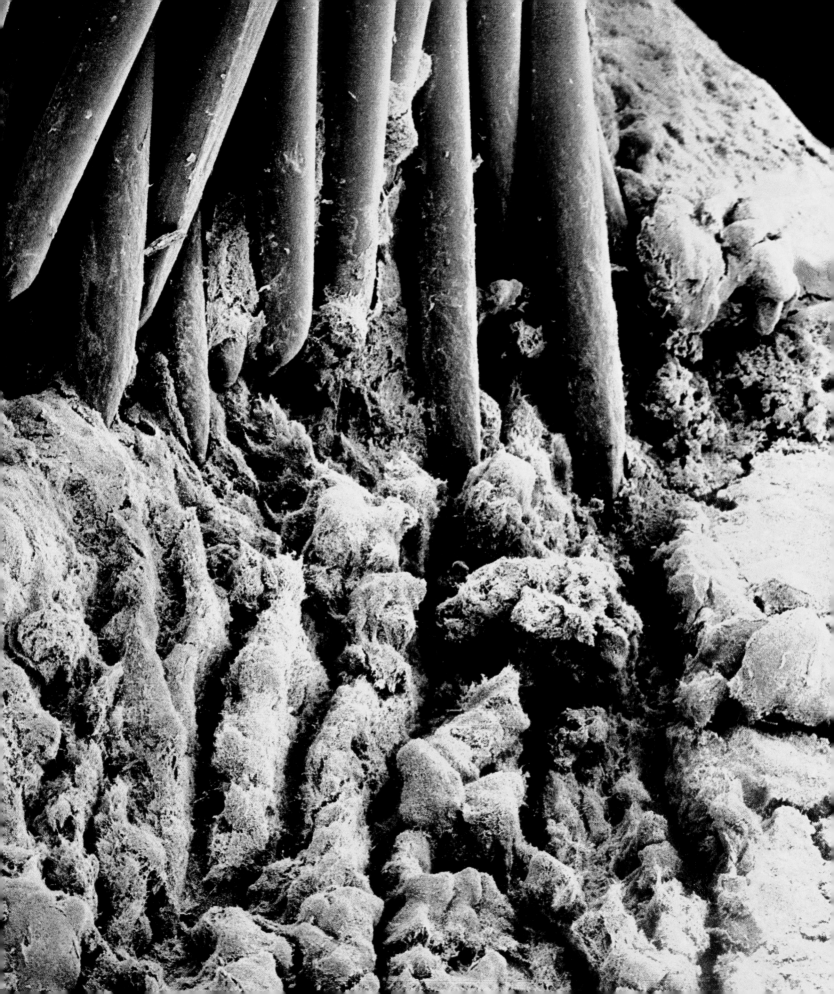

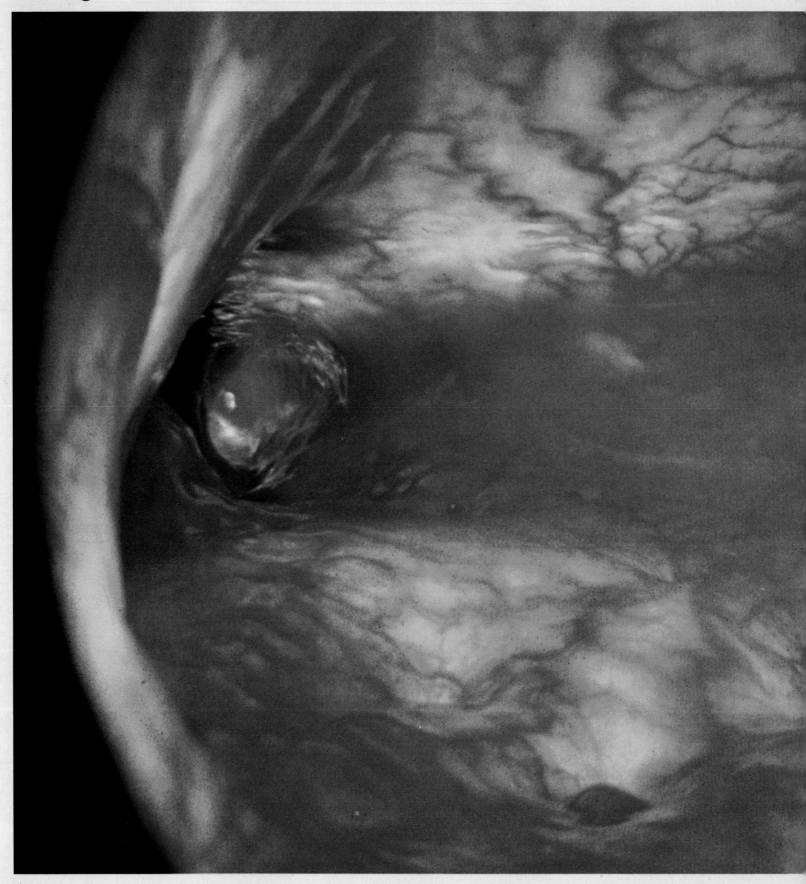

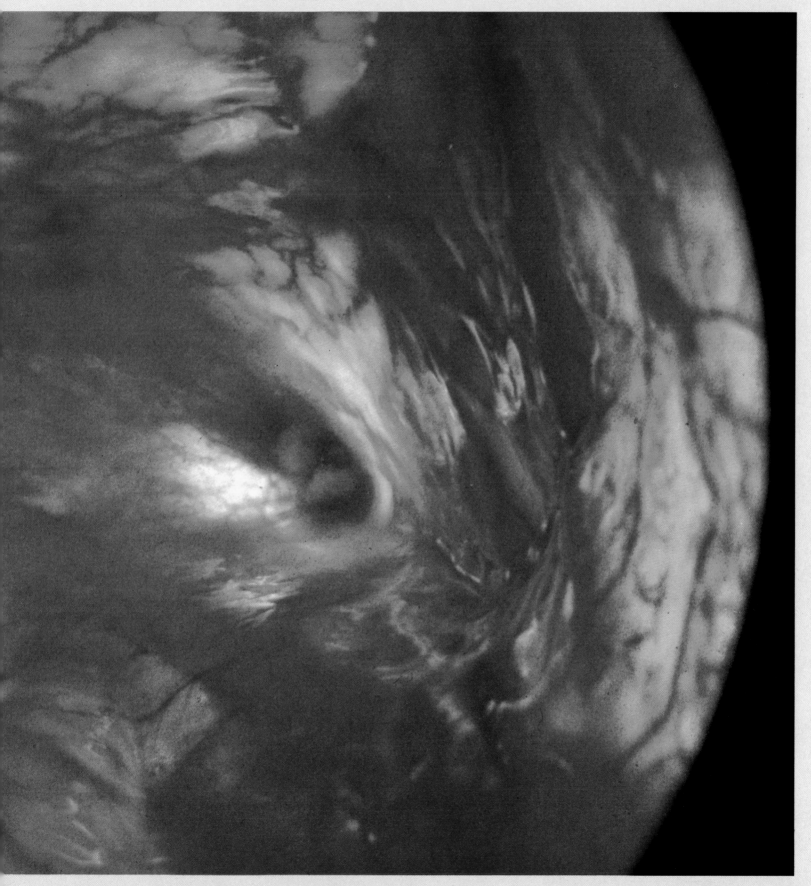

Inside the stomach. Lower exit is to the left, upper to the right. Glands produce hydrochloric acid, which fights bacteria.

The digestive tract

In the fetus, the digestive tract is entirely unused and therefore sterile. The fetus obtains all its nourishment (and oxygen) from the mother's blood, via the placenta and umbilical cord. The intestinal contents (meconium) of the newborn baby are not the remains of digested food but a mixture of mucus, glandular secretions, and swallowed amniotic fluid. Meconium may be regarded as one of the many instances of how the body, in the fetal stage, "tests" its systems before birth. Everything must be in perfect working order at the moment when the small satellite is launched from the mother craft.

The newborn child's digestive tract thus contains neither bacteria nor viruses. Nor has it any effective immune defences against the world of microbes into which the baby is precipitated at birth. This hazardous situation is one shared by the young of all other mammals. Like human babies, they are totally dependent on rapidly ingesting the mother's milk, and thereby getting a dose of antibodies. In man, these are of the IgA (immunoglobulin A) type, which during breast-feeding are dispersed throughout the surface of the gastrointestinal tract, from the mouth to the anus, where they form an initial protection against microbial assaults.

Antibodies of another type IgG, are transferred from the mother to the fetus via the blood. One might well ask why the same does not occur where IgA is concerned. The hiatus in defences between birth and the first suckling occasion is indeed a risky phase. The explanation lies in the fact that IgA antibodies are too large. They cannot pass through the placental filter, which also shuts out the mother's blood cells, bacteria, and larger viruses.

As soon as the infant receives its first dose of the mother's milk, a local defence force of IgA antibodies is established in the digestive tract. Trained by the mother's immune system, they are ready to identify and attack incoming microorganisms without delay.

The digestive tract is particularly rich in lymph node tissue, which is part of the immune system. The stomach, moreover, produces strongly bactericidal hydrochloric acid, in such a high concentration that the stomach must protect itself so as not to incur damage. The protection consists of a layer of tough, viscous mucus lining the sensitive gastric membrane.

If for any reason this layer is damaged—for example, if we happen to swallow emulsifying agents such as soap or washing powder—the membrane is laid open to attack by the acid. If countermeasures are not taken in time, the stomach's protein-dissolving enzyme, pepsin, can complete the assault by corroding the gastric membrane. Thus, a gastric ulcer is formed. (Most ulcers affect the duodenum, the part of the intestine below the pyloric sphincter, the stomach's lower exit.) However, glands in the stomach produce not only hydrochloric acid but also sodium bicarbonate, which has the capacity to moderate and neutralise the acid.

By means of hydrochloric acid and pepsin, the stomach produces chemical substances responsible for the dissolution and breakdown of meat and other proteins. They would also dissolve the stomach's own muscles if it were not for the protective layer of mucus, which is continually being renewed in response to signals both from the food itself and, via the vagus nerve, from the brain. The mere thought of food prompts the brain to send impulses that promote the production of both protective mucus, on the one hand, and hydrochloric acid and pepsin on the other.

Chemicals in the digestive tract, like the mechanical work of kneading and squeezing the food, rapidly wear down both the glandular cells and the membrane, which must be constantly reinforced by new cells. There is a complete turnover of such cells every four to six days. Investigations show that the formation of new cells starts to increase about eight hours after a meal and reaches its peak after sixteen hours.

If we eat three times a day, the formation of new cells is fairly constant. Regular eating habits are thus an important element in the defences of the digestive tract. Gulping down fast snacks now and again, when it suits us—a hamburger, potato chips, or coffee and a bun—undermines these defences. On the one hand, such a diet is monotonous and nutritionally dubious; on the other, it upsets the rhythm of the digestive organs. Modern man, with his stressful life-style, needs a tranquil break to settle down to an appetising and well-cooked meal.

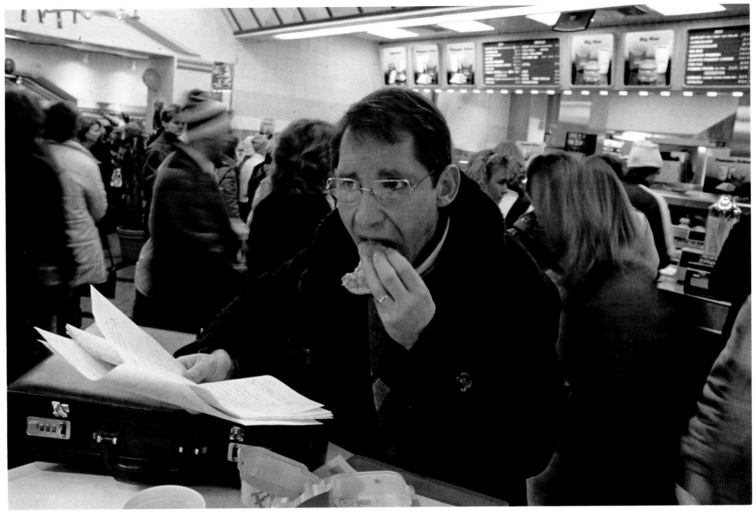

Modern man often lives dangerously, rushing from one meeting to the next, hastily devouring a hamburger or Danish pastry at convenient times—and thereby often paving the way for diseases of the gastrointestinal tract.

For people with sensitive stomachs, more frequent and smaller meals may be advantageous: a period of two hours between meals requires less gastric juice than four hours.

Food rich in protein stimulates the production of hydrochloric acid and pepsin, while fatty foods curb it. In the West, our protein intake is extremely high. A protein-rich diet promotes growth in young people, but there is also reason to believe that such a diet can damage certain organs, particularly the kidneys.

Alcohol, large quantities of strong coffee, and tobacco smoke involve hazards for the stomach. The same applies to medicines of the salicylic acid (aspirin) type, which can even provoke small hemorrhages in the stomach wall. People who have, or have had, a stomach ulcer must avoid pain relievers and antipyretics of this kind. There are alternatives with no such side effects.

Vomiting and diarrhea are also among the defence mechanisms of the digestive tract. Vomiting is a reflex-controlled emptying of the stomach, while diarrhea is caused by intestinal activity proceeding at a rate at which the large intestine is unable to absorb the water in feces. The causes include irritant or toxic food and infections of the gastrointestinal tract.

Autopsies show that numerous men and women have suffered from a gastric ulcer—in many cases without being aware of it. The underlying reason is not known for certain, but hereditary factors, stress, and faulty dietary habits play an important part. In the initial phase of the illness, the protective membrane is damaged by hydrochloric acid, whereupon pepsin can attack, and even corrode, the stomach wall. Through the hole thus formed, the contents of the stomach may leak out into the abdominal cavity and give rise to peritonitis, a life-threatening condition that requires immediate surgery.

The normal functioning of the stomach

Above left (1), a healthy gastric membrane: the glandular ducts, through which mucus, hydrochloric acid, and pepsin are delivered. *Above right (2)*, the "eruption" in a mucus gland cell, with the mucus being explosively ejected (× 2,500). *Below left (3)*, two glandular ducts in a microscopic cross-section through the gastric membrane. At their base are cells which produce hydrochlo-ric acid and pepsinogen and, higher up, the goblet cells that produce mucus. *Below right (4)*, is a magnification of a glandular duct, in which the hydrochloric acid–producing cell has emptied itself. *Opposite (5)*, cells in the surface layer of the gastric membrane (foreground) and, above, fat partly covered by mucus (× 9,000)

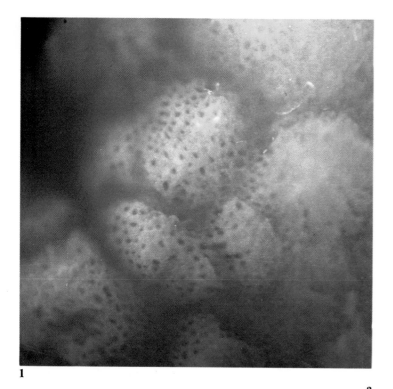

1

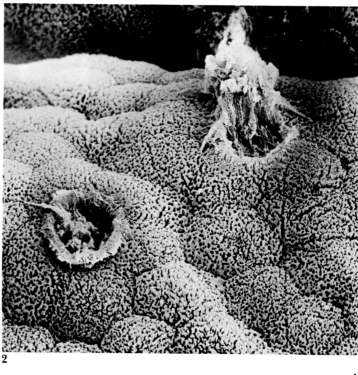

2

3

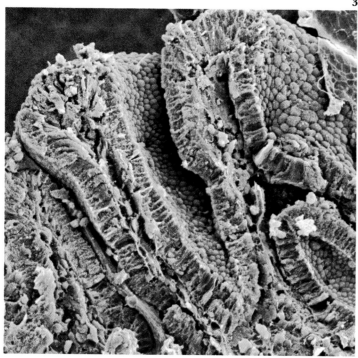

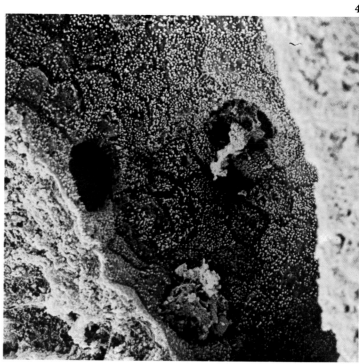

4

5

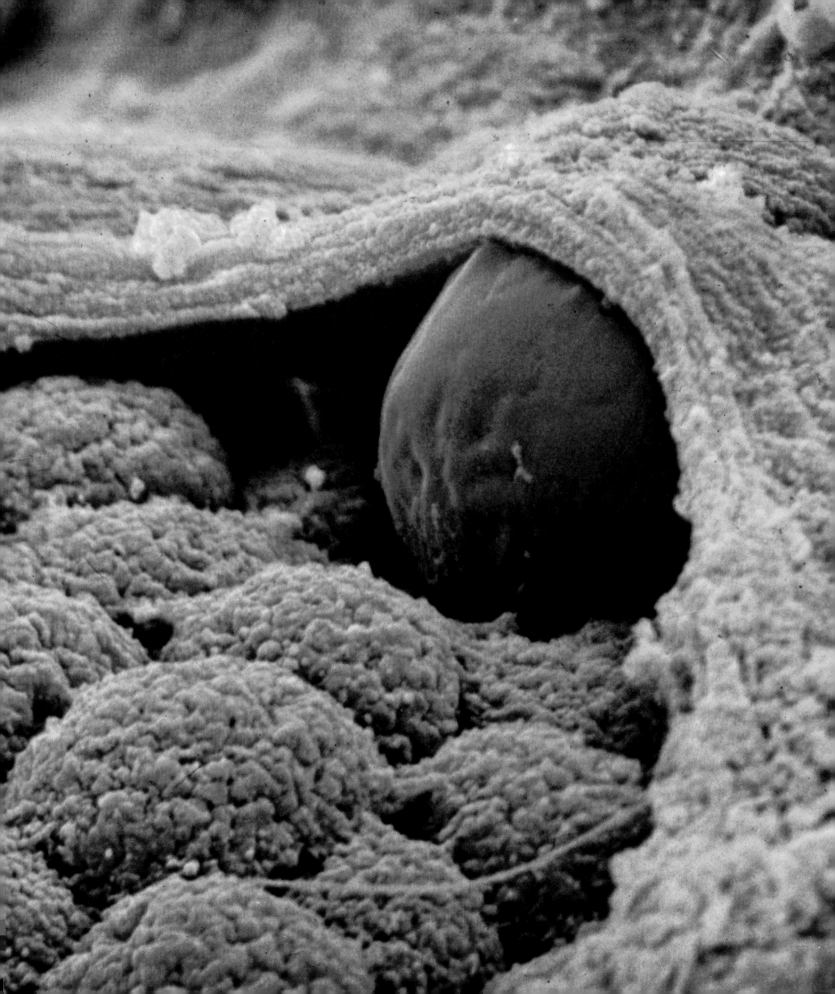

The normal functioning of the intestine

Below, the puckered membrane of the large intestine, with the glandular ducts, in which mucus threads hang like curtains. When the intestinal contents reach the large intestine, most of the nutrients have been absorbed—what remains is water, which is removed and stored. The large intestine is an important fluid regulator. *Opposite right,* the magnificent "volcanic eruption" of a mucus-producing cell in the duodenum, the part of the intestine contiguous to the stomach. The surface is clad with velvety, finger-like projections that absorb nutrients from the passing chyme (pulp). Their blood capillaries absorb fructose and amino acids (building blocks of protein), while their lymph capillaries absorb fat. There are millions of villi, each 0.5 to 1.5 mm long: their surface area has been estimated at ten square metres.

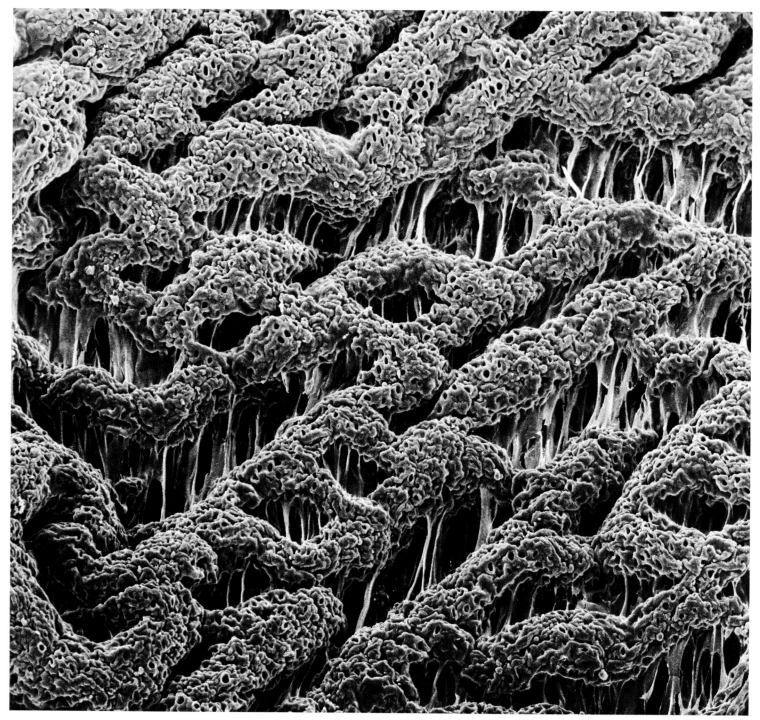

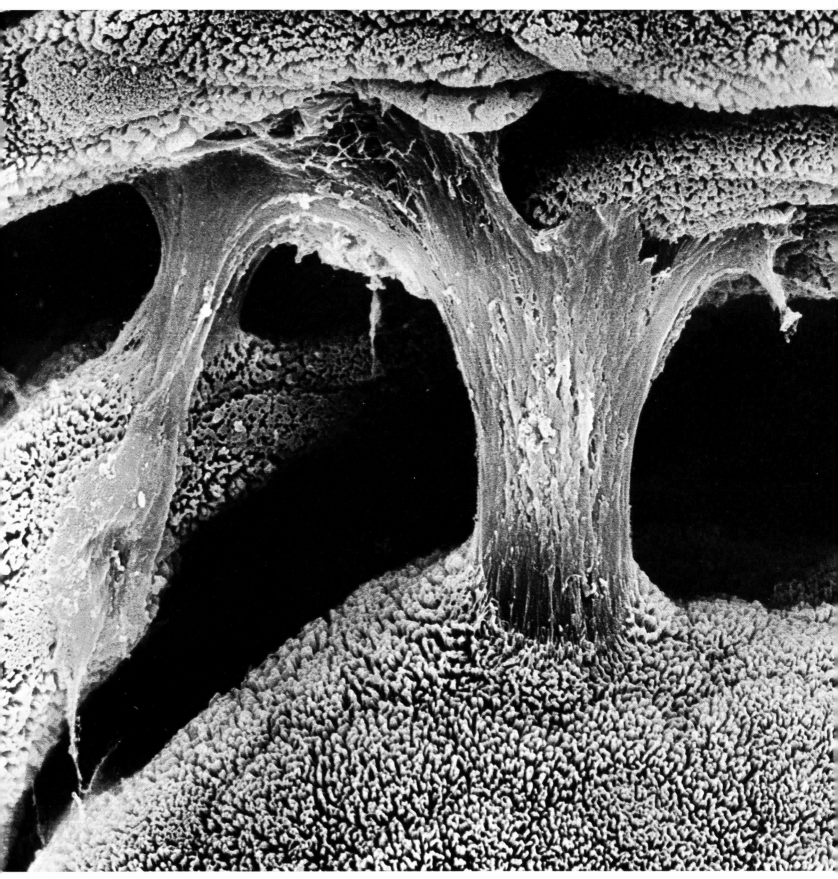

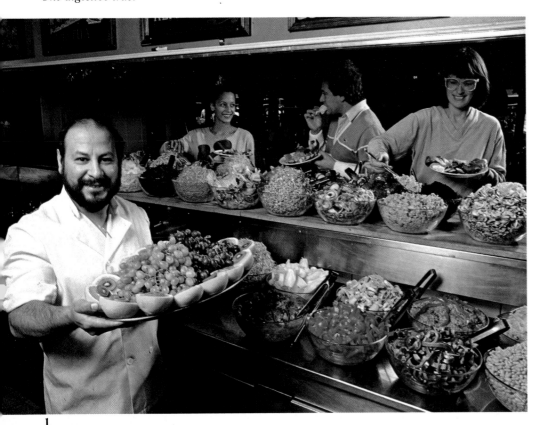

Crucial food balance

Below left, a section of the membrane in the small intestine: the villi, or projections, in the upper part show signs of excessive sensitivity to some foodstuff, for example, gluten. The *adjacent* picture shows the gastric membrane, with bacteria in the mucus. The hydrochloric acid kills virtually all bacteria entering the stomach. *Opposite,* the remains of a lettuce leaf have reached the large intestine. Since gastric and intestinal juices are incapable of digesting cellulose, it is hardly touched as it passes through the digestive tract. Plant material is useful, however, in that its fibres stimulate the intestinal membrane and promote peristalsis—the waves of contraction that propel intestinal contents on their way.

A vegetarian diet *(above left)* is rich in vitamins. They are essential for health and may also contribute to the body's defences against diseases such as cancer.

1. *A bountiful salad bar.*
2. *Membrane in the small intestine.* ($\times$ *100*)
3. *Gastric membrane with bacteria.* ($\times$ *3,000*)
4. *Remains of lettuce in the intestine.* ($\times$ *300*)

1

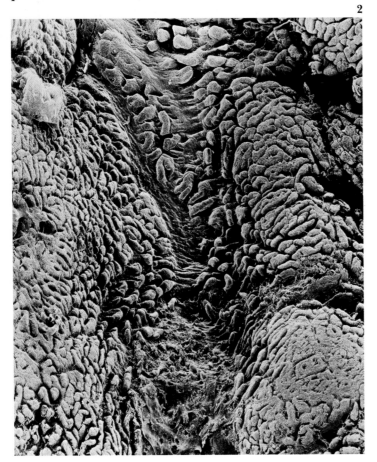

2

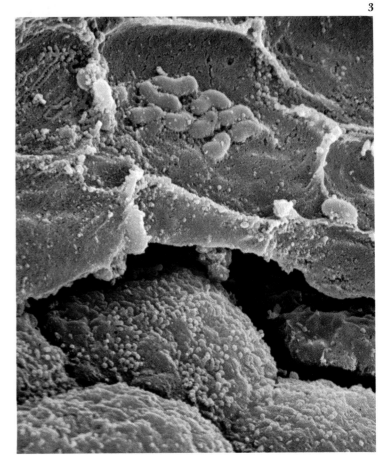

3

4

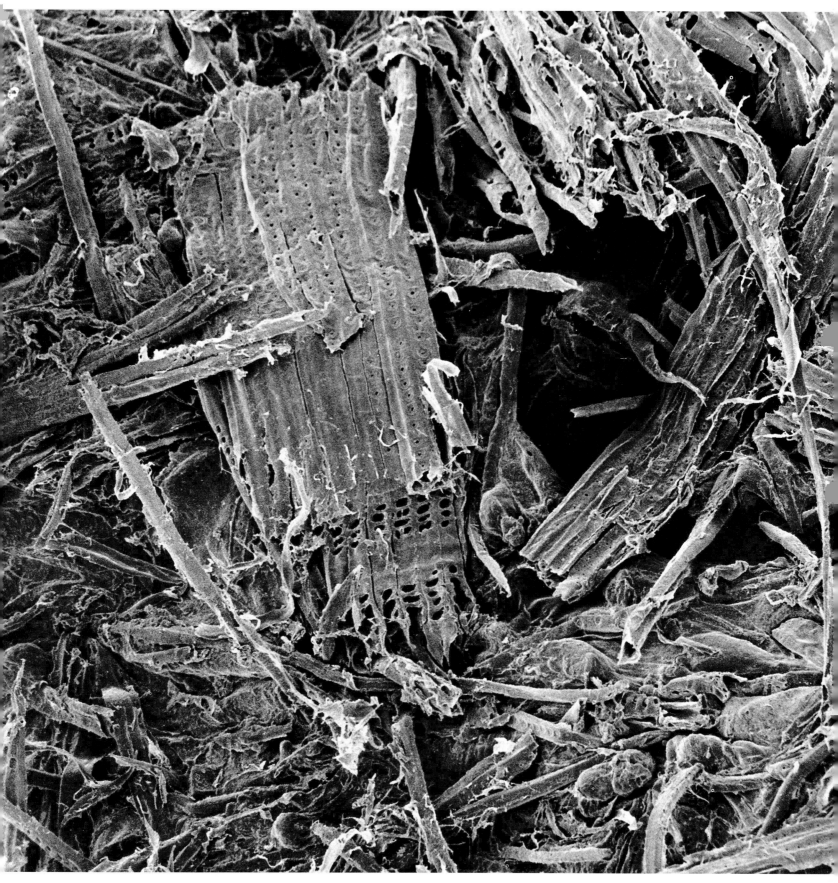

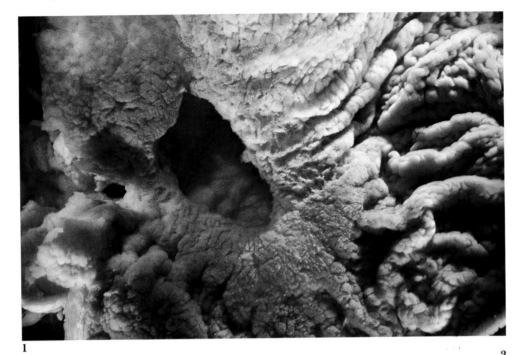

1

2

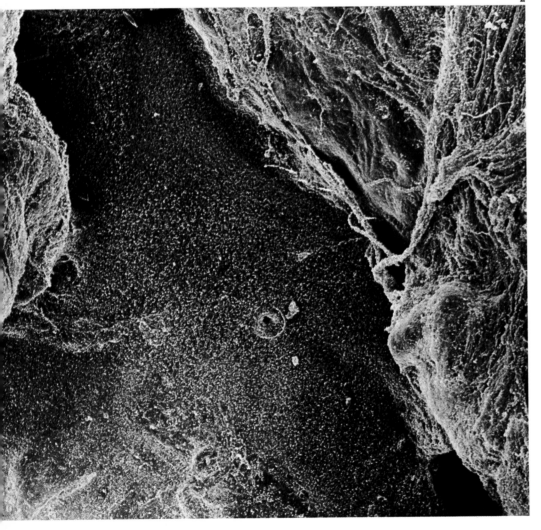

The stomach ulcer—a crater in the stomach wall

Right, a crater-like ulcer extends into the stomach wall. Around its edges are red blood cells. A deep hole like this leads to infected stomach contents extruding into the abdominal cavity and there possibly giving rise to peritonitis, a life-threatening condition.

Above left, the ulcer is surrounded by swollen membrane. *Below*, we see the initial phase of peritonitis: the ulcer has perforated the stomach wall, and there are fibrin threads and agglutinations.

Despite extensive research, the medical profession has not fully ascertained the mechanisms underlying gastric and duodenal ulcers. Hereditary disposition, weak points in the gastric membrane, and, above all, severe and prolonged mental stress all play a part. A person who has been involved in a traffic accident or a fire may develop an ulcer in a short time. Previously, a rise in hydrochloric acid production was considered an important cause of ulcers, but this does not occur in most cases. On the other hand, the gastric juice may attack the stomach wall when, for some reason, the protective mucous layer lays a portion of it bare.

About 10 percent of the adult population have stomach ulcers or their resulting scars. Considerably more men than women are affected. Half of all so-called stomach ulcers are in fact intestinal ulcers, since they arise in the duodenum. High consumption of alcohol and medicines such as those containing salicylic acid, as well as smoking, increase the risk of an ulcer. Medical treatment consists of dietary prescriptions and drugs to lower acidity in the stomach. In more severe cases, surgery is necessary: portions of the stomach wall containing a large number of the glands that produce gastric juice are removed. In some cases the nerves controlling the stomach's digestive glands are severed.

1. *A stomach ulcer, surrounded by swollen gastric membrane, seen from inside the stomach. Actual size.*
2. *The stomach ulcer has perforated the stomach wall: peritonitis is imminent. The picture was taken from the outside of the stomach. ($\times$ 15)*
3. *Detail of the crater-shaped stomach ulcer, magnified 600 times.*

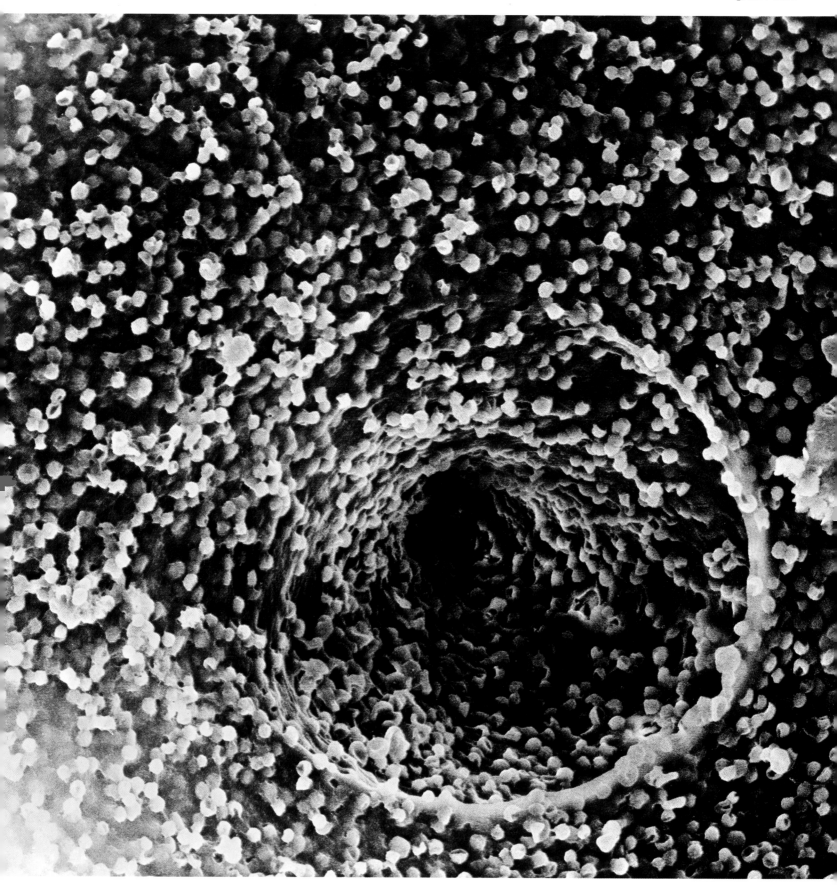

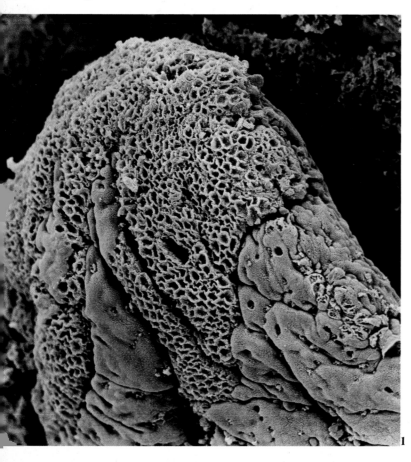

Damage to the digestive system

Large quantities of bacteria inhabit the large intestine. Most of them are innocuous, and do us no harm at all. *Above*, an example of the opposite kind: inflammation is in progress, and an ulcer is beginning to form. The membrane cells, *bottom right*, are healthy, but the overlying section is affected. Two (fairly common) intestinal infections with symptoms of this kind are Crohn's disease and ulcerative colitis; the underlying mechanisms of both are unknown. It is conceivable that harmful substances in the environment contribute to their incidence. Ulcerative colitis is treated with a particular sulfa drug, while surgery is usually resorted to in the case of Crohn's disease.

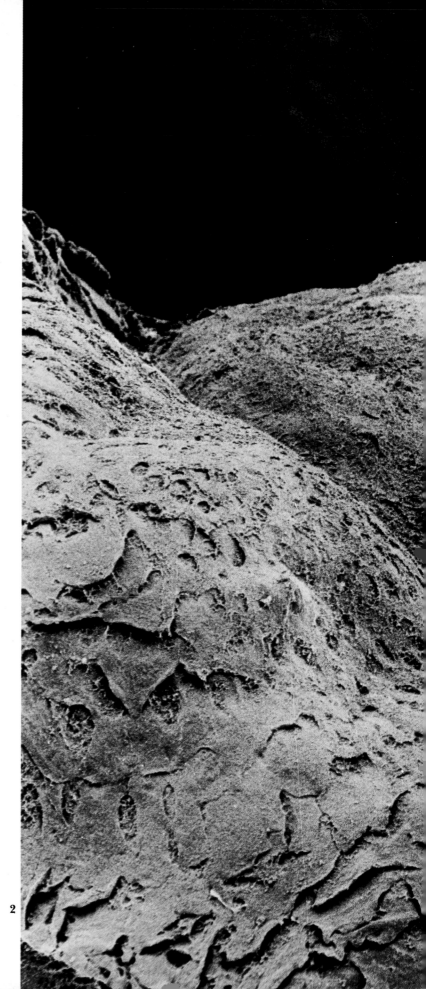

1. *Inflammation in progress in the membrane of the large intestine.*
2. *A crater-like stomach ulcer in the lunar landscape of the intestinal membrane. (× 230).*

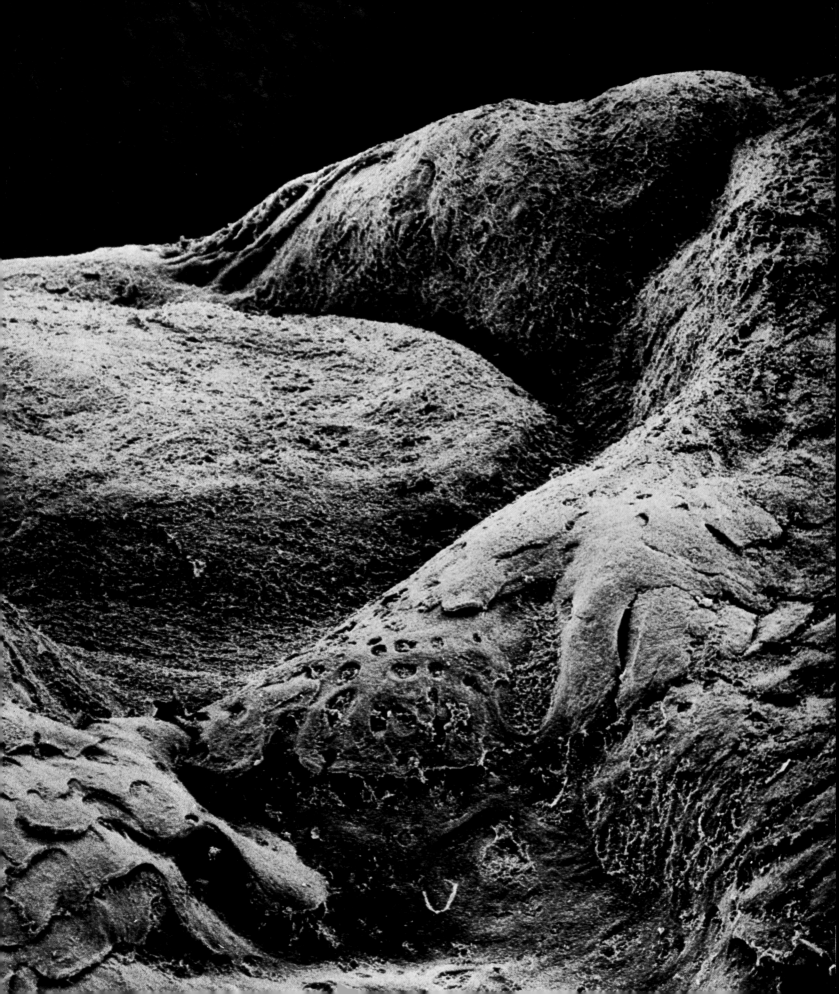

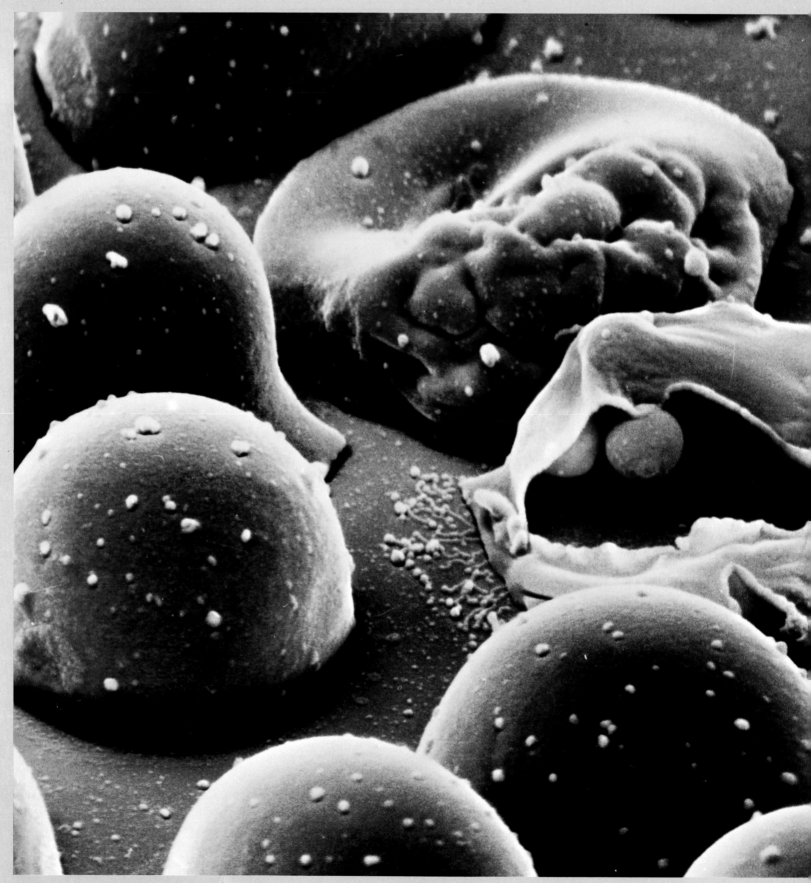

In the middle of the picture, a red blood cell ruptured by dividing malarial plasmodia.

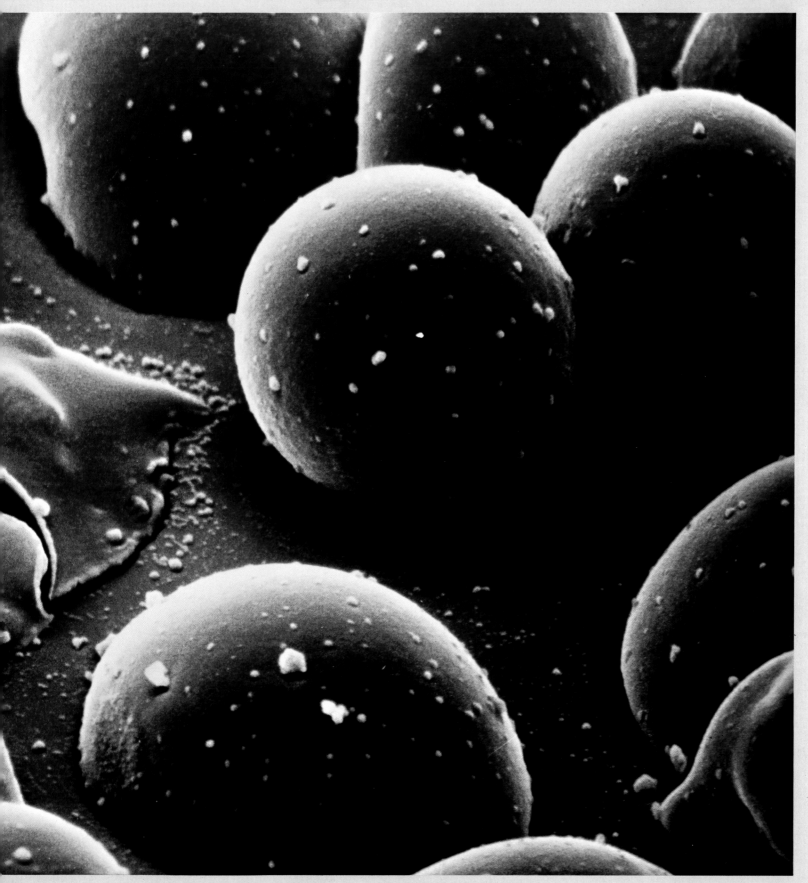

Parasites

Three widespread parasitic diseases—malaria, trypanosomiasis (sleeping sickness), and schistosomiasis (bilharzia)—plague hundreds of millions of people in the Third World today. Malaria alone, which occurs in Central Africa, Brazil, India, and the Far East, affects about 300 million people, and about 200 million suffer from schistosomiasis, which is common in Africa, South America, and China.

The remarkable life cycle of the malaria parasite
When the mosquito sucks blood from a nonimmune person, the parasite's sporozoites—smaller than bacteria—enter the blood, which conveys them to the liver. There, they occupy one liver cell each. After about twelve days, the cells burst—except in cases of slow infection, when it may take months—and the parasite now moves into red blood cells, in a new form: merozoites. In two or three days, the blood cells burst and large numbers of merozoites attack new blood cells. The fever attack comes when the blood cells burst. Sexual forms—male and female parasites (gametocytes)—develop. These are sucked up by the Anopheles *mosquito and mate in its intestinal canal; the progeny, sporozoites, migrate to the mosquito's salivary glands. When the mosquito bites a new human victim, a new cycle begins.*

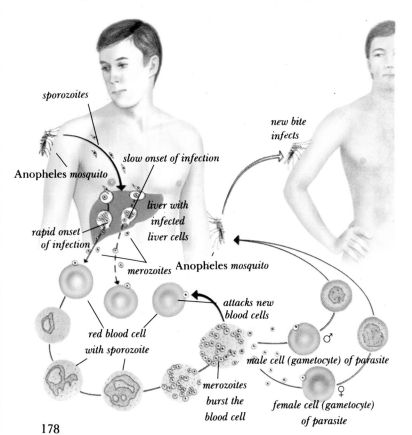

sporozoites

new bite infects

Anopheles *mosquito*

slow onset of infection

liver with infected liver cells

rapid onset of infection

merozoites Anopheles *mosquito*

attacks new blood cells

red blood cell with sporozoite

male cell (gametocyte) of parasite ♂

merozoites burst the blood cell

female cell (gametocyte) of parasite ♀

All organisms that live on plants or animals without giving anything in return are, in fact, parasites. For practical reasons, however, bacteria and viruses are regarded as distinct groups of pathogens, and the term "parasites" is reserved for such organisms as intestinal worms, blood-sucking insects, and insect-borne microorganisms.

Even with this limiting definition, parasitism is still one of the commonest life forms, with an ecological role. Man is included: he "parasitises" a number of organisms, and is himself exposed to about three hundred parasites. Most of them, though irritating, are not pathogenic: an equilibrium prevails between parasite and host. For the parasite, this situation is ideal. Killing the host is not to its advantage; all it wants is to suck the host's strength, for its own existence and reproduction. Low nutritional standards and poor hygiene, however, often tip the balance so that the parasite causes the host's death.

The relationship between the host and the parasitic organism is often extremely complicated. The tiny, sucking worms that cause schistosomiasis are, for example, dependent on their development on two host organisms: man and a freshwater snail that flourishes in stagnant water and is common in Egypt and elsewhere. When the peasant working in the fields wades across a canal, schistosome larvae in the water penetrate his skin and enter the circulatory system. There, the female lays her eggs, which in due course land in the intestines and bladder. When these are emptied, the eggs often return to the canal water and infect the snails. And so the life cycle starts again. In severe cases of schistosomiasis, it is primarily the liver and brain that are affected. The sufferer's general condition is debilitated and his powers of resistance reduced.

The cause of malaria is a microscopic protozoan called a *plasmodium*. There are three species, giving rise to malaria of varying degrees of severity. The plasmodia are dependent for their livelihood on two hosts: the *Anopheles* mosquito and man. They infest the mosquito's salivary glands and are transferred to man when the mosquito bites: the parasites then penetrate man's red blood cells, which burst when the plasmodia divide. The result is an attack of fever: the body temperature rises rapidly, the sufferer shivers violently and after a few hours breaks into a heavy sweat, whereupon his temperature falls. Plasmodia meanwhile force their way into new blood cells, bursting them and causing new, recurrent fever attacks every two or three days.

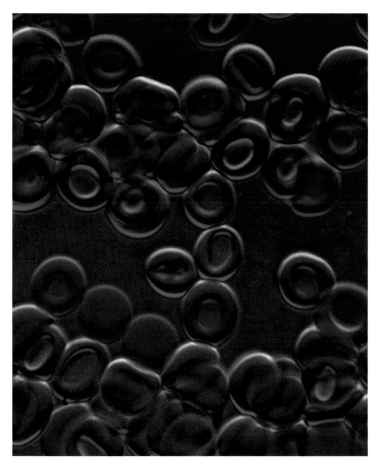

Healthy, biconcave red blood cells in man, bearing oxygen from the lungs to the body's many billions of cells. (Light microscope × 2,000)

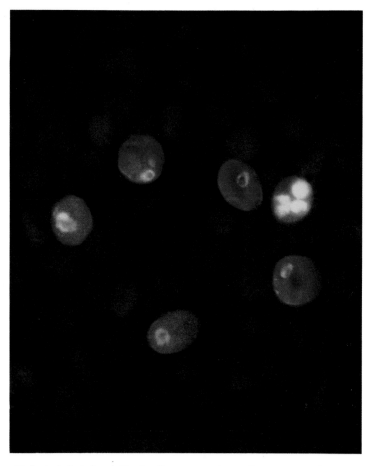

Malaria-infected red blood cells, seen under a fluorescence microscope. They contain merozoites, which divide in the blood cell. (× 2,000)

When the mosquito sucks blood from a person with malaria, the plasmodia settle in its stomach, where they develop into males and females. From the stomach, they move to the salivary glands and thereafter on to new victims. Human red blood cells thus function as incubators.

African sleeping sickness is caused by a genus of protozoa called *trypanosomes*. These are transmitted to man by the tsetse fly when it sucks his blood. Attacks of fever come after an incubation period of two to three weeks. Via the spinal fluid, trypanosomes migrate to the brain, where they attack tissue, including the sleep centres. Emaciated, apathetic, and subject to an ever-increasing need for sleep, the majority of victims die after a year or two.

In South America, trypanosomes cause Chaga's disease, which is transmitted from the armadillo family by an insect. It is thought that the inexplicable disease that plagued Charles Darwin after his voyage on the *Beagle,* for the rest of his life, may have been Chaga's disease, since during one excursion to the Andes he was so severely bitten by insects that he had to take to his bed for a while.

When so many hundred million people are incapaci-

tated or killed by schistosomes, plasmodia, and trypanosomes, one may well ask what the immune system is really doing. Researchers answer that parasites have lived with man for countless millennia, and that in this time they have succeeded in adapting themselves to human immune defences. Those that have not done so have gone under.

It is known that both malaria plasmodia and trypanosomes have a suppressive effect on the immune system. The trypanosomes are also capable of changing their coats, as it were—altering their surface antigens—and even doing so several times. When the host has developed antibodies against the first antigen layer, it is replaced by a new one, with new irritant properties; and when antibodies are developed against this layer, it is replaced by yet another.

Schistosomes can "kidnap" protective antigens from the host organism's cells, thus evading the immune system's attacks. Many protozoa also allow the macrophages to swallow them so as to be able to continue their reproduction therein, undisturbed. Parasites are thus past masters at deceiving the immune system.

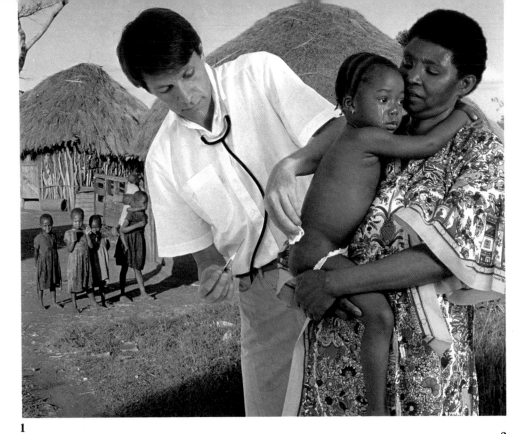

Playing hide-and-seek with the immune system

Plasmodium, a one-celled organism, is responsible for causing malaria. Its various phases of development take place partly in a mammal, such as man, and partly in the *Anopheles* mosquito. There are four different species of plasmodia, causing different symptoms; all, however, attack the red blood cells.

When the mosquito sucks blood from the malaria sufferer, it ingests the plasmodium's *gametocytes*, that is, the equivalents of sperm and eggs. The eggs, fertilised in the mosquito's intestine, migrate to the mosquito's salivary glands in the form of *sporozoites*. When the mosquito then sucks blood from a person not suffering from malaria, the sporozoites are transferred to that person's blood. They settle in the liver, where they divide, causing the liver cells to burst, and enter the blood as *merozoites*.

Some of the merozoites penetrate red blood cells, while others live freely in the blood, developing into sexual cells, gametocytes. In due course the gametocytes are sucked up by new mosquitoes, soon to infest new human hosts.

The merozoites that infect blood cells divide inside them, making them burst. When they enter the blood by the million, the sufferer begins to shiver and sweat, to be nauseous and feverish, every other or every third day, according to which plasmodium species has caused the infection.

In the course of its long evolution, the plasmodium has learned to deceive the immune system. If it confronts antibodies in the host's blood, it can change antigens, thus avoiding their attacks. Moreover, antibodies do not have long to attack sporozoites that have just entered the body: within minutes, they conceal themselves in the liver cells. There, they are protected by a sheath which the immune system interprets as indigenous to the body. The same applies to the merozoites, which hide in red blood cells.

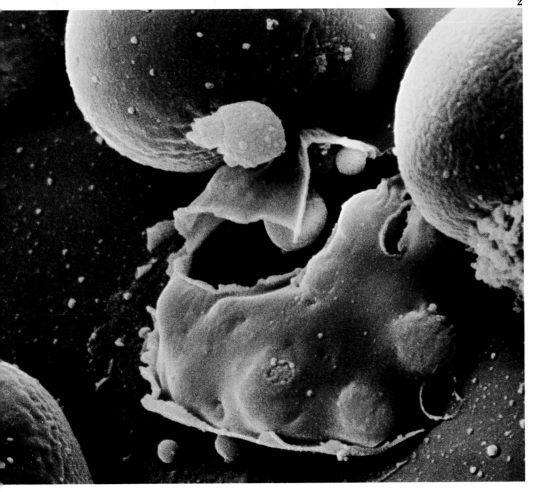

1. *Acute malaria often requires chloroquin injections. The parasites have become resistant and research is now directed toward developing a vaccine.*

2. *A red blood cell ravaged by one of the malarial merozoites, among intact cells. (× 8,000)*

3. *A merozoite emerges from the shell of the blood cell it has destroyed and heads immediately for a new, healthy blood cell. (× 40,000)*

1

2

3

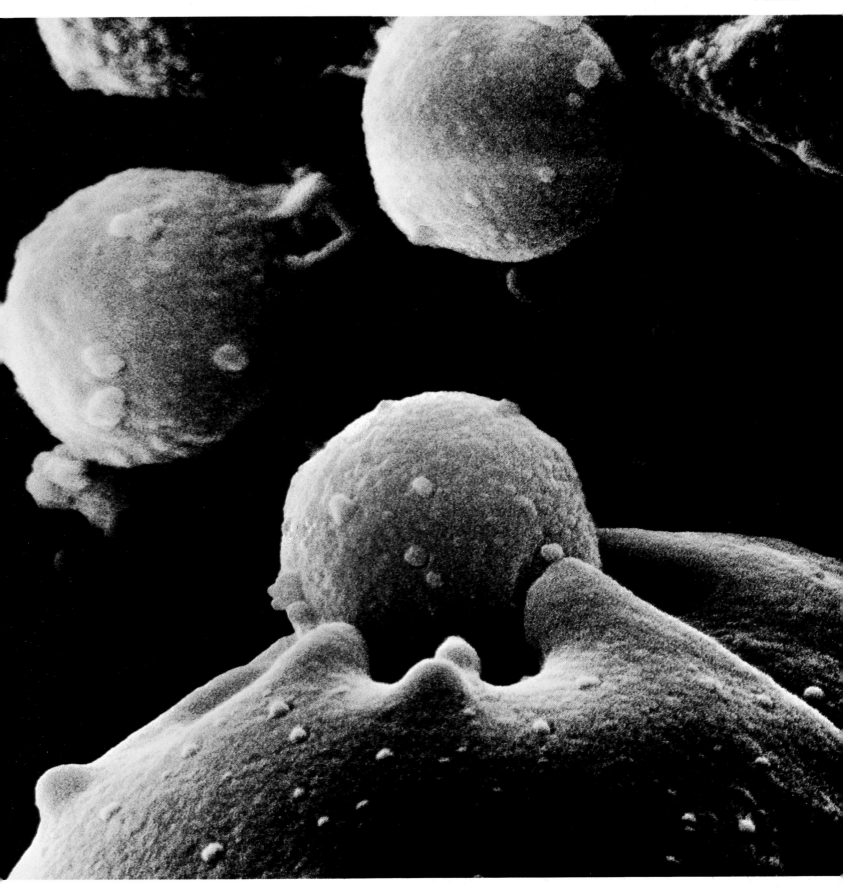

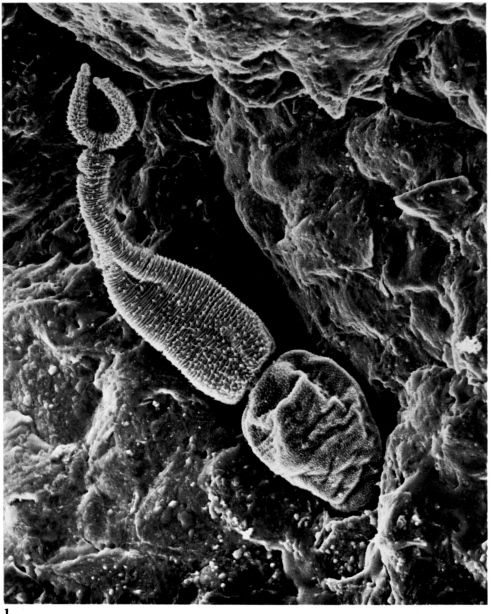

Bilharzia, scourge of the tropics

One of the worst scourges of mankind is the parasitic disease bilharzia (schistosomiasis), which in acute or chronic form affects about 200 million people in tropical and subtropical countries today. Malaria alone claims more victims.

The disease spreads via infected water, when larvae of the schistosome worm penetrate human skin. The larva, or *cercaria*, swims freely by means of its tail, shedding it as soon as the larva becomes attached to the skin. After penetration, it travels in the bloodstream to its chosen destination, the veins of the bladder or intestines.

Establishing itself there, the parasite develops male and female forms. At this stage the worms are one to four centimetres long. Adhering firmly to the blood vessel walls, they feed on the blood as it flows past. The male encloses the female in a long groove on his body, and thus the lifelong process of mating begins—one which may continue for several decades, and which prompts each female to deliver thousands of eggs into the blood daily.

1. *The schistosome larva, the* cercaria, *has just come into contact with human skin.*
2. *The* cercaria *sheds its tail and penetrates the skin.*
3. *Freshwater snails are the intermediate host of the worm.*
4. *Sexually mature worms adhering firmly to a blood vessel.*

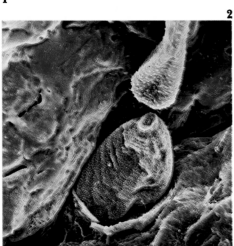

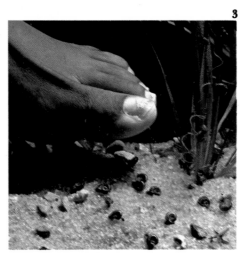

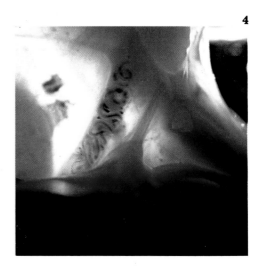

Schistosome eggs pass out of the body in urine and feces, whereupon they often enter rivers and lakes. On contact with fresh water, they hatch into minute swimming miracidia, equipped with cilia, which seek out certain snails to be their intermediate hosts. Here, they develop into cercariae, and the life cycle enters a new phase, in which they penetrate human skin.

In the acute form of the disease, the symptoms are inflammation with fever, cough, urticarial weals, and abdominal pain. Blood is present in urine and feces. Chronic bilharzia is characterised by the destruction of blood vessel and liver tissue and lowered resistance to infections, among other symptoms. The immune system's attacks, above all on parasite eggs deposited on the blood vessel walls, provokes an autoimmune reaction: feeding cells destroy tissues around the eggs, giving rise to ulcers.

Bilharzia is difficult to treat. If the infection is a mild one, detected at an early stage, an antimony preparation may be of use. However, preventive hygiene and sanitation measures are most important. Attempts have been made to eradicate the intermediate host, the freshwater snail, but with discouraging results.

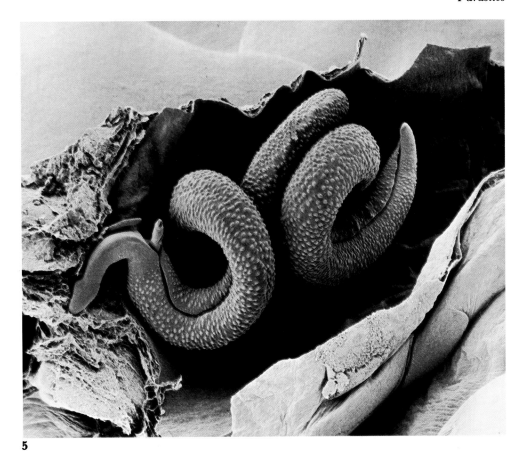

5

6

5. The male worm, about 4 cm long (here magnified approximately 25 times), embraces the female in a groove on his body. Her head protrudes.

6. The suction pads of the male, magnified 250 times.

7. The hooked edge of the suction pad. (× 3,000)

7

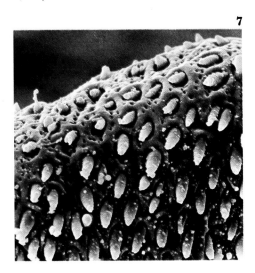

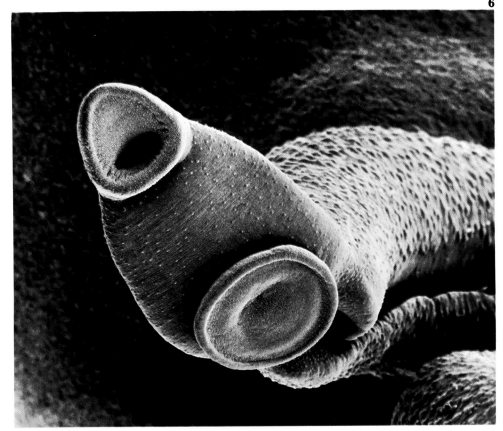

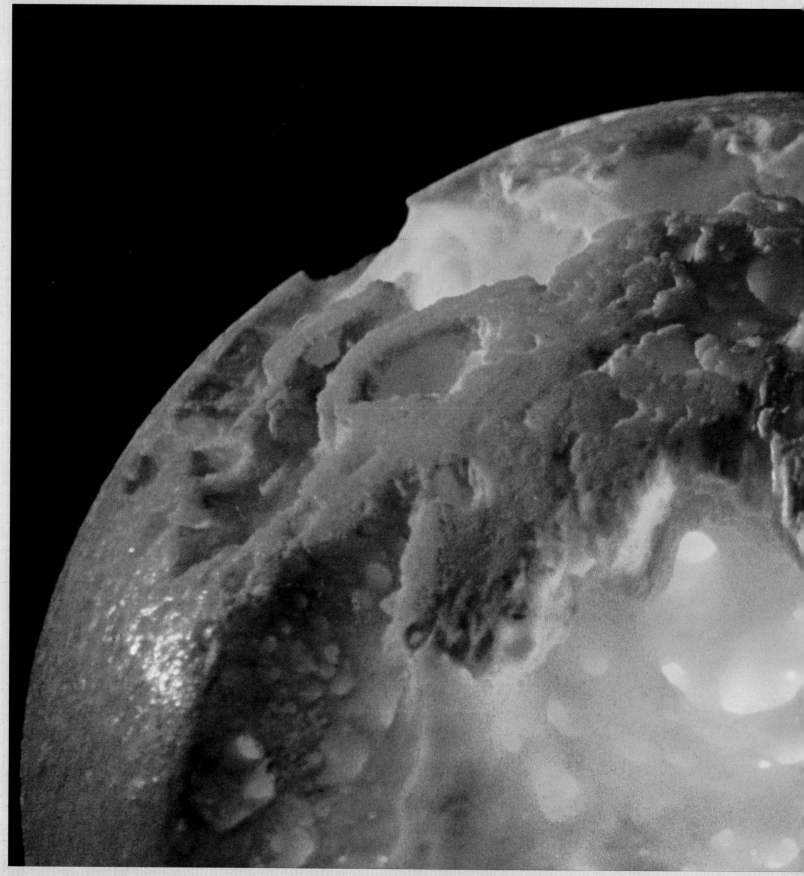

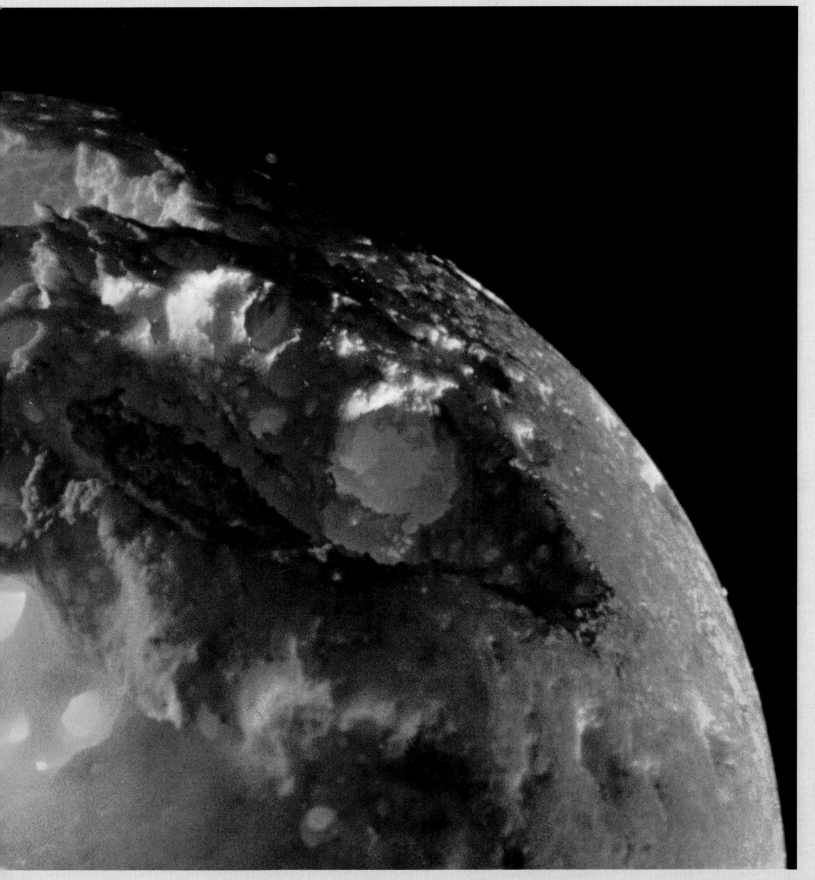

Corroded ball of the femur. The sufferer's own immune system plays some part in the destruction of joint surfaces.

Autoimmune disease

The idea that the immune system could sometimes err and turn against the body's own tissues seemed fanciful until as recently as the 1950s. A group of immunologists then discovered that chronic inflammation of the thyroid gland—also called Hashimoto's syndrome—had a clear connection with antibodies produced by the body's own immune system.

Today, thirty years later, we know—or in some cases suspect—that numerous diseases whose mechanisms of genesis are hard to explain have appeared to be characterised by a mistaken response on the immune system's part. Such diseases include the widespread ailment rheumatoid arthritis, the chronic disease of the connective tissue lupus erythematosus, multiple sclerosis, weakness of the muscles (myasthenia gravis), juvenile diabetes, and certain diseases of the gastrointestinal tract.

This phenomenon may appear paradoxical, but its existence has been confirmed by research in recent years. The causal chain of events is often highly complex, but it is clear that the equilibrium of the immune system may in some circumstances be disturbed, with negative effects: the immune system then itself *creates* disease instead of protecting the body against it.

Immunologists postulate the three following principal mechanisms underlying autoimmune disease:

• The immune system develops during childhood, learning to recognise the cells and tissues with which it is in unceasing contact, and becoming tolerant of these. But there are tissues in the body that either appear after the immune system reaches "maturity," or that develop in relative isolation from the immune system. Examples of the former are male sperm, which are first produced during puberty; examples of the latter are the ocular lens and the brain.

In men, antibodies may be formed against sperm: during their patrols of the tissues, the lymphocytes of the immune system may identify sperm as "foreign" to the body. In some cases, the result is sterility.

A mechanical injury to the eye may expose hidden antigens that the immune system has not encountered previously and therefore has not developed tolerance toward. The result is that antibodies are formed against these antigens, and the immune system launches an attack against them in the undamaged, healthy eye. The tissues of the brain may be subject to a similar course of events.

Moreover, it has been discovered that heart surgery can prompt the production of antibodies against the heart muscle. The explanation of this is either that hidden antigens have been released, or that the operation has altered the antigens in such a way as to endow them with the guise of alien intruders, to be repelled at all cost.

• Normally, every cell displays the right colour or "nationality" when the immune system demands proof of identity. Immunologically speaking, this means that the cells lack surface antigens which prompt the immune system to produce antibodies. The body's defences tolerate "indigenous" cells. This tolerance may, however, be transformed into its opposite. When viruses occupy cells, the cell surface changes. It acquires new antigen characteristics that make the immune system open fire. The same occurs in treatment with certain drugs or, sometimes, X rays. The immune system then no longer recognises the cells as indigenous; instead, it attacks. T-lymphocytes whose special task is to stimulate the B-lymphocytes to produce antigens step up their activity.

Many immunologists studying autoimmune diseases are convinced that they are often triggered by microorganisms—not only viruses, but also bacteria and parasites. These organisms may bear on their surfaces elements and structures that also occur on the body's cells. Helper T-cells boost the antibody-producing activities of the B-cells, which then attack not only the microorganism but also those body cells which happen to share some of their surface characteristics. In fact, this is quite logical. Chaga's disease is an example of this phenomenon: the same antigen occurs on the parasite, in heart muscle and on nerve cells, and the immune system indiscriminately seeks to destroy them all.

• A third mechanism in this context is a disturbance in the immune system's finely balanced regulatory system. Here, T-cells play a dominant role, since they act both as helper cells and as suppressor cells. The latter promote activity, while the former restrain it; by definition, if promotion or restraint are inopportune, untoward consequences will follow. Too much is as bad as too little.

If, for example, the activity of the suppressor cells declines, some researchers suspect that autoimmune diseases such as multiple sclerosis, lupus erythematosus, and rheumatoid arthritis arise as a result. If, on the other hand, the suppressor cells step up their activity, the leeway for infectious diseases such as measles, viral leukemia, and leprosy may increase.

Rheumatoid arthritis, one of the most widespread diseases and one that afflicts women more often than men, is thought to start with an infection. After some time, rheumatoid factors, or antibodies of various kinds united with immune complexes, are formed. The more complexes there are, the more diseased the joints become.

Autoimmune disease is a civil war between the body's cells. Research in recent years has shown that it is commoner than was previously believed. As causation has gradually become clearer, more effective forms of treatment have been successively adopted—for example, suppression of the immune system in lupus erythematosus and myasthenia gravis. The primary hope now is that immunologists will find improved methods of tackling the widespread, often severely disabling disease rheumatoid arthritis. Increasingly, autoimmune diseases are being seen as one of the great challenges facing immunological research.

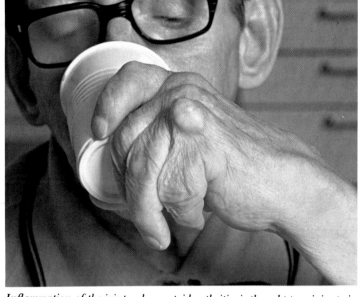

Inflammation of the joints, rheumatoid arthritis, is thought to originate in the immune system's assaults on joint cartilage. For some reason, the antibodies apprehend the cartilage cells as foreign, and attack them. This leads to joint injuries, with characteristic deformations of, for example, the hand (picture above*). Below left* is an X-ray picture of a healthy hand and,* right*, a hand deformed by rheumatoid arthritis.*

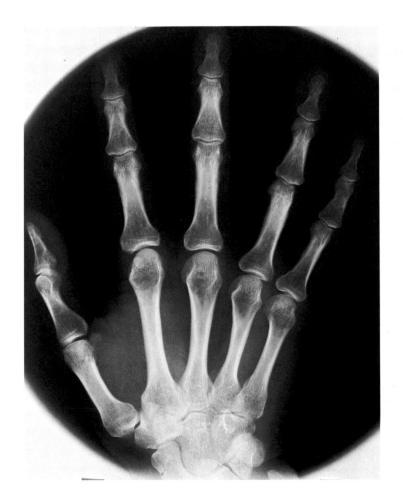

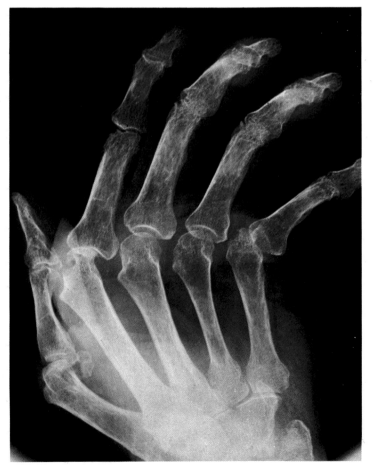

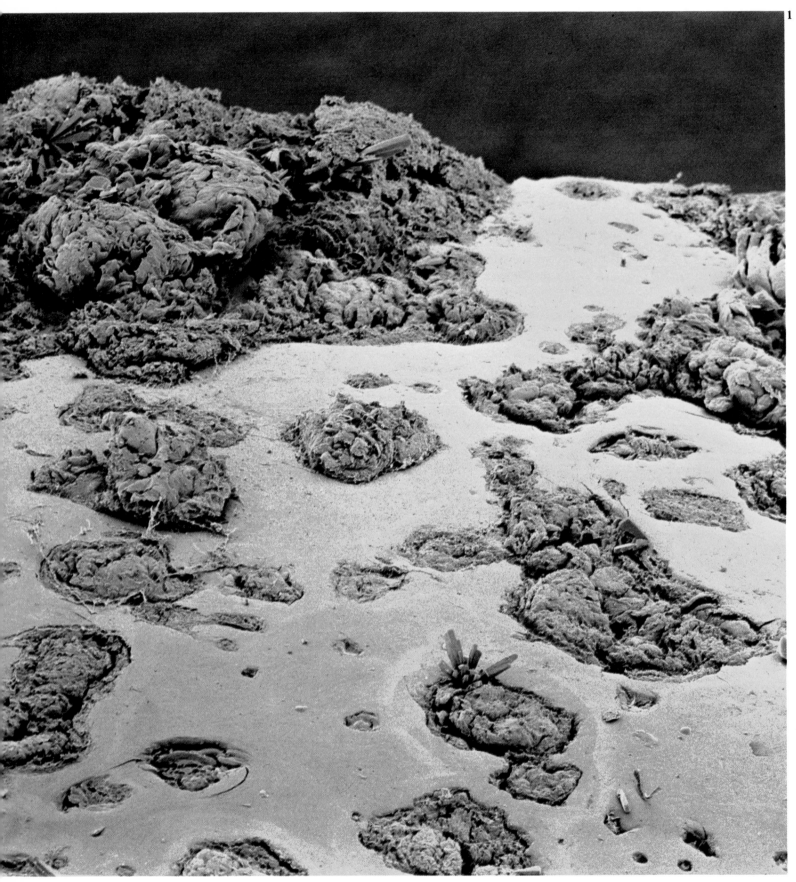

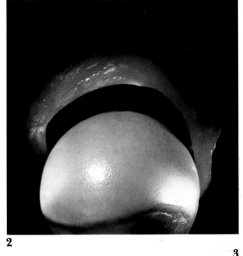

2

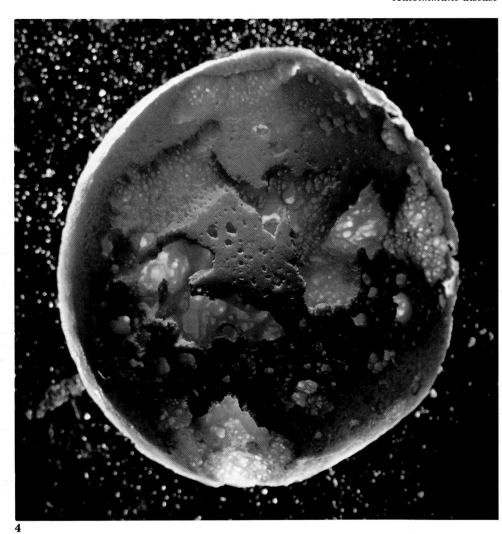

3

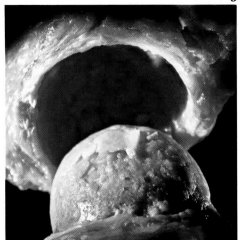

4

The ragged lunar landscape of rheumatoid arthritis

The upper of the two pictures *above, left* (**2**), shows the ball of the humerus (the bone in the upper arm) in a young, healthy individual. Normally, it is embedded in the socket of the shoulder blade. *Below* (**3**), the same joint in a person with rheumatoid arthritis. Beneath the cartilage attacked by antibodies (which has been removed), cavities in the ball's surface are visible. The brown portions are musculature, the yellow, cartilage. *Above right* (**4**), cavities in the ball of the femur.

Opposite (**1**), changes in the joint surface as a result of an autoimmune response, as seen under the scanning electron microscope. The boulder-like formations in the upper part of the picture are outgrowths from the joint membrane which normally produces lubricating (synovial) fluid. The flat structure in the foreground is cartilage, with crater-like injuries extending down into the underlying bone. A joint that looks like this is extremely painful. In a rapidly growing number of cases, damaged hip joints in particular are replaced by prostheses of plastic and metal. The picture to the *right* (**5**) shows a few macrophages attacking and damaging joint cartilage.

5

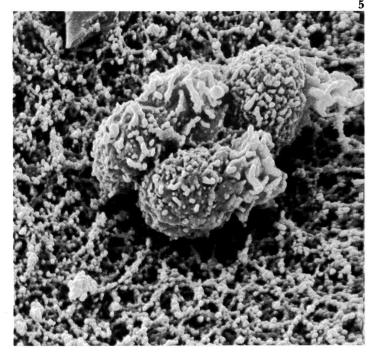

The Future

Few branches of medical science have developed as rapidly as immunology. This statement holds true even if we consider the spectacular successes of genetic engineering and transplantation technology in recent years. What we are witnessing in modern immunology can best be described as a snowball effect: greater insight into the complex functioning of the immune system will in the near future result in new, more effective vaccines; improved methods of combating infection, immune system defects, and autoimmune diseases; new knowledge of microorganisms, fetal development, and tumours; and the potential for both reinforcing and restraining the immune system.

One concrete example is the 1984 Nobel prize-winning technique (now well established) of fusing together a tumour cell and an antibody-producing lymphocyte to create a mixed cell—an "immortal" hybridoma—and a never-ending flow of antibodies, termed "monoclonal" because they originate from a single genetic source. By its division, this cell begets an ever-increasing clone of identical cells. No one had believed a fusion of this kind to be feasible—until it was suddenly achieved. The environmental requirements of a lymphocyte alone mean that there is no nutrient solution adequate to support its growth, and its life is brief. The tumour cell is less demanding. Its unstable genetic composition permits development in various directions, and in the laboratories there is always some cell variant that develops the desired traits. One important trait is the defect in the tumour cell's genetic blueprint which makes it capable of surviving and dividing only when nourished with a particular growth factor.

This slightly handicapped tumour cell is placed in a test tube with the antibody-producing lymphocyte. In due course the test tube contains three types of cells: lymphocytes, tumour cells, and mixed (hybrid) cells. Since only the hybrids are needed, the research worker cuts off the tumour cells' growth factor supply. Soon the tumour cells die; meanwhile, the lymphocytes die unaided.

Only the hybrid cells remain. Their genetic blueprint, with its combination of characteristics from lymphocytes and tumour cells, renders a special growth factor superfluous. The hybrid cell has no difficulty in surviving and dividing in the nutrient solution, in theory forever, producing the desired type of antibodies indefinitely.

An antibody has, of course, a narrowly specific target: it reacts only with a single antigen molecule on the surface of a cell, bacterium, or virus. But there are millions of different antibodies in the human immune system. Tests enable us to select those which interest us, and with the hybridoma technique we can obtain them in unlimited quantities. This fact has already had wide repercussions in many fields, and there are many more to come.

Nowadays interferon is purified from a soup-like mix of biological products by means of monoclonal antibodies. They are applied to viruses a few millionths of a millimetre in diameter, enabling us to dissect them. They help us to make a rapid diagnosis of infections, distinguish between different forms of leukemia, and locate tumour cells that have metastasised, that is, dispersed in the body.

As yet undiscovered is a means of preventing rejection when organs are transplanted between unrelated individuals. Rejection is the greatest threat to a transplant. Although the new organ, be it kidney, liver, pancreas, or heart, is necessary for the continuation of life, the body cannot induce its immune system

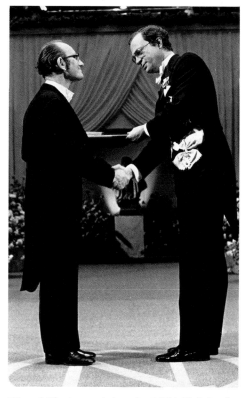

César Milstein receiving the 1984 Nobel prize for medicine from the hand of the Swedish king, Carl XVI Gustaf, for his achievements in immunology. On the same occasion, Niels Jerne and Georges Köhler were also awarded prizes.

to issue a safe conduct. The reason is that the organ's tissues are immunologically incompatible with those of the recipient, and are therefore treated as inimical. Antibodies, killer cells, granulocytes, and macrophages cast themselves frenziedly on the intruder, destroying its cells. At present, we resort to immunosuppressive drugs such as prednisolone and cyclosporin to restrain the immune system and save the transplant. The disadvantage is that in so doing we simultaneously pave the way for hostile activity of various kinds, such as infections and tumours.

Where transplantation is concerned, therefore, the aim is a method of specifically destroying the transplant recipient's lymphocytes, which, with all their might, are striving to get rid of the new organ. These lymphocytes—and they alone—must be eliminated. Immunologists are working on two solutions to the problem. One of these utilises the immune system's ability to form antibodies even against its own antibodies. The other is based on the discovery of special lymphocytes, called lymphokines, which stimulate or counteract both T-lymphocytes (or T-cells) and the antibody-generating B-lymphocytes (B-cells). The object is thus to force the recipient's immune system to obstruct itself.

The fact that a defence system develops weapons against its own weapons may seem remarkable, and paradoxical, but that is what the immune system does. The benefit is that it thereby gains access to a tremendous range of antibody specificities, that is, antibodies that recognise and combat all conceivable antigens and can save a person's life.

The principle is as follows: When an antigen enters the body, it selects an antibody that is its exact counterpart and, in so doing, initiates mass production of those antibodies. Since they are to a certain extent reflections of the antigen, they are, however, apprehended as foreign substances by the immune system. They circulate in the blood with their antigen-binding prehensile claws extended—and the immune system at once starts producing a second generation of antibodies to attack the original antibody.

In this way an anti-antibody comes into being. This, too, is interpreted as an intruder, and thus the third generation—the anti-anti-antibody—is born. And so the process continues, a torrent of antibodies being produced and, with them, the great advantage of an untold number of antibody specificities.

To save the transplant, immunologists are now testing a method of helping the immune system make anti-antibodies against the recipient's lymphocytes which attack the foreign tissue. Once they succeed in identifying these antibodies, the hybridoma technique will come into play and mass production will begin of monoclonal antibodies targeted on those lymphocytes which try to destroy the transplant. After being purified, these antibodies can be injected into the recipient's body, where they block and destroy hostile lymphocytes.

The other method, that of lymphocyte hormones, works as follows: The various constituents of the immune system communicate with each other by means of these hormones. Among the substances secreted by the large feeding cells, the macrophages, is one called interleukin 1, which stimulates the assistant T-cells. These in turn secrete a hormone, called interleukin 2, which gives a boost to the killer cells and antibody-producing B-cells.

Other lymphocyte hormones have the opposite effect, particularly relevant to transplants: They affect the suppressor T-cells, causing them to secrete substances with a suppressive capacity. The immune system demobilises its forces. The extraction of suitable lymphocytes from the recipient's blood and their mass-production in a nutrient solution by means of the hybridoma technique will make it possible in future to produce immunosuppressive lymphocyte hormones which, when injected, cause the attack on the transplant to peter out. The same technique may conceivably be used against those antibodies which

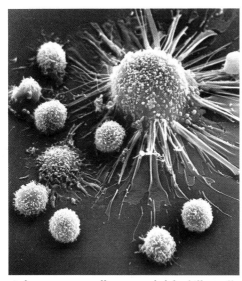

A large cancer cell surrounded by killer cells. Research is now focused on finding means of promoting the efficiency of the body's own immune defences.

Kidney transplantation. When any organ is transplanted, the recipient's immune system reacts by trying to reject it. Scientists are now looking for better ways to deal with this: the reaction has to be curbed, but the immune system must not be totally put out of action in the process—a difficult balancing act.

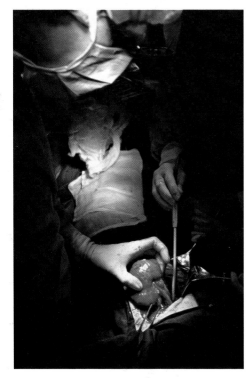

AIDS

When drug addicts and people with a large number of sexual contacts expose their bodies to massive doses of toxins and microbes, an additional severe infection may be all that is required for the immune forces to capitulate. When the insidious AIDS virus, HTLV-III, infects the T-lymphocytes, it may therefore deliver the coup de grace to the immune system. The microorganisms are given free scope: what begins as a fungal growth in the mouth may end in terminal cancer and death. AIDS is the greatest and most serious challenge so far posed to immunologists. But they have managed to identify the virus in record time, and to create tests that identify persons infected. Interferon and other agents are being tested to counteract the reproduction of the virus, and antibiotics are being tried to deal with the infections. Reconstruction of the immune defences is being attempted by bone marrow transplants and stimulation by means of interleukin and other substances.

1. *The AIDS virus can be transferred from one person to another via saliva, blood, and sperm. Blood used in transfusions must be checked.*

2. *A technique called cytometry enables the pathologist to determine whether T-lymphocytes have been infected by the AIDS virus.*

3. *The AIDS virus sheds particles on the surface of a T-cell.*

4. *HTLV-III virus, greatly magnified, coloured by means of computer technology.*

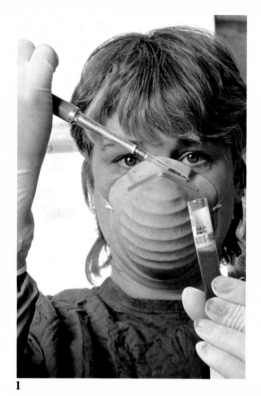

1

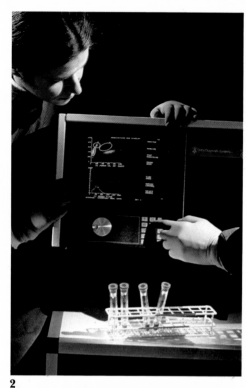

2

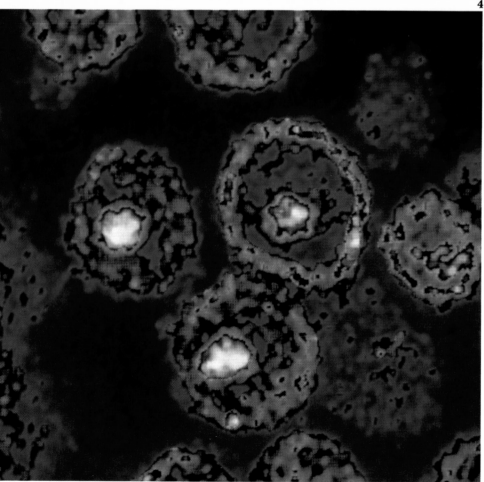

4

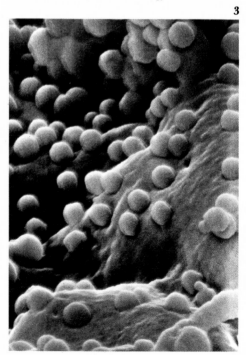

3

cause allergic responses or autoimmune disease: specific, suppressive lymphocyte hormones that neutralise the injurious powers of the immune system.

Among the conditions which might be treated are several rheumatic ailments such as rheumatoid arthritis; nerve diseases such as Chaga's disease, MS (multiple sclerosis), and myasthenia gravis (a disorder causing muscle weakness); skin diseases such as psoriasis, lupus erythematosus, herpes, patchy hair loss (alopecia areata); hormonal diseases such as juvenile diabetes and chronic inflammation of the thyroid gland; celiac disease, a condition of childhood; inflammations and ulcers of the colon; allergies such as hay fever and asthma; and certain congenital heart and lung diseases. The basic question of why the immune system attacks its own tissues still lacks a definitive answer in the majority of cases, but it is clear that a hereditary disposition, in the form of certain transplant antigens on the body's own cells, plays an important role. In addition, certain antigens on the surface of invasive microorganisms are so similar to antigens on the body's own cells that the immune system fails to distinguish between them. Rheumatoid arthritis, for example, is thought to fall into this category: an infection in joint cartilage in effect "opens the door" to T-cells and the autoimmune response.

The anti-antibody, produced by means of the hybridoma technique, also means a new vaccination principle. Modern vaccines are based on the injection of detoxified infectious matter into the body, whereupon the immune system generates antibodies against these antigens. When we are later infected with the natural, genuine infectious substance, we already have in our blood antibodies that can render it harmless. We are immune.

If we now produce anti-antibodies against this antibody, they will be immunologically identical with the bacterium or virus which caused the infection. Experiments show that these anti-antibodies can easily be injected into the body, and immunity created, without the process being via foreign antigens. One advantage is that it is possible, using the anti-antibody method, to obtain a considerably purer vaccine directed against exactly those (usually few) bacterial or viral antigens that are really crucial for the culprit's elimination.

Such anti-antibodies also make it feasible to vaccinate the fetus, inside the womb. Injected into the pregnant woman, they will pass through the placental filter, and cause the fetal immune system to produce antibodies specifically against them. Thus the child is immune to the disease by the time it is born.

Advancing knowledge of the immune system also paves the way for other forms of treatment in the future. Immunologists, for example, expect to be able to reinforce immune reactions in various ways. Lymphocyte hormones, which stimulate the body's powers of defence, have already been mentioned, but they are not the only means. As early as the 1960s, the body's defences were given a powerful boost by the injection of BCG vaccine containing mycoplasmas (the smallest free-living microorganisms), in a weakened state, into children suffering from leukemia. The result was an enhanced capacity to combat feeding cells and increased production of killer cells.

It is also important to make correct use of the existing arsenal of medicines. Certain antibiotics, for example, have proved deleterious to the immune system and must, of course, be avoided. Other antibiotics attack bacteria in one way while the immune system combats them in another, which means an enhanced striking power against severe infections such as blood poisoning. Thus research on the effects of different antibiotics is essential.

Alongside the treatment aspect, there is a need to discover new, unsuspected capacities of the immune system. Radioimmunological analysis (for which a Nobel prize was awarded in 1977) has in this context acquired a central role. It is based on a combination of immunological methods and isotope technology.

Using radioactively tagged antibodies, it is possible to detect in the body substances that occur in such minuscule amounts as billionths of a gram. Radioimmunology makes possible the identification of everything an antibody can bind itself to and the discovery—as in the case of certain mental disturbances—of deficiencies in signaling substances in the brain.

When considering the spectacular future prospects of immunology, we easily lose the retrospective thread. We may let ourselves be lulled into the fancy that mankind is in control of the natural environment. But the idea is a false one. Instead, man is catching up with nature, that patient experimenter. For millions of years, nature has proceeded by trial and error, step by step building up the richly varied immune system we possess. That system is the prototype, which has been there all the time but which we only now can perceive—and begin to understand.

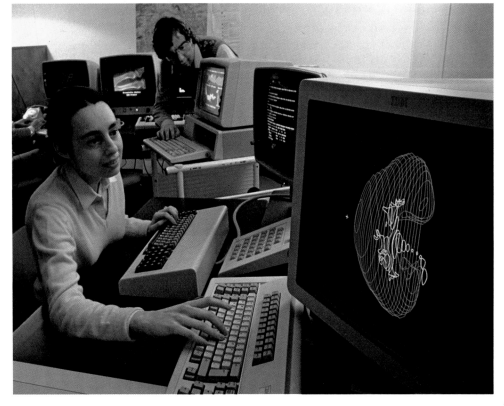

In medicine, as in other research fields, more and more assistance is being provided by computers. The computer makes it possible to obtain an overview and synthesise complex data. Important decisions are thus easier to make.

The nearest screen shows a computer-drawn kidney, which enables the surgeon to determine in advance where he can best make his incision in the operation. In the middle, a program that helps deaf children to control their voices is being tested. When their pronunciation is correct, the computer projects onto the screen a sharp-focus picture of the object named. If the pronunciation is wrong or indistinct, the picture of the object is correspondingly blurred. The far picture shows a computer which analyses and imparts colour to X-ray pictures, to increase the information yield and facilitate the detection of hairline bone fractures.

The pictures are from IBM's computer technology centre in Paris.

CREDITS

A large number of people, institutions, and companies have kindly assisted in work on this book. They are listed below, and I hope that no one has been inadvertently overlooked. My hearty thanks to all.

LN

Dr. Razzak Alsheikly, Department of Immune Biology, University of Stockholm. Jan-Åke Andersson, engineer, AGEMA Infrared Systems. Assoc. Prof. Gert Auer, Department of Pathology, Karolinska Hospital.

Margareta Berggren, laboratory assistant, Department of Toxicology, Karolinska Institute. Assoc. Prof. Lars Berghem, Cell and Tissue Biology Unit, Division of Experimental Medicine, National Defence Research Institute, Umeå. Kerstin Bernholm, senior laboratory assistant, Department of Bacteriology, Karolinska Institute. Prof. Gunnel Biberfeld, Department of Immunology, National Bacteriological Laboratory. Assoc. Prof. Peter Biberfeld, Immune Pathology Unit, Department of Pathology, Karolinska Hospital. Anders Björkman, M.D., Department of Infectious Diseases, Roslagstull Hospital, Karolinska Institute; Department of Parasitology, National Bacteriological Laboratory. Birgitta Björkroth, research engineer, Department of Medical Cell Genetics, Karolinska Institute, Prof. Birger Blombäck, Department of Blood Coagulation Research, Karolinska Institute; Department of Plasma Protein, The New York Blood Center. Kristina Borgedahl, head of department, Maternity Department, Söder Hospital. Assoc. Prof. Göran Bredberg, Ear, Nose and Throat Clinic, Söder Hospital. Jan-Inge Bäckström, autopsy technician, Nyköping Hospital. Dr. Blenda Böttiger, Department of Immunology, National Bacteriological Laboratory.

Kerstin Carlson, laboratory engineer, Lipoprotein Laboratory, King Gustaf V Research Institute, Karolinska Hospital. Prof. Lars A. Carlson, Department of Medicine, Karolinska Hospital.

Kjell Edh, autopsy technician, Nyköping Hospital. Assoc. Prof. Stig Ekeström, Department of Thoracic Surgery, Karolinska Hospital. Marianne Ekman, laboratory assistant, Immune Pathology Unit, Department of Pathology, Karolinska Hospital. Assoc. Prof. Ingemar Ernberg, Department of Tumour Biology, Karolinska Institute. Assoc. Prof. Ulf Ernström, Department of Histology, Karolinska Institute. Prof. Åke Espmark, Department of Virology, National Bacteriological Laboratory. Assoc. Prof. Gösta Ewert, Ear, Nose and Throat Clinic, Sabbatsberg Hospital.

Assoc. Prof. Per Flood, Department of Anatomy, University of Bergen, Norway. Dr. Flemming Frandsen, Danish Bilharziosis Laboratory, Copenhagen, Denmark, Dr. Tage Frisk, IBM Computer Science Center, Paris. Friskis & Svettis IF, St. Eriksgatan, Stockholm.

Prof. Robert Gallo, Laboratory of Tumor Cell Biology, National Cancer Institution, Bethesda, Maryland. Assoc. Prof. Hans Glaumann, Department of Pathology, Karolinska Institute, Huddinge Hospital. Assoc. Prof. Roland Grafström, Department of Toxicology, Karolinska Institute. Assoc. Prof. Monica Grandien-Kövamees, Department of Virology, National Bacteriological Laboratory. Prof. Carl-Gustav Groth, Transplant Surgery Unit, Karolinska Institute, Department of Surgery, Huddinge Hospital. Prof. Ragnhild Gullberg, Department of Rheumatology, Karolinska Hospital. Prof. Jan-Åke Gustafsson, Department of Medical Nutrition, Karolinska Institute, Huddinge Hospital.

Assoc. Prof. Hans Hebert, Department of Medical Physics, Karolinska Institute. Prof. Carl-Göran Hedén, Department of Bacteriology, Karolinska Institute. Vera Lindahl-Hohlfelt, senior laboratory assistant, Department of Bacteriology, Karolinska Institute. Prof. Tord Holme, Department of Bacteriology, Karolinska Institute. Department of Dermatology, Söder Hospital.

Assoc. Prof. Conni Jarstrand, Department of Bacteriology, Roslagstull Hospital. Prof. Björn V. Johansen, National Institute of Public Health, Oslo, Norway. Prof. Gunnar Johansson, Department of Forensic Odontology, National Institute of Forensic Medicine, Solna. Gert Jonsson, dentist, Faculty of Odontology, Karolinska Institute.

Department of Surgery, Karolinska Hospital. Department of Surgery, Nyköping Hospital.

Assoc. Prof. Bo Lambert, Department of Clinical Genetics, Karolinska Institute. Ulf Larsson, B.Sc., Department of Blood Coagulation Research, Karolinska Institute. Assoc. Prof. Ewert Linder, Department of Parasitology, National Bacteriological Laboratory. Prof. Jan Lindsten, Department of Clinical Genetics, Karolinska Hospital. Ann-Marie Lundberg, laboratory assistant, Research Unit of the Ear, Nose and Throat Clinic, King Gustav V Research Institute, Karolinska Hospital. Maija-Leena Lyssarides, research engineer, Department of Pharmacology, Karolinska Institute.

McDonald's Svenska AB.

The late Assoc. Prof. Magnus Nasiell, Departments of Pathology and Cytology, Sabbatsberg Hospital. Assoc. Prof. Bo A. Nilsson, Department of Gynaecology, Söder Hospital. Prof. Kenneth Nilsson, Department of Cell and Tumour Pathology, Wallenberg Laboratory, Uppsala. Prof. Siwert Nilsson, Palynology Laboratory, Stockholm. Rolf Nybom, research engineer, Wallenberg Laboratory Stockholm.

Prof. Per Olsson, Department of Experimental Surgery, Karolinska Institute. Assoc. Prof. Kari Ormstad, Department of Forensic Medicine, Karolinska Institute. Prof. Sten Orrenius, Department of Toxicology, Karolinska Institute, Dr. Karin Österman, Department of Thoracic Medicine, Karolinska Hospital.

Hedvig Perlmann, laboratory engineer, Institute of Immune Biology, University of Stockholm. Prof. Peter Perlmann, Institute of Immune Biology, University of Stockholm. Pinocchio Restaurant, Stockholm.

Radiumhemmet (Department of Non-Surgical Oncology), High Voltage Unit, Karolinska Hospital. Assoc. Prof. Jovan Rajs, Department of Forensic Medicine, Karolinska Institute. Prof. Nils Ringertz, Department of Medical Cell Genetics, Karolinska Institute. Anders Rosén, M.D., Department of Pharmacology, Karolinska Institute. Prof. Lars Rutberg, Department of Bacteriology, Karolinska Institute. The National Smoking and Health Association (NTS), Wenner-Gren Center. X-ray Department, Nyköping Hospital.

Prof. Bengt Samuelsson, Department of Physiological Chemistry, Karolinska Institute. Mr. Charles Serhan, Ph.D., Department of Medicine, New York University Medical Center. Assoc. Prof. Lennart and Dr. Brita Silverstolpe. Dr. Kjell Stenberg, Antiviral Chemotherapy Research and Development, Astra Läkemedel AB. Sundbyberg Hospital. Kristina Sundqvist, B.Sc., Department of Toxicology, Karolinska Institute. Assoc. Prof. Jesper Swedenborg, Surgical Clinic, Karolinska Hospital. Lennart Svensson, senior laboratory assistant, Department of Virology, National Bacteriological Laboratory, Inger Söderlund, laboratory assistant, Department of Physiology, Karolinska Institute; Andrology Unit, Sophiahemmet Hospital.

Prof. K. Tanaka, Institution of Anatomy, University of Tottori, Yonago, Japan. Tove Tengesdal, engineer, AGEMA Infrared Systems, Stockholm. Hjördis Thor, research engineer, Department of Toxicology, Karolinska Institute. Assoc. Prof. Johan Thyberg, Department of Histology, Karolinska Institute.

Prof. Börje Uvnäs, Department of Pharmacology, Karolinska Institute.

Assoc. Prof. Johan Wallin, Department of Venereology, University Hospital, Uppsala. Prof. Milan Valverius, National Institute of Forensic Medicine, Solna. Sirkka Vene, laboratory engineer, Department of Virology, National Bacteriological Laboratory. Anna Wiernik, laboratory assistant, Department of Bacteriology, Bacteriological Laboratory, Roslagstull Hospital. Prof. Hans Wigzell, Department of Immunology, Karolinska Institute. Birgitta Vogel, laboratory assistant, Departments of Pathology and Cytology, Sabbatsberg Hospital.

Dr. Jan Zabielski, Department of Medical Genetics, Biomedical Centre, Uppsala, Assoc. Prof. Olle Zetterström, Department of Thoracic Medicine, Karolinska Hospital.

Birgitta Åsjö, M.D., Department of Virology, Karolinska Institute; National Bacteriological Laboratory.

Assoc. Prof. Anders Ånggårdh, Ear, Nose and Throat Clinic, Karolinska Hospital.

Prof. Bo Öberg, Antiviral Chemotherapy Research and Development, Astra Läkemedel AB.

Special thanks to Catharina Fjellström, Bonnier Fakta Bokförlag AB, for her assistance in connection with several of the photographic sessions and her editorial help.

TECHNICAL INFORMATION

Scanning electron microscope images: *Jeol*, Japan. Light microscope images: *Zeiss*, West Germany. Custom-made endoscopes: *Karl Storz*, West Germany. Custom-made camera lenses: *Georg Vogl* and *Bo Möller*, engineers, Stockholm.

To enhance clarity in some photographs taken with a very high degree of magnification through the scanning electron microscope, colour has been artificially added using a method developed by *photographer Gillis Häägg*, Gothenburg. This applies to the pictures on the following pages: pp. 18–19, 20, 21, 26 (top), 48–49, 53 (top), 66, 70–71, 90, 148–149, and the front cover.

Some pictures have been coloured with the aid of a computer, by a method known as the image analysis system. Such pictures are the images of cholesterol on p. 67, the four virus portraits on p. 91, the herpes virus on p. 93 (bottom) and the AIDS virus on p. 192.

Index

acreolin, 135
adenitis, 91
adrenaline, 12
AIDS, 43, 192
air pollution, 124, 125
allergy, 31, 113, 119, 193
allergy test, 122
alveoli, 112, 126, 142
amino acids, 45
amniotic sac, 33
Anopheles mosquito, 178, 181
anti-antibody, 191, 193
antibiotics, 73, 82, 194
antibodies, 22, 24, 26, 27, 30, 38, 119, 121, 122, 150, 154, 164, 190, 191
antigens, 24, 26, 27, 30, 97, 100, 109, 123, 186, 190, 191, 193
antihemophilic factor, 68
antihistamine, 123
arteriosclerosis, 51, 64, 66, 147
asbestos, 129
asthma, 31, 113, 193
autoimmune diseases, 31, 184–189

bacteria, 39, 70–85
benzopyrene, 135
bilharzia, 178, 182, 183
blood clot (thrombus), 50, 51, 63, 64, 147
blood clotting, 13, 31, 48–69
blood plasma, 30, 56
blood poisoning, 73
B-lymphocytes, 22, 24, 27, 28, 30, 38, 43, 186, 191
bone marrow, 22, 26
breast cancer, 108, 109
breast milk, 34, 35, 36, 37, 145
breast-feeding, 34, 35, 36
bronchoscopy, 141, 142
bursa equivalents, 26

cancer, 17, 94–109, 138, 191
carbon monoxide, 135
caries, 150, 151, 155, 156, 159
celiac disease, 193
cell, the, 20, 21, 24
cell changes, 136
cercaria, 182, 183
Chagas' disease, 179, 186, 192
chemotaxis, 72
chickenpox, 93
Chlamydia bacterium, 26
cholera, 13, 15, 16, 17
cholesterol, 67
chromatin, 42
chromosomes, 21, 40, 41, 42, 47
cilia, 28, 112, 115, 117
clone, 27
coagulation, 13, 31, 51, 69
cocarcinogens, 138
colostrum, 35, 37
complement system, 22, 27, 29, 35
computer-aided research, 194
cough, 141
Crohn's disease, 174
cytomegalovirus, 89, 93
cytometry, 192
cytoplasm, 25
cytostatics, 109

dentine, 151
deoxyribonucleic acid (DNA), 42
diabetes, 193
DNA, 42, 45, 47, 88
Down's syndrome, 47

E. coli, 76
eczema, 31
elephantiasis, 13
endoplasmic reticulum, 21
enzymes, 25, 30, 45, 88
estrogen (oestrogen), 109

fatty acids, 138
feeding cells, 22, 29, 30, 35, 54, 55, 76, 80, 126, 183
fibrin, 30, 49, 50, 51, 57
fibrin threads, 59
fibrin web, 60, 63
fibrinogen, 50, 56
fibrinogen molecule, 57
fluoride, 151

gametocytes, 181
gangrene, 134, 147
gastric juice, 154
gastric ulcer, 164, 172
genes, 42, 45
genetic engineering, 43
genetic traits, 42, 45
German measles (rubella), 89
Golgi body, 20, 21
granulocytes, 22, 24, 25, 30, 35, 54, 122, 128, 132, 191

Hashimoto's syndrome, 31
hay fever, 31, 119, 193
HDL (high-density lipoprotein), 67
healing (of a wound), 53
heart infarction (attack), 66, 147
helper cells, 22, 28, 186
hemophilia, 50, 51, 68
herpes, 193
herpes simiae, 93
herpes simplex virus, 92, 93
histamine, 121, 122, 123
histiocytes, 25
hormones, 67, 193
"Hospital disease," 73, 84
HTLV-III, 192
hybrid-DNA techniques, 190
hybridoma, 190
hybridoma techniques, 190

IgA, 150, 154, 164
IgE, 113, 119, 122
IgG, 34, 36, 164
immune competence, 34
immunoglobulin A (IgA), 150, 164
immunoglobulin E (IgE), 113
immunoglobulin G (IgG), 34
inflammation, 28, 29, 156
influenza, 15, 87, 91
interferon, 89, 96, 190, 192
interleukin, 191

kidney transplants, 191
killer cells, 22, 26, 28, 98, 105, 106, 109, 191

LDL (low-density lipoprotein), 67

leprosy, 15, 87
leukemia, 187
leukotrienes, 109, 113
lipoprotein, 67
lung cancer, 140–143
lung emphysema, 142
lupus erythematosus, 186, 187, 193
lymph nodes, 38
lymphocyte hormones, 194
lymphocytes, 26, 28, 34, 35, 38, 186, 190, 191, 193
lymphoid tissues, 38
lymphokines, 191
lysosomes, 89
lysozyme, 28, 150

macrophages, 22, 24, 25, 30, 31, 35, 55, 71, 72, 76, 78, 81, 126, 128, 129, 130, 132, 138, 179, 191
malaria, 176–181
mammography, 109
mast cells, 113, 121, 122, 123
maternal milk, 34, 35, 36, 37, 145
measles, 88, 187
megakaryocytes, 55
melanoma, 96
merozoites (malaria), 179, 181
metastases, 109
microphages, 25
mitochondria, 20, 21, 106
mongolism, 47
monoclonal antibodies, 105, 109, 190, 193
monocytes, 22, 25, 30, 128
mucus, 112, 155, 121, 136, 138, 141, 166
multiple sclerosis (MS), 186, 187, 193
mumps, 89
myasthenia gravis, 186, 187, 193

narcotic drugs, 17
nephritis, 31
nicotine, 134, 135, 145, 146
nitrogen dioxide, 135
NK (natural killer) cells, 105, 109

oncogenes, 96
opsonins, 72, 78

pain, 29, 30
parasites, 176–183
passive smoking, 134
penicillin, 82, 83, 84
pepsin, 164, 165, 166
pepsinogen, 166
periodontal disease, 151, 156, 159
peritonitis, 165, 172
phagocytes, 72, 128
phagocytosis, 25, 81
phagosome, 72
phenols, 138
picogram, 194
pituitary gland, 12
placenta, 34, 38, 145, 164
plague, 12, 15, 16
plaque, 150, 154, 155, 156, 160
plasma cells, 22, 26, 27, 35, 54
plasmin, 56
plasmodium (malaria), 178, 179, 181
platelets (thrombocytes), 54, 59
pneumococci, 24

polio virus, 89, 91
pollen allergy, 119, 121
pseudopodia, 25, 132
psoriasis, 193
pulp, 156

rabies, 88, 89, 91
radiotherapy, 109
redness, 29, 30
respiratory tract, 113–147
rheumatoid arthritis, 186, 187, 189
ribosomes, 42, 106
rickettsias, 20
RNA, 88
rubella (German measles), 89

saliva, 150, 152, 154, 155, 156
schistosomes, 179
schistosomiasis, 178, 182
sepsis, 173
serotonin, 113
shingles, 93
smallpox, 15, 16, 88, 89
smoking, 67, 134–147
spirochetes, 154
spleen, 28
sporozoites (malaria), 181
spotted fever, 16
staphylococci, 80, 82, 83
stomach, 162–175
stomach ulcer, 164, 172
Streptococcus mutans, 150, 151, 155
stress reaction, 12
stroke, 147
sulfa drugs, 73
suppressor cells, 22, 28
surface antigens, 179
sweat glands, 13
swelling, 29, 30
syphilis, 16

tartar, 151
taste buds, 136
T-lymphocytes, 13, 24, 28, 31, 43, 96, 97, 98, 102, 105, 109, 191, 192
thrombin, 50, 56
thrombocytes (platelets), 54, 59
thrombus (blood clot), 50, 51, 63, 64, 147
thymus gland, 22, 27, 38, 97
thyroid gland, chronic inflammation of, 31, 193
tonsils, 112
transplant surgery, 25
transplants, 34
trypanosomes, 179
trypanosomiasis, 178
tsetse fly, 179
typhus, 15

ulcerative colitis, 174
umbilical cord, 38

vascular damage, 134
vascular disease, 17
viruses, 86–93, 192
von Willebrand's disease, 68

yellow fever, 89
yolk sac, 34

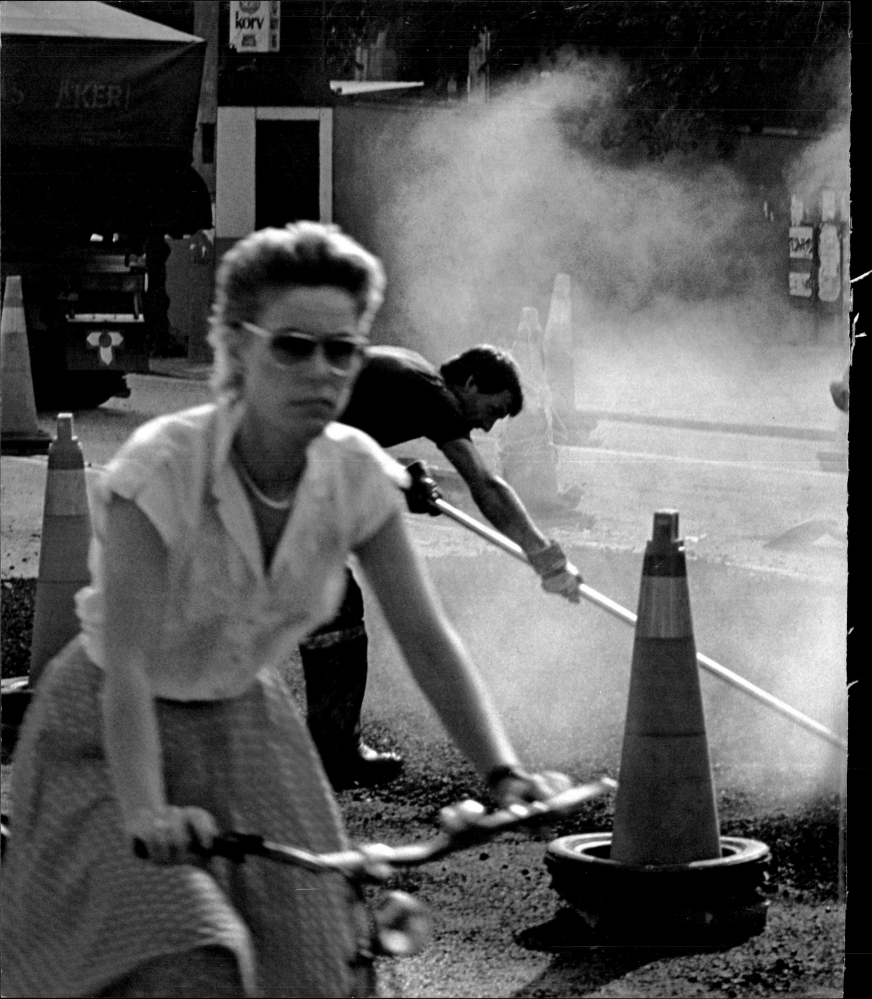